Atherosclerosis: Technologies of Personalized Medicine

Atherosclerosis: Technologies of Personalized Medicine

Editor

Yuliya I. Ragino

MDPI • Basel • Beijing • Wuhan • Barcelona • Belgrade • Manchester • Tokyo • Cluj • Tianjin

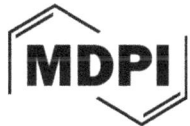

Editor
Yuliya I. Ragino
Laboratory of Biochemistry
Institute of Internal and
Preventive Medicine–Branch
of Institute of Cytology and
Genetics, Siberian Branch of
Russian Academy of Sciences
Novosibirsk
Russia

Editorial Office
MDPI
St. Alban-Anlage 66
4052 Basel, Switzerland

This is a reprint of articles from the Special Issue published online in the open access journal *Journal of Personalized Medicine* (ISSN 2075-4426) (available at: www.mdpi.com/journal/jpm/special_issues/Atherosclerosis_Technologies_Medicine).

For citation purposes, cite each article independently as indicated on the article page online and as indicated below:

LastName, A.A.; LastName, B.B.; LastName, C.C. Article Title. *Journal Name* **Year**, *Volume Number*, Page Range.

ISBN 978-3-0365-3528-9 (Hbk)
ISBN 978-3-0365-3527-2 (PDF)

© 2022 by the authors. Articles in this book are Open Access and distributed under the Creative Commons Attribution (CC BY) license, which allows users to download, copy and build upon published articles, as long as the author and publisher are properly credited, which ensures maximum dissemination and a wider impact of our publications.

The book as a whole is distributed by MDPI under the terms and conditions of the Creative Commons license CC BY-NC-ND.

Contents

About the Editor vii

Preface to "Atherosclerosis: Technologies of Personalized Medicine" ix

Yuliya Ragino, Evgeniia Striukova and Elena Shakhtshneider
Basic Research in Atherosclerosis: Technologies of Personalized Medicine
Reprinted from: *J. Pers. Med.* **2022**, *12*, 367, doi:10.3390/jpm12030367 1

Olga I. Afanasieva, Alexandra V. Tyurina, Elena A. Klesareva, Tatiana I. Arefieva, Marat V. Ezhov and Sergei N. Pokrovsky
Lipoprotein(a), Immune Cells and Cardiovascular Outcomes in Patients with Premature Coronary Heart Disease
Reprinted from: *J. Pers. Med.* **2022**, *12*, 269, doi:10.3390/jpm12020269 5

Victoria A. Metelskaya, Natalia E. Gavrilova, Maria V. Zhatkina, Elena B. Yarovaya and Oxana M. Drapkina
A Novel Integrated Biomarker for Evaluation of Risk and Severity of Coronary Atherosclerosis, and Its Validation
Reprinted from: *J. Pers. Med.* **2022**, *12*, 206, doi:10.3390/jpm12020206 19

Olga V. Gruzdeva, Yulia A. Dyleva, Ekaterina V. Belik, Maxim Y. Sinitsky, Aleksandr N. Stasev and Aleksandr N. Kokov et al.
Relationship between Epicardial and Coronary Adipose Tissue and the Expression of Adiponectin, Leptin, and Interleukin 6 in Patients with Coronary Artery Disease
Reprinted from: *J. Pers. Med.* **2022**, *12*, 129, doi:10.3390/jpm12020129 29

Marina Shapkina, Andrey Ryabikov, Ekaterina Mazdorova, Anastasia Titarenko, Ekaterina Avdeeva and Elena Mazurenko et al.
The Determinants of the 13-Year Risk of Incident Atrial Fibrillation in a Russian Population Cohort of Middle and Elderly Age
Reprinted from: *J. Pers. Med.* **2022**, *12*, 122, doi:10.3390/jpm12010122 47

Sofia Malyutina, Olga Chervova, Taavi Tillmann, Vladimir Maximov, Andrew Ryabikov and Valery Gafarov et al.
The Relationship between Epigenetic Age and Myocardial Infarction/Acute Coronary Syndrome in a Population-Based Nested Case-Control Study
Reprinted from: *J. Pers. Med.* **2022**, *12*, 110, doi:10.3390/jpm12010110 59

Victoria Korneva, Tatyana Kuznetsova and Ulrich Julius
The Role of Cumulative LDL Cholesterol in Cardiovascular Disease Development in Patients with Familial Hypercholesterolemia
Reprinted from: *J. Pers. Med.* **2022**, *12*, 71, doi:10.3390/jpm12010071 73

Viktoriya S. Shramko, Eugeniia V. Striukova, Yana V. Polonskaya, Ekaterina M. Stakhneva, Marina V. Volkova and Alexey V. Kurguzov et al.
Associations of Antioxidant Enzymes with the Concentration of Fatty Acids in the Blood of Men with Coronary Artery Atherosclerosis
Reprinted from: *J. Pers. Med.* **2021**, *11*, 1281, doi:10.3390/jpm11121281 85

Elena Shakhtshneider, Dinara Ivanoshchuk, Olga Timoshchenko, Pavel Orlov, Sergey Semaev and Emil Valeev et al.
Analysis of Rare Variants in Genes Related to Lipid Metabolism in Patients with Familial Hypercholesterolemia in Western Siberia (Russia)
Reprinted from: *J. Pers. Med.* **2021**, *11*, 1232, doi:10.3390/jpm11111232 . . . . **101**

Hamzah Khan, Shubha Jain, Reid C. Gallant, Muzammil H. Syed, Abdelrahman Zamzam and Mohammed Al-Omran et al.
Plateletworks® as a Point-of-Care Test for ASA Non-Sensitivity
Reprinted from: *J. Pers. Med.* **2021**, *11*, 813, doi:10.3390/jpm11080813 . . . . **115**

Yana V. Polonskaya, Elena V. Kashtanova, Ivan S. Murashov, Evgenia V. Striukova, Alexey V. Kurguzov and Ekaterina M. Stakhneva et al.
Association of Matrix Metalloproteinases with Coronary Artery Calcification in Patients with CHD
Reprinted from: *J. Pers. Med.* **2021**, *11*, 506, doi:10.3390/jpm11060506 . . . . **129**

About the Editor

Yuliya I. Ragino

Ph.D. and Sc.D. in medicine, Main Accreditation Commission (VAK) professor, Russian Academy of Sciences (RAS) professor, corresponding member of the RAS, head of the Institute of Internal and Preventive Medicine—a branch of a federal publicly funded scientific institution, the federal research center Institute of Cytology and Genetics, the Siberian Branch of the RAS (IIPM—a branch of the ICG SB RAS)

Ragino Yu.I. is an expert in the fields of medical biochemistry and pathophysiology and an author or coauthor of more than 400 scientific publications, including 8 books, 10 patents of the Russian Federation, and 4 patents of the Eurasian Patent Organization. In the Russian Scientific Citation Index (RSCI): h-index 24. In Scopus: h-index 10. In the Web of Science: h-index 8.

The main basic-research accomplishments of Ragino Yu.I.: A study on the key biochemical markers and mechanisms of formation of unstable atherosclerotic plaquesand of their various types in atherosclerosis. The development of methods for early biochemical diagnosis of atherosclerosis and risk assessment of acute coronary syndrome. Conceptualization of the one-directionality of highly atherogenic changes of oxidation-modified and structurally altered lipoproteins of the blood, including small high-density atherogenic subfractions of lipoproteins, in clinically significant atherosclerosis and in the presence of its major risk factors; in this regard, novel evaluation criteria of pharmacotherapy effectiveness have been proposed. Research into atherogenic properties of oxidized proteins and their role in atherogenesis. Creation and investigation of experimental animal models (in vitro, in vivo), new lipid-containing coordination compounds of HMG-CoA reductase inhibitors with glycyrrhizin. Significant antiatherogenic effects of the obtained compounds have been demonstrated.

Preface to "Atherosclerosis: Technologies of Personalized Medicine"

The first national conference with international participation, "Fundamental aspects of atherosclerosis: scientific research for improving the technologies of personalized medicine", was held in Novosibirsk on 15 October, 2021. The purpose of this conference was to disseminate the latest basic and clinical findings in the fields of etiology, clinical characteristics, and modern diagnostics and treatments of atherosclerosis among various relevant specialists. The conference was intended for practicing cardiologists, primary care physicians, medical geneticists, and physician–scientists. The conference included plenary sessions, specialty sessions, satellite symposia, an open competition for young scientists.

The scientific topics included experimental research in the field of atherosclerosis; biochemical studies of atherosclerosis; genomics, GWAS and population genetics of atherosclerosis; epigenetics and miRNA of atherosclerosis; hereditary dyslipidemia; proteomic studies of atherosclerosis; etiopathogenetic aspects of atherosclerosis; lipids, lipoproteins, apolipoproteins; macrophages and atherosclerosis; vascular wall remodeling and atherosclerosis; inflammation and atherosclerosis; oxidative stress and atherosclerosis; immunology of atherosclerosis; climatic-geographical and ethnic features of atherosclerosis development; therapy with antisense oligonucleotides and miRNAs.

Scientists from Siberian cities (Novosibirsk, Kemerovo, Tomsk, Barnaul), from Moscow, St. Petersburg, Samara, Chelyabinsk, and from Great Britain (London), delivered presentations at the conference. The conference was organized by the Institute of Internal and Preventive Medicine –a branch of the Institute of Cytology and Genetics,the Siberian Branch of the Russian Academy of Sciences (IIPM—a branch of the ICG SB RAS). The objectives and subject areas of the IIPM are basic, exploratory, and applied scientific studies in priority areas of molecular medicine and human genetics, as well as safeguarding and improvement of human health, the development of health care and medical science, and preparation of advanced specialists in science and medicine.

Yuliya I. Ragino
Editor

Editorial

Basic Research in Atherosclerosis: Technologies of Personalized Medicine

Yuliya Ragino *, Evgeniia Striukova and Elena Shakhtshneider

Institute of Internal and Preventive Medicine—Branch of Institute of Cytology and Genetics, Siberian Branch of Russian Academy of Sciences (SB RAS), 175/1 Borisa Bogatkova Str., 630089 Novosibirsk, Russia; stryukova.j@mail.ru (E.S.); 2117409@mail.ru (E.S.)
* Correspondence: ragino@mail.ru

The first national conference with international participation, "Fundamental aspects of atherosclerosis: scientific research for improving the technologies of personalized medicine", was held in Novosibirsk on 15 October 2021. The purpose of this conference was to disseminate the latest basic and clinical findings in the fields of etiology, clinical characteristics, and modern diagnostics and treatments of atherosclerosis among various relevant specialists. The conference was intended for practicing cardiologists, primary care physicians, medical geneticists, and physician–scientists. The conference included plenary sessions, specialty sessions, satellite symposia, an open competition for young scientists.

This Special Issue on "Atherosclerosis: Technologies of Personalized Medicine" includes a review and ten original studies about epidemiologic, genetic aspects of atherosclerosis, antioxidant system, biomarkers of atherosclerosis. Four of the special-issue articles, Metelskaya et al. [1], Gruzdeva et al. [2], Shramko et al. [3], Polonskaya et al. [4], focus on the various biomarkers of atherosclerosis. Metelskaya et al. [1] evaluated the feasibility of a combination of biochemical and imaging parameters for estimation of risk and severity of coronary atherosclerosis (CA), and to verify the created integrated biomarker (i-BIO) on the independent cohort. They determined that the i-BIO > 4 detected CA (GS > 0) with sensitivity of 87.9%, i-BIO ≥ 9 excluded patients without severe CA (GS < 35), specificity 79.8%. Validation of i-BIO confirmed the feasibility of i-BIO > 4 to separate patients with any CA with sensitivity 76.2%, and of i-BIO ≥ 9 to exclude atherosclerosis-free subjects with a specificity of 84.0%. Gruzdeva et al. [2] investigated the expression and secretion of adipocytokine genes in the adipose tissue (AT) of patients with coronary artery disease (CAD) and patients with aortic or mitral valve replacement. The study included 84 patients with CAD and 50 patients with aortic or mitral valve replacement. The authors revealed the pathogenetic significance of alterations in the adipokine and cytokine status of adipocytes of epicardial (EAT) and perivascular (PVAT) in patients with CAD. Shramko et al. [3] researched associations of fatty acids (FAs) with the antioxidant enzymes in the blood of men with coronary atherosclerosis and ischemic heart disease (IHD). The study included 80 patients: control group—20 men without IHD, the core group—60 men with IHD. The core group was divided into subgroups: subgroup A—with the presence of vulnerable atherosclerotic plaques, subgroup B—with the absence of vulnerable atherosclerotic plaques. The authors analyzed the levels of FAs, free radicals, superoxide dismutase (SOD), catalase (CAT), and glutathione peroxidase (GPx) in the blood and revealed that changes in the levels of antioxidant enzymes, and a disbalance of the FAs profile, probably indicate active oxidative processes in the body and may indicate the presence of atherosclerotic changes in the vessels. Polonskaya et al. [4] investigated the relationship of matrix metalloproteinases with calcification of the coronary arteries. The study included 78 people with coronary heart disease (CHD) and 36 without CHD. Blood and samples of coronary arteries obtained as a result of endarterectomy were examined. Serum levels of metalloproteinases (MMP) MMP-1, MMP-2, MMP-3, MMP-7, MMP-9, MMP-10, MMP-12, and MMP-13 were determined by multiplex analysis. In blood vessel samples, MMP-1, MMP-3, MMP-7, and MMP-9 were determined by enzyme immunoassay; MMP-9 expression was evaluated by immunohistochemistry. The results obtained indicate the participation of some MMPs, and especially MMP-9, in the calcification processes. The study can serve as a basis for the further study of the possibility of using MMP-1, MMP-7 and MMP-12 as potential biomarkers of CHD.

Afanasieva et al. [5] focused on the relationship between Lp(a), immune blood cells and major adverse cardiovascular events (MACE) in patients with the early manifestation of coronary heart disease (CHD). The study included 200 patients with chronic CHD, manifested up to the age of 55 in men and 60 in women. An increased Lp(a) concentration [hyperLp(a)] was shown to predict cardiovascular events in patients with premature CHD with long-term follow-up. The combination of an increased monocyte count and hyperLp(a) significantly increased the proportion of patients with early CHD with subsequent development of MACE. The odds of cardiovascular events in patients with early CHD manifestation were highest in patients with an elevated lymphocyte-to-monocyte ratio and an elevated Lp(a) level. A higher neutrophil blood count and an elevated neutrophil-to-lymphocyte ratio determined the faster development of MACE in patients with a high Lp(a) concentration. The authors suggested that the high atherothrombogenicity of Lp(a) is associated with the "inflammatory" component and the innate immune cells' involvement in this process. The easily calculated immunological ratios of blood cells and Lp(a) concentrations can be considered simple predictors of future cardiovascular events.

Shapkina et al. [6] investigated the determinants of the 13-year risk of incident atrial fibrillation (AF) in a Russian population cohort of middle and elderly age. A random population sample (n = 9360, age 45–69 years) was examined at baseline in 2003–2005 and reexamined in 2006–2008 and 2015–2017 in Novosibirsk (the HAPIEE study). Incident AF was being registered during the average follow-up of 13 years. The final analysis included 3871 participants free from baseline AF and cardiovascular disease (CVD) who participated in all three data collections. In a multivariable-adjusted Cox regression model, the 13-year risk of AF was positively associated with the male sex, age, body mass index (BMI), systolic blood pressure (SBP), and it was negatively associated with total cholesterol (TC). In women, the risk of AF was more strongly associated with hypertension (HT) and was also negatively related to total cholesterol (TC) level. No independent association was found with mean alcohol intake per drinking occasion.

Malyutina et al. [7] evaluated the relationship between 'epigenetic age' (EA) derived from DNA methylation (DNAm) and myocardial infarction (MI)/acute coronary syndrome (ACS). A random population sample was examined in 2003/2005 (n = 9360, 45–69, the HAPIEE project) and followed up for 15 years. From this cohort, incident MI/ACS (cases, n = 129) and age- and sex-stratified controls (n = 177) were selected for a nested case-control study. Baseline EA (Horvath's, Hannum's, PhenoAge, Skin and Blood) and the differences between EA and chronological age (CA) were calculated (ΔAHr, ΔAHn, ΔAPh, ΔASB). EAs by Horvath's, Hannum's and Skin and Blood were close to CA (median absolute difference, MAD, of 1.08, −1.91 and −2.03 years); PhenoAge had MAD of −9.29 years vs. CA. The adjusted odds ratios (ORs) of MI/ACS per 1–year increments of ΔAHr, ΔAHn, ΔASB and ΔAPh were 1.01 (95% CI 0.95–1.07), 1.01 (95% CI 0.95–1.08), 1.02 (95% CI 0.97–1.06) and 1.01 (0.93–1.09), respectively. When classified into tertiles, only the highest tertile of ΔAPh showed a suggestion of increased risk of MI/ACS with OR 2.09 (1.11–3.94) independent of age and 1.84 (0.99–3.52) in the age- and sex-adjusted model. The authors concluded that in a prospective population-based cohort there were no strong associations between accelerated epigenetic age markers and risk of MI/ACS.

Korneva et al. [8] analyzed the contribution of "cum LDL-C for all life" and the index "cum LDL-C/age" to the development of coronary heart disease (CHD), myocardial infarction (MI), and a combined endpoint: MI, stroke, unstable angina in FH patients. The study included 188 patients (mean age 49.2 years, males 45.7%) with FH were examined (Dutch Lipid Clinic Criteria). The authors had evaluated cumulative LDL-C and index "cum DL-C/age" along with other classical risk factors. Cum LDL-C was calculated as LDL-Cmax × (age at initiating of hypolipidemic therapy) + LDL-C at inclusion age at initiation/correction therapy). Cumulative LDL-C and "cum LDL-C/age" were calculated as the ratio cum LDL-C to age. The follow-up period was 5.4 (from 3 to 10) years. The index "cum LDL-C/age" was higher in patients with CHD 58.7 ± 10.4 mmol/L/years vs. 40.1 ± 11.7 mmol/L/years in patients without CHD. According to their data based on the results of the logistic regression analysis in patients with FH, cumulative LDL-C and the cumulative index "cum LDL–C/age" played a strong predictive role in the development of CHD in FH patients; it was greater than the role of TC and LDL-C concentrations. The authors suggest that cumulative LDL-C level plays an important role in the development of CHD in FH patients.

Shakhtshneider et al. [9] focused on the genetic variants potentially involved in familial hypercholesterolemia in 43 genes associated with lipid metabolism disorders. Targeted high-throughput sequencing of lipid metabolism genes was performed (80 subjects with a familial-hypercholesterolemia phenotype). For patients without functionally significant substitutions in the above genes, multiplex ligation-dependent probe amplification was conducted to determine bigger mutations (deletions and/or duplications) in the *LDLR* promoter and exons. A clinically significant variant in some genes associated with familial hypercholesterolemia was identified in 47.5% of the subjects. Clinically significant variants in the *LDLR* gene were identified in 19 probands (73.1% of all variants identified in probands); in three probands (11.5%), pathogenic variants were found in the *APOB* gene; and in four probands (15.4%), rare, clinically significant variants were identified in genes *LPL*, *SREBF1*, *APOC3*, and *ABCG5*. In 12 (85.7%) of 14 children of the probands, clinically significant variants were detectable in genes associated with familial hypercholesterolemia. The use of clinical criteria, targeted sequencing, and multiplex ligation-dependent probe amplification makes it possible to identify carriers of rare clinically significant variants in a wide range of lipid metabolism genes and to investigate their influence on phenotypic manifestations of familial hypercholesterolemia.

Khan et al. [10] evaluated how ASA non-sensitivity can be diagnosed using Plateletworks®, a point-of-care platelet function test. Patients prescribed 81 mg of ASA were recruited in a series of two successive phases—a discovery phase and a validation phase. In the discovery phase, a total of 60 patients were recruited to establish a cut-off point (COP) for ASA non-sensitivity using Plateletworks®. Each sample was simultaneously cross-referenced with a light transmission aggregometer (LTA). Their findings demonstrated that >52% maximal platelet aggregation using Plateletworks® had a sensitivity, specificity, and likelihood ratio of 80%, 70%, and 2.67, respectively, in predicting ASA non-sensitivity. This COP was validated in a secondary cohort of 40 patients prescribed 81 mg of ASA using Plateletworks® and LTA. The data demonstrated that established COP had a 91% sensitivity and 69% specificity in identifying ASA non-sensitivity using Plateletworks®. The authors suggested that Plateletworks® is a point-of-care platelet function test that can appropriately diagnose ASA non-sensitive patients with a sensitivity exceeding 80%.

The articles in this special issue cover interesting topics in lipidology that are also related to cardiology, internal medicine, genetics, and epidemiology. The presented data expand our knowledge about atherosclerosis.

Author Contributions: E.S. (Elena Shakhtshneider) and Y.R. were responsible for the preparation of the scientific program and overall organization of the conference; E.S. (Evgeniia Striukova) chaired the sessions and was in charge of the conference content; Y.R. conceived the conference. All authors have read and agreed to the published version of the manuscript.

Funding: This work received no external funding.

Conflicts of Interest: The authors declare that they have no conflict of interest.

References

1. Metelskaya, V.A.; Gavrilova, N.E.; Zhatkina, M.V.; Yarovaya, E.B.; Drapkina, O.M. A Novel Integrated Biomarker for Evaluation of Risk and Severity of Coronary Atherosclerosis, and Its Validation. *J. Pers. Med.* **2022**, *12*, 206. [CrossRef] [PubMed]
2. Gruzdeva, O.V.; Dyleva, Y.A.; Belik, E.V.; Sinitsky, M.Y.; Stasev, A.N.; Kokov, A.N.; Brel, N.K.; Krivkina, E.O.; Bychkova, E.E.; Tarasov, R.S.; et al. Relationship between Epicardial and Coronary Adipose Tissue and the Expression of Adiponectin, Leptin, and Interleukin 6 in Patients with Coronary Artery Disease. *J. Pers. Med.* **2022**, *12*, 129. [CrossRef] [PubMed]
3. Shramko, V.S.; Striukova, E.V.; Polonskaya, Y.V.; Stakhneva, E.M.; Volkova, M.V.; Kurguzov, A.V.; Kashtanova, E.V.; Ragino, Y.I. Associations of Antioxidant Enzymes with the Concentration of Fatty Acids in the Blood of Men with Coronary Artery Atherosclerosis. *J. Pers. Med.* **2021**, *11*, 1281. [CrossRef] [PubMed]
4. Polonskaya, Y.V.; Kashtanova, E.V.; Murashov, I.S.; Striukova, E.V.; Kurguzov, A.V.; Stakhneva, E.M.; Shramko, V.S.; Maslatsov, N.A.; Chernyavsky, A.M.; Ragino, Y.I. Association of Matrix Metalloproteinases with Coronary Artery Calcification in Patients with CHD. *J. Pers. Med.* **2021**, *11*, 506. [CrossRef] [PubMed]
5. Afanasieva, O.I.; Tyurina, A.V.; Klesareva, E.A.; Arefieva, T.I.; Ezhov, M.V.; Pokrovsky, S.N. Lipoprotein(a), Immune Cells and Cardiovascular Outcomes in Patients with Premature Coronary Heart Disease. *J. Pers. Med.* **2022**, *12*, 269. [CrossRef] [PubMed]
6. Shapkina, M.; Ryabikov, A.; Mazdorova, E.; Titarenko, A.; Avdeeva, E.; Mazurenko, E.; Shcherbakova, L.; Pikhart, H.; Bobak, M.; Malyutina, S. The Determinants of the 13-Year Risk of Incident Atrial Fibrillation in a Russian Population Cohort of Middle and Elderly Age. *J. Pers. Med.* **2022**, *12*, 122. [CrossRef] [PubMed]
7. Malyutina, S.; Chervova, O.; Tillmann, T.; Maximov, V.; Ryabikov, A.; Gafarov, V.; Hubacek, J.A.; Pikhart, H.; Beck, S.; Bobak, M. The Relationship between Epigenetic Age and Myocardial Infarction/Acute Coronary Syndrome in a Population-Based Nested Case-Control Study. *J. Pers. Med.* **2022**, *12*, 110. [CrossRef] [PubMed]
8. Korneva, V.; Kuznetsova, T.; Julius, U. The Role of Cumulative LDL Cholesterol in Cardiovascular Disease Development in Patients with Familial Hypercholesterolemia. *J. Pers. Med.* **2022**, *12*, 71. [CrossRef] [PubMed]
9. Shakhtshneider, E.; Ivanoshchuk, D.; Timoshchenko, O.; Orlov, P.; Semaev, S.; Valeev, E.; Goonko, A.; Ladygina, N.; Voevoda, M. Analysis of Rare Variants in Genes Related to Lipid Metabolism in Patients with Familial Hypercholesterolemia in Western Siberia (Russia). *J. Pers. Med.* **2021**, *11*, 1232. [CrossRef] [PubMed]
10. Khan, H.; Jain, S.; Gallant, R.C.; Syed, M.H.; Zamzam, A.; Al-Omran, M.; Rand, M.L.; Ni, H.; Abdin, R.; Qadura, M. Plateletworks® as a Point-of-Care Test for ASA Non-Sensitivity. *J. Pers. Med.* **2021**, *11*, 813. [CrossRef] [PubMed]

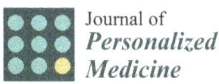

Article

Lipoprotein(a), Immune Cells and Cardiovascular Outcomes in Patients with Premature Coronary Heart Disease

Olga I. Afanasieva [1], Alexandra V. Tyurina [2,*], Elena A. Klesareva [1], Tatiana I. Arefieva [1], Marat V. Ezhov [2] and Sergei N. Pokrovsky [1]

[1] Institute of Experimental Cardiology, National Medical Research Center of Cardiology, Ministry of Health of the Russian Federation, 121552 Moscow, Russia; afanasieva.cardio@yandex.ru (O.I.A.); hea@mail.ru (E.A.K.); tiarefieva@cardio.ru (T.I.A.); dr.pokrovsky@mail.ru (S.N.P.)

[2] A.L. Myasnikov Institute of Clinical Cardiology, National Medical Research Center of Cardiology, Ministry of Health of the Russian Federation, 121552 Moscow, Russia; marat_ezhov@mail.ru

* Correspondence: alex.tyurina.cardio@yandex.ru

Citation: Afanasieva, O.I.; Tyurina, A.V.; Klesareva, E.A.; Arefieva, T.I.; Ezhov, M.V.; Pokrovsky, S.N. Lipoprotein(a), Immune Cells and Cardiovascular Outcomes in Patients with Premature Coronary Heart Disease. *J. Pers. Med.* **2022**, *12*, 269. https://doi.org/10.3390/jpm12020269

Academic Editors: Yuliya I. Ragino and Akinori Nakamura

Received: 29 December 2021
Accepted: 10 February 2022
Published: 12 February 2022

Publisher's Note: MDPI stays neutral with regard to jurisdictional claims in published maps and institutional affiliations.

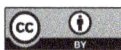

Copyright: © 2022 by the authors. Licensee MDPI, Basel, Switzerland. This article is an open access article distributed under the terms and conditions of the Creative Commons Attribution (CC BY) license (https://creativecommons.org/licenses/by/4.0/).

Abstract: The detection of lipoprotein(a) [Lp(a)] in the artery wall at the stage of lipid-bands formation may indicate that it participates in the atherosclerosis local nonspecific inflammatory process. Innate immune cells are involved in atherogenesis, with monocytes playing a major role in the initiation of atherosclerosis, while neutrophils can contribute to plaque destabilization. This work studies the relationship between Lp(a), immune blood cells and major adverse cardiovascular events (MACE) in patients with the early manifestation of coronary heart disease (CHD). The study included 200 patients with chronic CHD, manifested up to the age of 55 in men and 60 in women. An increased Lp(a) concentration [hyperLp(a)] was shown to predict cardiovascular events in patients with premature CHD with long-term follow-up. According to the logistic regression analysis results, an increase in the monocyte count with OR = 4.58 (95% CI 1.04–20.06) or lymphocyte-to-monocyte ratio with OR = 0.82 (0.68–0.99), ($p < 0.05$ for both) was associated with MACE in patients with early CHD, regardless of gender, age, classical risk factors, atherogenic lipoproteins concentration and statin intake. The combination of an increased monocyte count and hyperLp(a) significantly increased the proportion of patients with early CHD with subsequent development of MACE ($p = 0.02$, $p_{trend} = 0.003$). The odds of cardiovascular events in patients with early CHD manifestation were highest in patients with an elevated lymphocyte-to-monocyte ratio and an elevated Lp(a) level. A higher neutrophil blood count and an elevated neutrophil-to-lymphocyte ratio determined the faster development of MACE in patients with a high Lp(a) concentration. The data obtained in this study suggest that the high atherothrombogenicity of Lp(a) is associated with the "inflammatory" component and the innate immune cells involvement in this process. Thus, the easily calculated immunological ratios of blood cells and Lp(a) concentrations can be considered simple predictors of future cardiovascular events.

Keywords: lipoprotein(a); immune cells blood count; coronary heart disease

1. Introduction

Atherosclerotic cardiovascular diseases (ASCVDs) have remained the leading cause of death worldwide over the past 15 years, despite continued advances in pharmaceuticals and technology [1]. Although there is some progress in the treatment of cardiovascular disease, a trend towards the earlier development of ASCVD and associated cardiovascular events can be observed [2–5]. A significant proportion of major adverse cardiovascular events (MACE) could be avoided via the correction of modifiable risk factors [6], but despite this, the residual risk of CVD development remains [7].

Signs of the local nonspecific inflammatory process in atherosclerosis are traced from the earliest stages of the vessel-wall-lesion development to the stage of destabilization and atherosclerotic plaque damage [8,9]. There is a growing body of evidence supporting the idea that lipoprotein(a) [Lp(a)] and inflammation are important factors in residual risk of ASCVD development [10]. The structural organization of Lp(a), the genetic nature of Lp(a) levels inheritance and its presence in the walls of the arteries already at the stage of lipid-band formation suggested it can participate in this inflammatory process. Several types of immune cells are involved in the atherosclerotic process, such as monocytes, T and B lymphocytes, neutrophils. The results of some studies have shown that enhanced myelopoiesis plays a central role in increasing monocyte and neutrophil numbers in cardiovascular disease and intensifies the formation of atherosclerotic lesions [11]. Despite exploring Lp(a) for several decades, many aspects regarding its role in the development of atherosclerosis are still unclear. There are data that Lp(a) is able to enhance the production of inflammatory monocytes in the bone marrow [12]. We have recently shown that in patients with an elevated Lp(a) level, the absolute and relative content of non-classical CD14+CD16++ monocytes is significantly higher [13], indicating the ability of Lp(a) to influence monocytes. Residual cardiovascular risk in patients with atherosclerosis, despite adequate hypolipidemic therapy, could be related to the increased concentration of Lp(a) and, therefore, the possible relationship between Lp(a) and the vascular wall inflammation deserves further evaluation. Thus, the aim of this study is to investigate the association between Lp(a) concentration, immune blood cells count, and cardiovascular outcomes in patients with early manifestation of coronary heart disease (CHD).

2. Materials and Methods

This retrospective study included consecutive patients who underwent a repeat examination at the National Medical Research Center of Cardiology of the Ministry of Health of the Russian Federation between 2019 and 2021 (Figure A1). The study was carried out in accordance with Good Clinical Practice and the principles of the Declaration of Helsinki. The study protocol was approved by the local ethics committee and written informed consent was obtained from all the patients before their enrollment. We included 200 patients aged 59 ± 9 years with a history of early CHD manifestation (before 55 and 60 years in men and women, respectively). Clinical charts were available from the time of manifestation of CHD for all the included patients. Exclusion criteria were severe comorbidities affecting the prognosis; dementia; alcohol abuse; autoimmune and infectious diseases; and treatment with any hormones, PCSK9 inhibitors, and apheresis. All the patients were examined and interviewed to evaluate the course of the disease and the presence of classical atherosclerosis risk factors. Arterial hypertension was diagnosed if the patient took antihypertensives, or in cases of of systolic blood pressure level being above 140 mmHg and/or diastolic blood pressure being above 90 mmHg according to two blood-pressure measurements on two different visits. Smoking status was assessed as never smoker, former smoker or current smoker [14]. Type 2 diabetes was diagnosed according to the World Health Organization criteria [15,16]. Body mass index (BMI) was calculated for all the participants and obesity was recorded at BMI $\geq$ 30 kg/m^2.

The lipids (total cholesterol (C), triglyceride (TG) and high-density lipoprotein cholesterol (HDL-C)) were determined by enzymatic colorimetric method on Hitachi 912 biochemical analyzers (Roche Diagnostics, Basal, Switzerland) and Architect C-8000 (Abbott, Abbott Park, Illinois, USA). The quality control of the studies was accomplished with the control sera Precinorm and Precipat (Roche Diagnostics, Basal, Switzerland). The low-density lipoprotein cholesterol (LDL-C) level was calculated with Martin–Hopkins's formula:

$$\text{LDL–C} = \text{TC} - \text{HDL–C} - \frac{\text{TG}}{f}, \qquad (1)$$

where f is an adjustable factor from 3.1 to 11.9 (result in mg/dL).

The concentration of LDL-C corrected for Lp(a)-cholesterol (LDL-C corr.) was calculated by Dahlen modification [17]:

$$\text{LDL–C corr} = \text{LDL–C} - 0.3 \times \frac{\text{Lp}(a)}{38.7}, \text{ (result in mmol/L)}, \qquad (2)$$

Lp(a) concentration was determined using an enzyme immunoassay with sheep monospecific polyclonal antibodies against human Lp(a), as previously described [18]. The sensitivity of the method was 0.2 mg/dL, the intra-plate and between experiments variation coefficients were 3.8% and 9.8% in the Lp(a) concentration ranged from 5 to 190 mg/dL. The method was validated with two kits, TintElize Lp(a) (Biopool AB, Umea, Sweden) and Immunozym Lp(a) (Progen Biotechnik GmbH, Heidelberg, Germany). The control serum (Technoclone, Vienna, Austria) was approved by the International Federation of Clinical Chemistry and was used to standardize the ELISA.

In addition, a routine blood test with the absolute count of leukocytes, the absolute and relative counts of lymphocytes, neutrophils, and monocytes was performed in all the patients. The lymphocyte-to-monocyte ratio (LMR) and neutrophil-to-lymphocyte ratio (NLR) were calculated as the ratios of the absolute count of lymphocyte to absolute count of monocyte and absolute count of neutrophil to absolute count of lymphocyte.

A statistical analysis was performed using a MedCalc 20.022. (MedCalc Software Ltd., Ostend, Belgium). The results were presented as a mean value ± standard deviation or median with 25th and 75th percentiles for normal or abnormal distribution according to Kolmogorov–Smirnov test, respectively. Student's parametric t-test and non-parametric Mann–Whitney test were used when comparing the quantitative data of the two groups. Fischer's exact test was used to estimate frequency data between groups. The Spearman rank correlation and multiple regression or logistic analysis were used. Odds ratio (OR) and 95% confidence intervals (CI) were calculated to evaluate associations between outcomes and study parameters. ROC-analysis was conducted to determine the cut-off criterion of Lp(a) level or lymphocyte-to-monocyte or neutrophil-to-lymphocyte ratios and associated sensitivity and specificity for MACE. Apart from that, and the Kaplan–Meier survival curve was analyzed because parameters such as sex, age of CHD manifestation, statin medication, and hyperLp(a) ($\geq$30 mg/dL), remained unchanged during the whole time from CHD manifestation until now.

3. Results

Most of the patients were males (n = 166, 83%). Arterial hypertension was observed in 87% of the patients, type 2 diabetes in 30%, and 63% were current or former smokers. All the patients took statins at an adequate dose, the average dose equivalent to atorvastatin was 43.4 ± 21.3 mg. Another therapy is presented in the Table A1.

Over the median follow-up of 12 years, starting from the time of CHD manifestation in 121 out of 200 patients, the following major adverse cardiovascular events (MACE) were distinguished: non-fatal myocardial infarction (n = 57, 29%), coronary artery bypass grafting (n = 65, 33%), hospitalizations for unstable angina (n = 35, 18%), and ischemic stroke (n = 14, 7%).

There were no differences in terms of age, gender, classical risk factors frequency, baseline levels of TC, TG, HDL-C or LDL-C, hypolipidemic and antiplatelet therapy in the studied groups (Table 1).

The concentration of Lp(a) was higher in the patients with MACE in comparison with the group without MACE: 44 [13; 98] mg/dL and 25 [8; 79] mg/dL, respectively, $p < 0.05$ (Figure 1).

According to ROC-analysis, the concentration of Lp(a) $\geq$ 30 mg/dL was associated with MACE with 60% sensitivity and 54% specificity (area under the curve 0.59; 95% CI 0.51–0.65; $p < 0.05$). The ROC analysis for the two cut-off points—30 and 50 mg/dL—showed no significant differences, but the AUC was slightly higher for the cut-off point 30 mg/dL vs. 50 mg/dL: 0.57; 0.50–0.64 vs. 0.56; 0.49–0.63, $p > 0.05$.

The level of Lp(a) $\geq$ 30 mg/dl detected in 60% of the patients with early manifestation of CHD and MACE in comparison with 45% of the patients without MACE is presented, with $p < 0.05$ (Figure 2). The OR of MACE in patients with Lp(a) concentration of $\geq$ 30 mg/dL was 1.25 (0.99 1.58), $p = 0.06$.

Table 1. The patients' characteristics depending on the occurrence of MACE.

	without MACE n = 79	MACE n = 121	p-Value
Men	61 (77%)	105 (87%)	0.1
Age, years	57.6 ± 8.5	59.5 ± 9.0	0.5
Age of CHD manifestation, years	47.7 ± 6.8	45.9 ± 7.9	0.2
BMI, kg/m^2	29.4 ± 6.3	30.0 ± 5.0	0.5
Follow-up, years	10 ± 7	13 ± 8	0.4
Obesity	45 (57%)	57 (47%)	0.2
Arterial hypertension	70 (89%)	102 (84%)	0.6
Smoking	47 (60%)	79 (65%)	0.5
Family history of CVD	32 (41%)	39 (32%)	0.3
Type 2 diabetes	25 (32.6%)	35 (29%)	0.8
TC, mmol/L	4.3 ± 1.2	4.3 ± 1.1	1.0
TG, mmol/L	1.5 [1.1; 2.1]	1.5 [1.1; 2.2]	1.0
HDL-C, mmol/L	1.1 ± 0.3	1.2 ± 0.3	0.9
LDL-C, mmol/L	2.5 ± 1.1	2.4 ± 1.0	0.4
LDL-C corr, mmol/L	2.2 ± 1.1	1.8 ± 1.1	0.1
Average dose of statins, mg	42 ± 20	45 ± 22	0.3
LDL-C < 1.4 mmol/L	10 (13%)	14 (12%)	0.8
Antiplatelet/anticoagulant	65 (82%)	101 (83%)	1.0

Data are presented as mean ± standard deviation, or median [25%; 75%], or n (%).

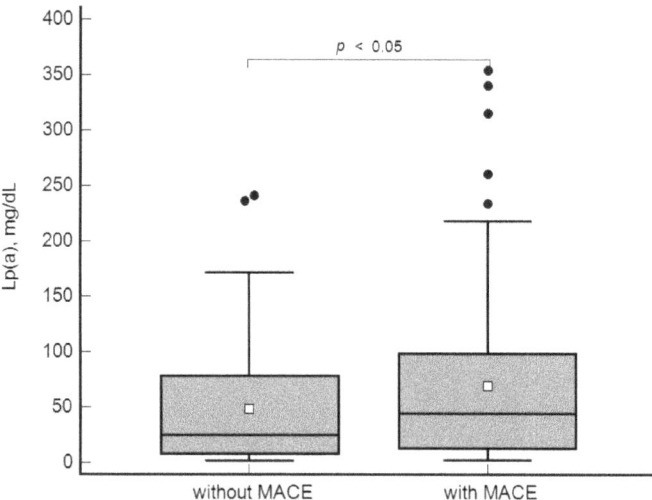

Figure 1. Concentration of lipoprotein(a) in patients with and without MACE. Data are presented as Box-and-Whisker plot: a grey box is drawn from the 25% and 75%; a horizontal line is a median (50%), a white square symbol is a mean, black points are values to the above of 1.5 × IQR (the Interquartile range (IQR) is calculated as 75%–25%).

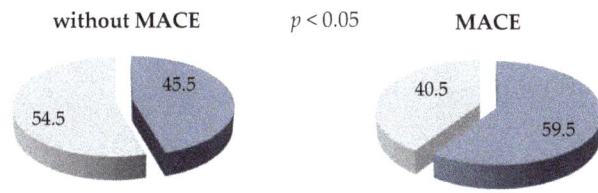

Figure 2. The proportion of patients with Lp (a) ≥ 30 mg/dL in groups with and without MACE.

A trend towards a more rapid development of MACE was detected in the patients with Lp(a) ≥ 30 mg/dL. The patients without MACE but with Lp(a) ≥ 30 mg/dL had a mean survival time of 143 ± 15 months versus 168 ± 18 months in those with Lp(a) < 30 mg/dL, $p < 0.01$ (Figure A2).

The blood-cells count did not significantly differ in the patients with and without MACE (Table 2).

Table 2. Blood cells counts in patients with and without MACE.

	without MACE $n = 79$	MACE $n = 121$	p-Value
Leukocytes, 10^9/L	7.8 [6.6; 9.2]	7.7 [6.3; 8.9]	0.64
Lymphocytes, 10^9/L	2.2 [1.7; 2.9]	2.0 [1.6; 2.5]	0.12
Lymphocytes, %	28.9 [24.4; 35.5]	27.5 [22.3; 33.2]	0.10
Neutrophils, 10^9/L	4.7 [3.7; 5.5]	4.5 [3.8; 5.7]	0.85
Neutrophils, %	59.8 [53.8; 64.9]	61.8 [55.8; 67.7]	0.14
Monocytes, 10^9/L	0.5 [0.4; 0.6]	0.6 [0.4; 0.7]	0.20
Monocytes, %	6.8 [5.4; 8.1]	7.0 [5.9; 9.2]	0.09
Basophiles, 10^9/L	0.07 [0.05; 0.09]	0.06 [0.05; 0.09]	0.50
Basophils, %	0.90 [0.68; 1.16]	0.87 [0.58; 1.10]	0.37
Eosinophils, 10^9/L	0.2 [0.1; 0.3]	0.14 [0.07; 0.21]	0.12
Eosinophils, %	2.2 [1.1; 3.2]	1.7 [1.0; 2.7]	0.20
Platelets, 10^9/L	220.0 [195.5; 268.0]	210.0 [177.0; 251.3]	0.04

Data are presented as median [25%; 75%].

A correlation analysis showed no significant associations between immune-blood cells count and Lp(a) concentrations or other atherogenic lipoproteins.

According to the logistic regression analysis, an increase in Lp(a) concentration by 10 mg/dL with OR = 1.06 (95% CI 1.00–1.14), age increase by one year with OR = 1.04 (1.00–1.08) and male sex of the patients with OR = 2.57 (1.07–6.19) were independently associated with MACE, regardless of other risk factors, lipids, and the monocytes count.

The combination of an elevated monocyte count (above median) in the presence of Lp(a) ≥ 30 mg/dL significantly increased the proportion of the patients with MACE ($p = 0.02$, $p_{trend} = 0.003$) (Figure 3).

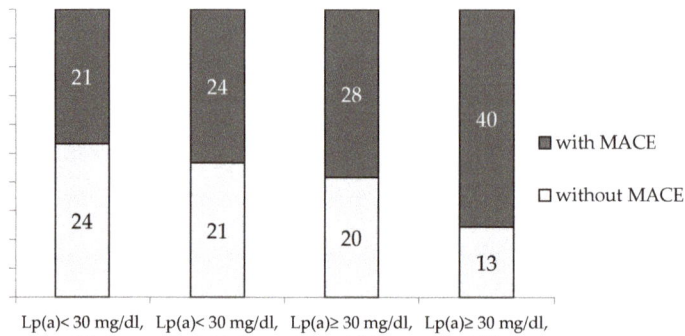

Figure 3. The proportion of CHD patients with and without MACE during observation period depends on blood monocyte count and Lp(a) concentration. Mon—monocytes. Median for Mon = 0.54×10^9/L.

The lymphocyte-to-monocyte ratio was lower in the group of the patients with MACE during the observation period 3.9 ± 2.5 vs. 4.6 ± 1.9, $p = 0.05$. According to the ROC analysis, the lymphocyte-to-monocyte ratio was significantly associated with MACE (AUC = 0.61, $p = 0.01$) and the cut-off value was calculated as <4.56 (a sensitivity of 69% and a specificity 49%). The median of the distribution for the lymphocyte-to-monocyte ratio was 4.18. This value discriminates MACE with a sensitivity of 60% and a specificity of 55% and was chosen as the most suitable for the proceeding calculations.

The combination of the reduced lymphocyte-to-monocyte ratio with Lp(a) ≥ 30 mg/dL was found in 34% of the patients with MACE vs. 19% in the patients without MACE (Figure 4) and significantly increased the chance of developing MACE in such patients (Table 3).

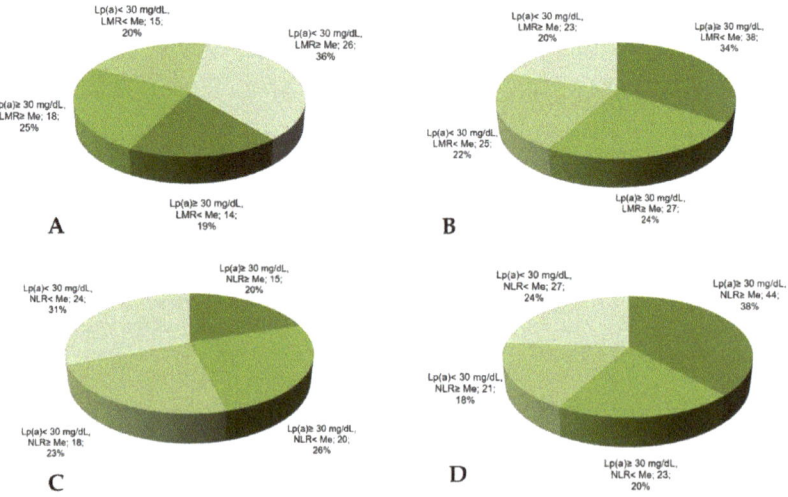

Figure 4. The proportion of CHD patients according to Lp(a) concentration, lymphocyte-to-monocyte ratio, or neutrophil-to-lymphocyte ratio in groups without (**A,B**) or with (**C,D**) MACE. LMR—lymphocyte-to-monocyte ratio, NLR—neutrophil-to-lymphocyte ratio, Me—median. Median for LMR = 4.18, for NLR = 2.66.

Table 3. MACE odds ratio in patients depending on Lp(a) concentration and blood immune cell distribution according to the median.

	Lp(a) < 30 mg/dL	Lp(a) ≥ 30 mg/dL
Monocytes < 0.54×10^9/L	1	1.22 (0.53–2.78)
Monocytes ≥ 0.54×10^9/L	1.0 (0.44–2.28)	2.69 (1.14–6.34) *
LMR ≥ 4.18	1	1.70 (0.75–3.85)
LMR < 4.18	1.88 (0.80–4.41)	3.07 (1.33–7.04) *
Neutrophils < 5.04×10^9/L	1	1.38 (0.59–3.21)
Neutrophils ≥ 5.04×10^9/L	0.76 (0.33–1.74)	1.65 (0.96–4.92)
NLR < 2.66	1	1.02 (0.45–2.30)
NLR ≥ 2.66	1.04 (0.45–1.10)	2.61 (1.17–5.82) *

* $p < 0.05$; LMR—lymphocyte-to-monocyte ratio, NLR—neutrophil-to-lymphocyte ratio.

The neutrophil-to-lymphocyte ratio has no significant association with MACE (AUC = 0.56, p = 0.07) according to the ROC analysis. Nevertheless, the proportion of the patients with Lp(a) ≥ 30 mg/dL and the neutrophil-to-lymphocyte ratio above the median was maximal in the patients with MACE (Figure 4).

According to the logistic-regression analysis, an increase in the lymphocyte-to-monocyte ratio per unit was associated with MACE in the patients with the early CHD manifestation regardless of their sex, age, risk factors (arterial hypertension, diabetes, smoking), lipid levels, and statin intake (OR = 0.8 (0.7–1.0), p = 0.04). The neutrophils count and neutrophil-to-lymphocyte ratio were not associated with MACE in the same model.

However, in the subgroup of the patients with neutrophil-to-lymphocyte ratio and neutrophils count above the median, the Lp(a) concentration ≥ 30 mg/dL significantly reduced the mean survival time for MACE, in contrast to the subgroup of the patients with neutrophils count below the median (Figures 5 and 6).

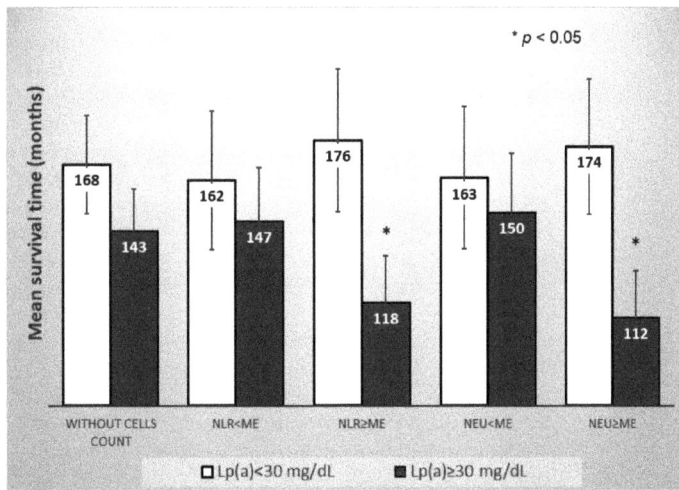

Figure 5. Mean survival time without MACE in subgroups of patients depending on the of Lp(a) concentration, the neutrophils blood count, or the neutrophil-to-lymphocyte ratio. NLR—neutrophil-to-lymphocyte ratio, NEU—neutrophil, Me—median. Median for NLR = 2.66, for Neu = 5.04×10^9/L.

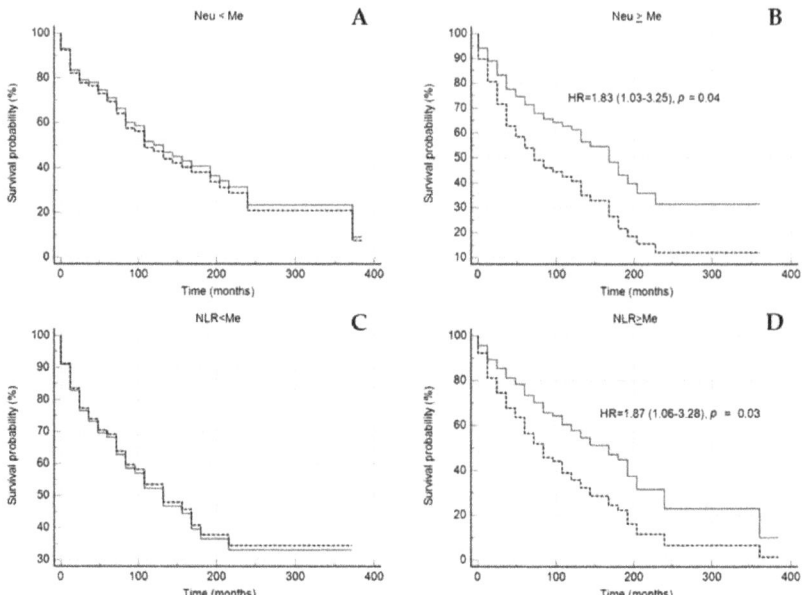

Figure 6. Kaplan–Meier survival without events curves in subgroups of patients with neutrophils count < median (**A**) or ≥ median (**B**), NLR < median (**C**) or ≥ median (**D**) depending on the of Lp(a) < 30 mg/dL (grey solid line) and Lp(a) ≥ 30 mg/dL (black dotted line). NLR—neutrophil-to-lymphocyte ratio, NEU—neutrophil, Me—median. Median for NLR 2.66, for Neu 5.04×10^9/L. Sex, age of CHD manifestation, statin medication was included in model of Cox proportional regression.

4. Discussion

The hypothesis that Lp(a) pathogenicity is associated with inflammation and that immune cells, and monocytes in particular, are involved, was expressed quite a long time ago [19]. The relationship between the innate immune system and Lp(a) is based on the fact that oxidized phospholipids localized on Lp(a) can be recognized by receptors of innate immunity [20].

Inflammation in the arterial vessel wall is detected in subjects with increased concentration of Lp(a). In contrast, monocytes isolated from the blood of patients with a high concentration of Lp(a) demonstrate an increased ability to transendothelial migration [21].

The activation of the innate immune system in patients with hyperlipoproteinemia(a) is consistent with our recent study, which demonstrated that in patients with an elevated Lp(a) concentration, there is a redistribution of monocyte subpopulations towards an increase in CD14+CD16++ monocytes [13]. Furthermore, the combination of hyperlipoproteinemia(a) and a higher content of intermediate monocytes was associated with a significant increase in stenotic plaques in all major coronary arteries.

The results of this retrospective study, in which patients with early CHD manifestation participated, showed that an increased monocyte count on the background of hyperlipoproteinemia(a) is associated with a 2.7-fold increase in the chance of MACE developing compared to those with Lp(a) < 30 mg/dl and the monocyte count below the median.

Experiments on apoE-/- mice demonstrated that myocardial infarction caused by artery ligation leads to an accelerated accumulation of innate immune cells, namely, an increase in both the total number of monocytes/macrophages in the aorta and a subpopulation of pro-inflammatory monocytes with a high content of Ly-6C as well as larger atherosclerotic lesions with a more advanced morphology relative to individuals without myocardial infarction [22]. The secreted pro-inflammatory cytokines by activated monocytes can accelerate the atherosclerotic process and contribute to the further destabilization of atherosclerotic plaques.

The neutrophil-to-lymphocyte ratio, as a possible marker of chronic systemic inflammation, is a simple predictor for both cardiovascular events and cardiovascular death in large prospective observational studies [23,24].

In our study, a neutrophil-to-lymphocyte ratio of more than 2.66 with an elevated Lp(a) concentration showed a twofold chance of MACE in patients with early CHD manifestation. A faster onset of MACE was demonstrated in patients with Lp(a) > 30 mg/dL and elevated neutrophil blood count or neutrophil-to-lymphocyte ratio. However, the correlation between Lp(a) concentration and neutrophils was not detected. Moreover, a correlation between HDL-C and neutrophil-to-lymphocyte ratio that has been described for healthy subjects, was not found in the patients with early manifestation of CHD [25].

Neutrophil-to-lymphocyte ratio as a marker of systemic inflammation has no specificity and is of prognostic value in oncology, sepsis, and other conditions [26,27]. However, a growing body of evidence demonstrates that neutrophils play an integral role in atherosclerotic cardiovascular disease development. The ability of neutrophils to enhance monocyte adhesion and transmigration to atherosclerotic plaques may contribute to a more severe atherosclerotic process in patients with an elevated Lp(a) level and early manifestation of CHD. There is evidence that neutrophils are localized near plaques that are prone to rupture [28]. Previously, it has been shown that the concentration of matrix metalloproteinase 9 was positively associated with the size of the necrotic core of atherosclerotic plaques and was inversely related to the fibrous tissue content of the plaques in patients with chronic CHD and Lp(a) level > 60 mg/dL [29]. The secretion of active proteases by neutrophils metalloproteinase 9, which degrades the fibrous capsule, may also explain the effects of neutrophils on MACE development in patients with elevated Lp(a) concentrations.

Despite the prominent role of both dyslipidemia and inflammation as crucial factors in atherogenesis [30], the diversity and sequence of inflammatory processes and the involvement of atherogenic lipoproteins are still unclear.

All the patients in the present study took statins, but most patients had MACE during a median of 12 years of follow-up, and the groups did not differ in terms of LDL-C concentration.

Patients with early CHD belong to the category of very high cardiovascular risk, which may explain the high percentage of cases with MACE during prolonged observation. In addition, in 78% of patients CHD has been manifested with myocardial infarction, which significantly worsens the prognosis. There are identical results for the high 15-year mortality in patients with early myocardial infarction in a long-term survival study [31]. Overall, 65% of patients had at least one serious cardiovascular event and/or death in the study Yagel and colleagues, examining cardiovascular outcomes in patients with early acute coronary syndrome [32]. More, than half (52.9%) of patients with early CHD had at least one cardiovascular event during 10 years of follow-up in another study of long-term prognosis [33]. The observation period in our study was more than 12 years for 50% and more than 18 years for 25% of included patients.

Male gender is a risk factor for cardiovascular diseases, especially for early CHD manifestation, and the number of men in our study was higher than the number of women. This corresponded with the prospective observational cohort study GENESIS-PROXY (Gender and Sex determinants of cardiovascular disease: from bench to beyond-Premature Acute Coronary Syndrome) [34] and another study devoted to the long-term prognosis in patients with early coronary heart disease [33]. In the study of risk profiles, sex-related differences, and outcomes in a contemporary population of young patients with CAD, men also made up 70% of the study group [5].

Although the existing effective methods of lipid-lowering therapy significantly reduce the burden of cardiovascular diseases, their effect on inflammation is contradictory. The results of a post hoc analysis of the FOURIER study showed that patients with a CRP level > 2 mg/L had a higher risk of MACE compared to participants with normal CRP levels, despite achieving the target LDL-C levels [35]. The risk associated with an increased Lp(a) concentration was also significantly higher in patients with more pronounced inflammation and higher CRP > 2 mg/L [36].

A reduction of cardiovascular events risk while taking anti-inflammatory drugs has been demonstrated in several clinical studies—Canakinumab Anti-inflammatory Thrombosis Outcome Study (CANTOS) that used therapeutic monoclonal antibodies against IL-1β (canakinumab), and LoDoCo2 study where low doses of colchicine in patients with chronic CHD were used [37,38].

We hypothesize a relationship between chronic inflammation processes, Lp(a) concentrations, and the development of MACE. The clinical significance of the present study results is related to the fact that patients with early CHD manifestation and elevated Lp(a) chronic inflammation, expressed as an increased ratio of immune blood cells, are associated with a more severe disease. The ratios could be calculated from a routine blood test, and their association with a prospective prognosis for various diseases has been shown above [24]. We propose assessing such ratios in patients with early CHD manifestation, especially in patients with elevated Lp(a) levels. Elevated levels of circulating monocytes and neutrophils in patients with early CHD manifestation and subsequent MACE can provide a pool of inflammatory cells available for recruitment into the growing arteries and their secreted pro-inflammatory cytokines and can accelerate the atherosclerotic process and thus, contribute to further destabilization of atherosclerotic plaques, leading to the subsequent MACE.

5. Study Limitation

Our study has some limitations. Patients had CHD manifestation in the past, prior to enrolling in the study (median 12 years). Currently, all the patients are taking statins at adequate doses, but we have no precise data on the regularity of intake from the beginning of the disease to the present time. Because our study was retrospective, we cannot say that the neutrophils count, and the neutrophil-to-lymphocyte ratio were elevated at CHD manifestation. However, we assumed the relative stability of neutrophil blood counts and neutrophil-to-lymphocyte ratio by dividing the patients into subgroups according to these parameters and analyzing survival curves [23].

The ELISA method for Lp(a) determination was sensitive to apolipoprotein(a) isoforms, resulting in a slight increase in the Lp(a) concentration in samples with high molecular weight apo(a) isoforms. The absolute bias (median [25%; 75%]) was ~1.5 [−0.4; 5.7] mg/dL. The high variability in the Lp(a) measurement, regardless of apo(a) isoforms, and the nonsignificant bias in the absolute Lp(a) concentration in our ELISA method makes it possible to assume that sensitivity of ELISA to apo(a) isoforms did not affect the results of the study. In addition, there were no significant differences in the Lp(a)-associated relative risk of CAD in studies using methods both sensitive and insensitive to the size of apo(a) isoforms, according to meta-analysis [39].

According to the results of a recent prospective ACCELERATE trial, the significant association between an elevated Lp(a) concentration and time to first MACE was found in patients with CRP levels $\geq$ 2 mg/L [36]. We did not determine interleukin or C-reactive protein concentrations, which is also a limitation of the study.

6. Conclusions

An elevated Lp(a) concentration was shown to be a predictor of cardiovascular events in patients with premature CHD with long-term follow-up. The likelihood of cardiovascular events in patients with early CHD manifestation were highest in patients with an elevated lymphocyte-to-monocyte ratio and an elevated Lp(a) level. A higher neutrophil blood count and an elevated neutrophil-to-lymphocyte ratio determine the faster development of MACE in patients with a high Lp(a) concentration. Thus, the easily calculated immunological ratios of blood cells and Lp(a) concentration can be considered as simple predictors of future cardiovascular events.

Author Contributions: Conceptualization, O.I.A., T.I.A., M.V.E.; writing—original draft preparation, O.I.A., A.V.T. investigation, A.V.T., E.A.K. writing—review and editing, T.I.A.; M.V.E., S.N.P. All authors have read and agreed to the published version of the manuscript.

Funding: The study was supported by Russian Science Foundation, project No. 22-25-00051.

Institutional Review Board Statement: The study was approved by the Ethics Committee of National Research Medical Center of Cardiology, Moscow, Russian Federation (protocol No. 251, 25 November 2019).

Informed Consent Statement: Informed consent was obtained from all subjects involved in the study.

Conflicts of Interest: The authors declare no conflict of interest.

Appendix A

Table A1. Therapy performed in the examined patients.

Therapy	MACE $n = 121$ (%)		without MACE $n = 79$ (%)		p-Value
Antiplatelet therapy	92	(76)	65	(82)	0.38
Anticoagulants	31	(26)	18	(23)	0.74
ACE- inhibitors	57	(47)	31	(39)	0.31
Angiotensin II receptor antagonists	36	(30)	25	(32)	0.87
Beta-blockers	107	(88)	70	(89)	1.00
Calcium channel antagonists	39	(32)	24	(30)	0.88
Nitrates	20	(17)	5	(6)	0.04
Diuretics	37	(31)	24	(30)	1.00

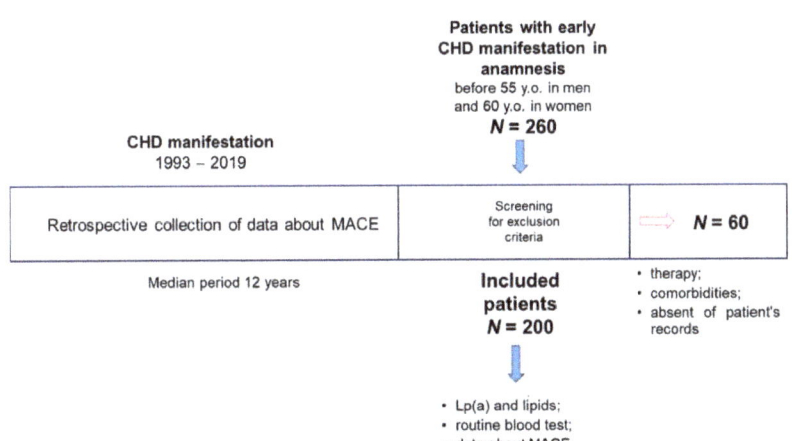

Figure A1. Design of the study. 260 patients with an early history of CHD hospitalized and screened between 2019 and 2021 were included during the screening phase. 60 people were expelled according to the exclusion criteria. The information about the presence or absence of any significant cardiovascular events as well as the date of each such event from the CHD manifestation was available for all patients according to medical records. All patients, after signing an informed consent, were re-examined, relevant medical data were collected, biochemical tests and routine blood tests were performed.

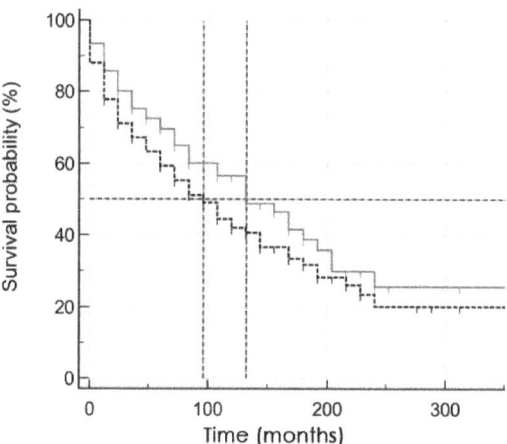

Figure A2. Kaplan–Meier survival curve in subgroups of patients Lp(a) < 30 mg/dL (grey solid line) and Lp(a) ≥ 30 mg/dL (black dotted line). 50% of patients in the group with elevated Lp(a) concentration lived to MACE after 96 (95% CI 60–144) months vs. 132 months (95% CI 84–192).

References

1. WHO. *The Top 10 Causes of Death*; World Health Organization: Geneva, Switzerland, 2018.
2. Andersson, C.; Vasan, R.S. Epidemiology of cardiovascular disease in young individuals. *Nat. Rev. Cardiol.* **2018**, *15*, 230–240. [CrossRef] [PubMed]
3. Maillet, A.; Desormais, I.; Rivière, A.B.; Aboyans, V.; Lacroix, P.; Mirault, T.; Messas, E.; Bataille, V.; Constans, J.; Boulon, C. Peripheral Atheromatous Arterial Disease in the Young: Risk Factors, Clinical Features, and Prognosis from the COPART Cohort. *Angiology* **2017**, *68*, 893–898. [CrossRef]
4. Tibæk, M.; Dehlendorff, C.; Jørgensen, H.S.; Forchhammer, H.B.; Johnsen, S.P.; Kammersgaard, L.P. Increasing Incidence of Hospitalization for Stroke and Transient Ischemic Attack in Young Adults: A Registry-Based Study. *J. Am. Heart Assoc.* **2016**, *5*, e003158. [CrossRef]
5. Vikulova, D.N.; Grubisic, M.; Zhao, Y.; Lynch, K.; Humphries, K.H.; Pimstone, S.N.; Brunham, L.R. Premature Atherosclerotic Cardiovascular Disease: Trends in Incidence, Risk Factors, and Sex-Related Differences, 2000 to 2016. *J. Am. Heart Assoc.* **2019**, *8*, e012178. [CrossRef]
6. Yusuf, S.; Joseph, P.; Rangarajan, S.; Islam, S.; Mente, A.; Hystad, P.; Brauer, M.; Kutty, V.R.; Gupta, R.; Wielgosz, A.; et al. Modifiable risk factors, cardiovascular disease, and mortality in 155,722 individuals from 21 high-income, middle-income, and low-income countries (PURE): A prospective cohort study. *Lancet* **2020**, *395*, 795–808. [CrossRef]
7. Cho, K.I.; Yu, J.; Hayashi, T.; Han, S.H.; Koh, K.K. Strategies to Overcome Residual Risk During Statins Era. *Circ. J. Off. J. Jpn. Circ. Soc.* **2019**, *83*, 1973–1979. [CrossRef] [PubMed]
8. Kaski, J.C.; Valenzuela Garcia, L.F. Therapeutic options for the management of patients with cardiac syndrome X. *Eur. Heart J.* **2001**, *22*, 283–293. [CrossRef]
9. Libby, P.; Ridker, P.M.; Maseri, A. Inflammation and atherosclerosis. *Circulation* **2002**, *105*, 1135–1143. [CrossRef]
10. Hoogeveen, R.C.; Ballantyne, C.M. Residual Cardiovascular Risk at Low LDL: Remnants, Lipoprotein(a), and Inflammation. *Clin. Chem.* **2021**, *67*, 143–153. [CrossRef]
11. Morgan, P.K.; Fang, L.; Lancaster, G.I.; Murphy, A.J. Hematopoiesis is regulated by cholesterol efflux pathways and lipid rafts: Connections with cardiovascular diseases. *J. Lipid Res.* **2020**, *61*, 667–675. [CrossRef]
12. Schnitzler, J.G.; Hoogeveen, R.M.; Ali, L.; Prange, K.H.M.; Waissi, F.; van Weeghel, M.; Bachmann, J.C.; Versloot, M.; Borrelli, M.J.; Yeang, C.; et al. Atherogenic Lipoprotein(a) Increases Vascular Glycolysis, Thereby Facilitating Inflammation and Leukocyte Extravasation. *Circ. Res.* **2020**, *126*, 1346–1359. [CrossRef] [PubMed]
13. Afanasieva, O.I.; Filatova, A.Y.; Arefieva, T.I.; Klesareva, E.A.; Tyurina, A.V.; Radyukhina, N.V.; Ezhov, M.V.; Pokrovsky, S.N. The Association of Lipoprotein(a) and Circulating Monocyte Subsets with Severe Coronary Atherosclerosis. *J. Cardiovasc. Dev. Dis.* **2021**, *8*, 63. [CrossRef] [PubMed]
14. Burki, T.K. WHO releases latest report on the global tobacco epidemic. *Lancet Oncol.* **2021**, *22*, 1217. [CrossRef]
15. *Classification of Diabetes Mellitus*; World Health Organization: Geneva, Switzerland, 2019; Available online: https://apps.who.int/iris/handle/10665/325182 (accessed on 1 December 2021).
16. *Use of Glycated Haemoglobin (HbA1c) in the Diagnosis of Diabetes Mellitus*; Abbreviated Report of a WHO Consultation (WHO/NMH/CHP/CPM/111); World Health Organization: Geneva, Switzerland, 2011.

17. Dahlen, G.H. Incidence of Lp(a) lipoproteins among populations. In *Lipoprotein(a)*; Scanu, A.M., Ed.; Academic Press: New York, NY, USA, 1990; pp. 151–173.
18. Afanasieva, O.I.; Ezhov, M.V.; Razova, O.A.; Afanasieva, M.I.; Utkina, E.A.; Pokrovsky, S.N. Apolipoprotein(a) phenotype determines the correlations of lipoprotein(a) and proprotein convertase subtilisin/kexin type 9 levels in patients with potential familial hypercholesterolemia. *Atherosclerosis* **2018**, *277*, 477–482. [CrossRef]
19. Kraaijenhof, J.M.; Hovingh, G.K.; Stroes, E.S.G.; Kroon, J. The iterative lipid impact on inflammation in atherosclerosis. *Curr. Opin. Lipidol.* **2021**, *32*, 286–292. [CrossRef]
20. Boffa, M.B.; Koschinsky, M.L. Oxidized phospholipids as a unifying theory for lipoprotein(a) and cardiovascular disease. *Nat. Rev. Cardiol.* **2019**, *16*, 305–318. [CrossRef]
21. van der Valk, F.M.; Bekkering, S.; Kroon, J.; Yeang, C.; Van den Bossche, J.; van Buul, J.D.; Ravandi, A.; Nederveen, A.J.; Verberne, H.J.; Scipione, C.; et al. Oxidized Phospholipids on Lipoprotein(a) Elicit Arterial Wall Inflammation and an Inflammatory Monocyte Response in Humans. *Circulation* **2016**, *134*, 611–624. [CrossRef]
22. Dutta, P.; Courties, G.; Wei, Y.; Leuschner, F.; Gorbatov, R.; Robbins, C.S.; Iwamoto, Y.; Thompson, B.; Carlson, A.L.; Heidt, T.; et al. Myocardial infarction accelerates atherosclerosis. *Nature* **2012**, *487*, 325–329. [CrossRef]
23. Adamstein, N.H.; MacFadyen, J.G.; Rose, L.M.; Glynn, R.J.; Dey, A.K.; Libby, P.; Tabas, I.A.; Mehta, N.N.; Ridker, P.M. The neutrophil-lymphocyte ratio and incident atherosclerotic events: Analyses from five contemporary randomized trials. *Eur. Heart J.* **2021**, *42*, 896–903. [CrossRef]
24. Balta, S.; Celik, T.; Mikhailidis, D.P.; Ozturk, C.; Demirkol, S.; Aparci, M.; Iyisoy, A. The Relation Between Atherosclerosis and the Neutrophil-Lymphocyte Ratio. *Clin. Appl. Thromb. Hemost.* **2016**, *22*, 405–411. [CrossRef]
25. Varol, E.; Bas, H.A.; Aksoy, F.; Ari, H.; Ozaydin, M. Relationship between neutrophil-lymphocyte ratio and isolated low high-density lipoprotein cholesterol. *Angiology* **2014**, *65*, 630–633. [CrossRef] [PubMed]
26. Guthrie, G.J.; Charles, K.A.; Roxburgh, C.S.; Horgan, P.G.; McMillan, D.C.; Clarke, S.J. The systemic inflammation-based neutrophil-lymphocyte ratio: Experience in patients with cancer. *Crit. Rev. Oncol./Hematol.* **2013**, *88*, 218–230. [CrossRef] [PubMed]
27. Ljungström, L.; Pernestig, A.K.; Jacobsson, G.; Andersson, R.; Usener, B.; Tilevik, D. Diagnostic accuracy of procalcitonin, neutrophil-lymphocyte count ratio, C-reactive protein, and lactate in patients with suspected bacterial sepsis. *PLoS ONE* **2017**, *12*, e0181704. [CrossRef] [PubMed]
28. Soehnlein, O. Multiple roles for neutrophils in atherosclerosis. *Circ. Res.* **2012**, *110*, 875–888. [CrossRef] [PubMed]
29. Ezhov, M.; Safarova, M.; Afanasieva, O.; Mitroshkin, M.; Matchin, Y.; Pokrovsky, S. Matrix Metalloproteinase 9 as a Predictor of Coronary Atherosclerotic Plaque Instability in Stable Coronary Heart Disease Patients with Elevated Lipoprotein(a) Levels. *Biomolecules* **2019**, *9*, 129. [CrossRef]
30. Libby, P.; Nahrendorf, M.; Swirski, F.K. Monocyte heterogeneity in cardiovascular disease. *Semin. Immunopathol.* **2013**, *35*, 553–562. [CrossRef] [PubMed]
31. Cole, J.H.; Miller, J.I., 3rd; Sperling, L.S.; Weintraub, W.S. Long-term follow-up of coronary artery disease presenting in young adults. *J. Am. Coll. Cardiol.* **2003**, *41*, 521–528. [CrossRef]
32. Yagel, O.; Shadafny, N.; Eliaz, R.; Dagan, G.; Leibowitz, D.; Tahiroglu, I.; Planer, D.; Amir, O.; Elbaz Greener, G.; Alcalai, R. Long-Term Prognosis in Young Patients with Acute Coronary Syndrome Treated with Percutaneous Coronary Intervention. *Vasc. Health Risk Manag.* **2021**, *17*, 153–159. [CrossRef]
33. Zeitouni, M.; Clare, R.M.; Chiswell, K.; Abdulrahim, J.; Shah, N.; Pagidipati, N.P.; Shah, S.H.; Roe, M.T.; Patel, M.R.; Jones, W.S. Risk Factor Burden and Long-Term Prognosis of Patients With Premature Coronary Artery Disease. *J. Am. Heart Assoc.* **2020**, *9*, e017712. [CrossRef]
34. Pilote, L.; Karp, I. GENESIS-PRAXY (GENdEr and Sex determInantS of cardiovascular disease: From bench to beyond-Premature Acute Coronary SYndrome). *Am. Heart J.* **2012**, *163*, 741–746. [CrossRef]
35. Bohula, E.A.; Giugliano, R.P.; Leiter, L.A.; Verma, S.; Park, J.G.; Sever, P.S.; Lira Pineda, A.; Honarpour, N.; Wang, H.; Murphy, S.A.; et al. Inflammatory and Cholesterol Risk in the FOURIER Trial. *Circulation* **2018**, *138*, 131–140. [CrossRef] [PubMed]
36. Puri, R.; Nissen, S.E.; Arsenault, B.J.; St John, J.; Riesmeyer, J.S.; Ruotolo, G.; McErlean, E.; Menon, V.; Cho, L.; Wolski, K.; et al. Effect of C-Reactive Protein on Lipoprotein(a)-Associated Cardiovascular Risk in Optimally Treated Patients With High-Risk Vascular Disease: A Prespecified Secondary Analysis of the ACCELERATE Trial. *JAMA Cardiol.* **2020**, *5*, 1136–1143. [CrossRef] [PubMed]
37. Nidorf, S.M.; Fiolet, A.T.L.; Mosterd, A.; Eikelboom, J.W.; Schut, A.; Opstal, T.S.J.; The, S.H.K.; Xu, X.F.; Ireland, M.A.; Lenderink, T.; et al. Colchicine in Patients with Chronic Coronary Disease. *N. Engl. J. Med.* **2020**, *383*, 1838–1847. [CrossRef]
38. Ridker, P.M.; Everett, B.M.; Thuren, T.; MacFadyen, J.G.; Chang, W.H.; Ballantyne, C.; Fonseca, F.; Nicolau, J.; Koenig, W.; Anker, S.D.; et al. Antiinflammatory Therapy with Canakinumab for Atherosclerotic Disease. *N. Engl. J. Med.* **2017**, *377*, 1119–1131. [CrossRef]
39. Erqou, S.; Kaptoge, S.; Perry, P.L.; Di Angelantonio, E.; Thompson, A.; White, I.R.; Marcovina, S.M.; Collins, R.; Thompson, S.G.; Danesh, J. Lipoprotein(a) concentration and the risk of coronary heart disease, stroke, and nonvascular mortality. *JAMA* **2009**, *302*, 412–423. [CrossRef] [PubMed]

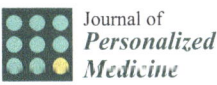

Article

A Novel Integrated Biomarker for Evaluation of Risk and Severity of Coronary Atherosclerosis, and Its Validation

Victoria A. Metelskaya [1,*], Natalia E. Gavrilova [2], Maria V. Zhatkina [3], Elena B. Yarovaya [1,4] and Oxana M. Drapkina [1]

1. National Medical Research Center for Therapy and Preventive Medicine, 101990 Moscow, Russia; yarovaya@mech.math.msu.su (E.B.Y.); odrapkina@gnicpm.ru (O.M.D.)
2. Scandinavian Health Center, 111024 Moscow, Russia; gavrilova_n@scz.ru
3. Filatov City Clinical Hospital No 15, 111539 Moscow, Russia; mvzhatkina@gmail.com
4. Department of Probability Theory, Faculty of Mechanics and Mathematics, Lomonosov Moscow State University, 119234 Moscow, Russia
* Correspondence: vmetelskaya@gnicpm.ru

Abstract: Objective: To assess the feasibility of a combination of biochemical and imaging parameters for estimation of risk and severity of coronary atherosclerosis (CA), and to verify the created integrated biomarker (i-BIO) on independent cohort. Methods: Two cohorts of patients admitted to the hospital for coronary angiography and ultrasound carotid dopplerography were enrolled into the study ($n = 205$ and $n = 216$, respectively). The extent of CA was assessed by Gensini Score (GS). Results: According to GS, participants were distributed as follows: atherosclerosis-free (GS = 0), CA of any stage (GS > 0), subclinical CA (GS < 35), severe CA (GS $\geq$ 35). Based on the analysis of mathematical models, including biochemical and imaging parameters, we selected and combined the most significant variables as i-BIO. The ability of i-BIO to detect the presence and severity of CA was estimated using ROC-analysis with cut-off points determination. Risk of any CA (GS > 0) at i-BIO > 4 was 7.3 times higher than in those with i-BIO $\leq$ 4; risk of severe CA (GS $\geq$ 35) at i-BIO $\geq$ 9 was 3.1 times higher than at i-BIO < 9. Results on the tested cohort confirmed these findings. Conclusions: The i-BIO > 4 detected CA (GS > 0) with sensitivity of 87.9%, i-BIO $\geq$ 9 excluded patients without severe CA (GS < 35), specificity 79.8%. Validation of i-BIO confirmed the feasibility of i-BIO > 4 to separate patients with any CA with sensitivity 76.2%, and of i-BIO $\geq$ 9 to exclude atherosclerosis-free subjects with specificity of 84.0%.

Keywords: circulating biochemical markers; coronary atherosclerosis presence and severity; integrated biomarker (i-BIO); validation; visual markers

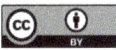

1. Introduction

Among the causes of premature death and disability, atherosclerosis-related cardiovascular diseases (ASCVDs), despite advances in their diagnostics and treatment, remain the leading cause worldwide, including in the Russian Federation [1–3].

Cardiovascular risk assessment, which is based on the identification of traditional risk factors, has a high prognostic value at the population level, but offers little information in terms of predicting individual risk [4]. Moreover, a significant number of acute coronary events are diagnosed in individuals with low or moderate risk calculated on the basis of epidemiological scores [5,6]. The effectiveness of noninvasive diagnostic tests (resting electrocardiography, echocardiography, computed tomography, or stress test) in evaluation of severity of ASCVD is not fully defined. For example, only 38% of patients without known heart disease who underwent elective invasive angiography had obstructive coronary heart disease [7], so better strategies for risk stratification are needed in order to increase the diagnostic power.

Understanding the molecular mechanisms of pathogenesis of atherosclerosis from subclinical to severe stages showed the high significance of biomarkers in ASCVD risks determination [8,9]. The increased interest in the study of cardiovascular risk markers in recent decades is largely due to advances in biomedicine, including both achievements in basic science and the development of new technologies to search for and study biomolecules [9–11]. In this connection, the problem of searching, validation and introduction into clinical practice of reliable, minimally invasive, and accessible to use markers, allowing assessment of the atherogenic potential of each individual at the early stages of the disease, i.e., before its clinical manifestations or development of complications, does not lose its relevance [11,12]. Indeed, the issue of using new biomarkers is widely discussed in the literature, including an analysis of the merits and demerits of both already known diagnostic and/or prognostic tools and the results of the latest developments using omics technologies [5,8,13,14].

Obviously, two different approaches might be used to improve the prediction of the risk of coronary atherosclerosis development and severity: either the use of additional biochemical markers or the use of noninvasive methods of imaging subclinical atherosclerotic vascular changes [15].

The analysis of the literature and our own data allowed us to conclude that it is expedient and relevant to study the possibility of applying a multi-marker approach to create diagnostic panels of biomarkers for individual risk assessment of ASCVDs and their complications. Indeed, novel complex or integrated biomarkers can include well-known metabolic parameters or combinations previously not considered for risk estimation. The clinical value of serum biomarkers for the diagnosis and prediction of manifestations of atherosclerosis has been assessed in numerous studies. A number of risk prediction models have been developed to assess ASCVD risk, but relatively modest prognostic power of individual biomarkers for risk prediction suggests that multiple biomarkers can be combined to improve their predictive power [13]. The multi-marker approach has been tested in several studies on circulating biomarkers [13,16–18].

An important step in the introduction of new biomarkers into clinical practice, in addition to the creation of new diagnostic panels themselves, is the assessment of their diagnostic/prognostic significance with the analysis of such characteristics as sensitivity and specificity, i.e., their validation [19]. Validation, or verification, of biomarkers involves their evaluation either in prospective follow-up of the original cohort (on which the biomarker was obtained) or in an independent cohort in a one-step analysis. Despite the large number of parameters claiming to be candidate biomarkers for cardiovascular risk assessment, few have passed the stages of clinical and analytical validation and have been recognized as real biomarkers [20]. Being in the era of personalized and preventive medicine, we have to understand that the main task of forming new biomarkers is to improve exactly the individual assessment of the probability of the presence and/or development of a disease and its prognosis.

Objective: To assess the feasibility of combination of biochemical and imaging markers for estimation of risk and severity of coronary atherosclerosis, and to verify a created integrated biomarker on an independent cohort.

2. Materials and Methods

The examined two cohorts consisted of patients admitted to the National Research Centre for Therapy and Preventive Medicine in Moscow for diagnostic coronary angiography: the initial cohort observed in 2012–2014 ($n = 205$, 66.0% males; mean age 62.8 ± 9.0 years), and the tested one observed in 2016–2019 ($n = 216$, 53.2% males; mean age 61.5 ± 10.7 years).

Inclusion criteria: consecutive inclusion of all patients over 18 years old who were admitted to the hospital for diagnostic angiography of coronary arteries. Exclusion criteria were: acute coronary syndrome within 6 months prior to the study; surgery within 6 months prior to the study; left ventricular ejection fraction below 40%; serious chronic or acute infectious diseases; chronic kidney diseases stages III and higher with glomerular filtration rate under 60 mL/min/1.73 m^2); type I and II diabetes mellitus (level of glycosylated hemoglobin over 7.5%); familial hypercholesterolemia; neoplastic conditions; pregnancy and lactation.

All patients underwent coronary angiography according to the method Judkins (1967) using, as a rule, transfemoral access in the radiology operating setting with an angiographic unit Philips Integris Allura and General Electric Innova 4100. The procedure was performed considering the presence of at least one of the following causes: angina pectoris, history of myocardial infarction, heart rhythm disorders.

Location and extent of coronary artery lesions were assessed by Gensini Score (GS) [21]. Preliminary analysis of the most commonly used angiographic scoring systems revealed a good correlation between two angiographic scores (SYNTAX and GS) and quantitative assessment of coronary arteries ($r = 0.87$, $p < 0.0001$). GS had been chosen because according to our previous data [22], it appeared to be superior in estimation of severity of coronary atherosclerosis. The following GS cut-off points were used to estimate overall severity of vascular lesions: GS = 0 corresponds to unaffected coronary arteries; GS > 0 corresponds to the presence of coronary atherosclerosis of any stage; GS ≥ 35 corresponds to severe coronary atherosclerosis [22].

Atherosclerosis of carotid arteries was diagnosed by duplex B-mode scanning with color Doppler flow mapping 3–9 MHz linear transducer of PHILIPS iU22 ultrasound system in supine position with measuring carotid intima-media thickness (CIMT), determining the presence of atherosclerotic plaques (AP) in carotid arteries, and estimation of the degree (per cent) of stenosis. According to the experts [23], the values of CIMT < 0.9 mm have been chosen as the normal ones. The increase of CIMT was considered to be values from 0.9 to <1.3 mm, and AP criterion was indicated as CIMT > 1.3 mm or local CIMT increase by 0.5 mm (or by 50%) compared to the CIMT of the nearby vascular wall.

Anthropometric and clinical data included age, body mass index, waist circumference, and systolic and diastolic blood pressure. Blood was drawn from the cubital vein after 12–14 h of fasting prior to invasive angiography. Serum and plasma were obtained by low-speed centrifugation at $900 \times g$, +4 °C; sample processing and storage were performed according to international guidelines [24]. Biochemical parameters were determined by standardized laboratory methods.

Statistical analysis was performed using the SPSS software version 20. Normal distribution of continuous variables was assessed using Shapiro–Wilk's test. For normally distributed variables, the results were expressed as mean (M) ± standard deviation (SD) and for variables with significant deviations from the normal distribution were expressed as median (Me) and interquartile range (Q25–Q75). The differences between mean values were assessed using Student's t-test. The nonparametric Mann–Whitney U-test was used to compare the medians of two independent groups. Multivariate logistic regression analysis with odds ratio calculations was used to screen for predictors of presence and severity of coronary atherosclerosis. The Receiver Operating Characteristic (ROC) curves were used to analyze the predictive power of integrated biomarker and to determine the optimal threshold values for the AP number and carotid stenosis degree, as well as for fibrinogen and adiponectin levels. The thresholds for all the rest of the parameters have been chosen according to the corresponding Guidelines [23,25,26]. p values < 0.05 were considered statistically significant.

3. Results

The first step of our study was devoted to creation of a novel integrated biomarker for estimation of risk of coronary atherosclerosis presence and severity. The total initial cohort was split into patients with unaffected coronary arteries (GS = 0; $n = 39$) and those with any stage of coronary atherosclerosis (GS > 0; $n = 166$). The extent of coronary lesion was estimated by Gensini Score [21]; all patients were split into two groups with no/subclinical atherosclerosis (GS < 35; $n = 112$) and severe coronary atherosclerosis (GS ≥ 35; $n = 93$). No differences in major anthropometric characteristics were found between groups. A wide range of circulating parameters was analyzed, including lipoprotein profile, markers of insulin-dependent glucose utilization, inflammatory and hemostasis markers, and parameters of visceral adipose tissue metabolism (Table 1).

Table 1. Circulating biochemical parameters of the patients from the initial cohort.

Characteristics Means ± SD; Median (Q25–Q75)	GS = 0 (n = 39)	GS > 0 (n = 166)	GS < 35 (n = 112)	GS ≥ 35 (n = 93)
TC, mmol/L	5.5 ± 1.3	5.1 ± 1.2	5.2 ± 1.2	5.1 ± 1.3
LDL-C, mmol/L	3.7 ± 1.3	3.1 ± 1.1 [a]	3.3 ± 1.0	3.2 ± 1.2
HDL-C, mmol/L	1.1 ± 0.3	1.0 ± 0.3 [a]	1.0 ± 0.3	1.0 ± 0.3
Triglycerides, mmol/L	1.6 (1.2–2.1)	1.6 (1.2–2.2)	1.6 (1.2–2.1)	1.6 (1.2–2.2)
apo AI, g/L	1.70 ± 0.29	1.55 ± 0.28	1.60 ± 0.32	1.54 ± 0.25
apo B, g/L	1.02 ± 0.24	0.89 ± 0.24 [a]	0.95 ± 0.23	0.87 ± 0.26 [b]
hsCRP, mg/L	2.8 (1.1–5.7)	2.8 (1.3–5.8) [a]	2.4 (1.1–5.1)	3.3 (1.5–6.6) [b]
Fibrinogen, g/L	3.7 (3.2–4.1)	3.6 (3.2–4.1)	3.6 (3.2–4.1)	3.7 (3.3–4.2)
Glucose, mmol/L	5.7 ± 1.1	6.0 ± 1.5	5.9 ± 1.5	6.0 ± 1.4
Insulin, µU/mL	10.1 (7.4–15.0)	10.5 (7.3–14.5)	10.2 (7.2–14.3)	10.7 (7.5–14.9)
Adiponectin, µg/mL	9.2 (7.1–11.8)	7.8 (5.4–11.5) [a]	8.0 (5.8–11.8)	7.8 (5.5–11.4)
Leptin, ng/mL	33.5 (15.9–49.5)	19.4 (10.6–32.5)	22.9 (10.6–36.9)	19.1 (11.9–33.8)

TC—total cholesterol; LDL-C—low-density lipoprotein cholesterol; HDL-C—high-density lipoprotein cholesterol; hsCRP—high-sensitive C-reactive protein; apo–apolipoprotein; $p < 0.05$: a—between GS = 0 and GS > 0; b—between GS < 35 and GS ≥ 35.

Preliminary analysis of various mathematical regression models included structure parameters of the arterial wall, biochemical markers, and their combinations allowed us to select the most significant variables (listed in the Table 2) which together represent a combined or integrated biomarker called i-BIO. For each parameter incorporated into i-BIO, the points were assigned depending on cut-off values indicating deviations from the normal conditions, and detailed scoring of these parameters was carried from minimal (no changes) to maximal (presence of marked changes).

Thus, imaging parameters included in i-BIO were: CIMT (≤0.9; >0.9 mm), the number of AP (<3; ≥3), and the degree of carotid stenosis (≤45; >45%). Metabolic parameters incorporated into i-BIO included levels of triglycerides (TG) (≤1.7; 1.8-1.9; ≥2.0 mmol/L), glucose (≤5.5; 5.6–6.0; 6.1–6.9; ≥7.0 mmol/L), fibrinogen (≤4.0; >4.0 g/L), high sensitive C-reactive protein (hsCRP) (<1.0; 1.0–2.9; ≥3.0 mg/L), and adiponectin (<8.0; ≥8.0 µg/mL) as shown in Table 2. The sum of points calculated for each patient represents individual i-BIO value.

To assess the discriminative power of i-BIO, we performed the ROC curve analysis and used the corresponding areas under curve (AUC) to determine the sensitivity and specificity of the i-BIO (Figure 1). Two threshold values of i-BIO to assess the risk of coronary atherosclerosis and its severity were found. The threshold i-BIO value over 4 points for patients with coronary atherosclerosis of any stage (GS > 0) was proposed for detection of this disease presence with a sensitivity of 87.9% and specificity of 50.0% (Figure 1A). Risk of coronary atherosclerosis (GS > 0) among patients with i-BIO > 4 points was 7.3 times higher than for patients with i-BIO ≤ 4 points (OR = 7.3; 95% CI 3.2–16.4,

$p = 0.0001$). In patients with GS $\geq$ 35 the threshold for i-BIO $\geq$ 9 points was proposed to be optimal for prediction of severity of coronary atherosclerosis with a relatively low sensitivity of 43.8% but with rather high specificity of 79.8% (Figure 1B). Risk of severe coronary atherosclerosis (GS $\geq$ 35) at i-BIO $\geq$ 9 points was 3.1 times higher than for patients with i-IBIO < 9 points (OR = 3.1; 95% CI 1.6–5.8, $p = 0.001$).

Table 2. Integrated biomarker (i-BIO).

Parameters	Points
Sex	0—female 1—male
Ultrasound carotid dopplerography parameters: CIMT, mm AP, n Extent of carotid stenosis, %	0—CIMT $\leq$ 0.9, AP < 3, Extent of carotid stenosis $\leq$45 1—CIMT > 0.9, AP < 3, Extent of carotid stenosis $\leq$45 2—CIMT $\leq$ 0.9, AP $\geq$ 3, Extent of carotid stenosis $\leq$45 3—CIMT > 0.9, AP $\geq$ 3, Extent of carotid stenosis $\leq$45 4—CIMT $\leq$ 0.9, AP < 3, Extent of carotid stenosis >45 5—CIMT > 0.9, AP < 3, Extent of carotid stenosis >45 6—CIMT $\leq$ 0.9, AP $\geq$ 3, Extent of carotid stenosis >45 7—CIMT > 0.9, AP $\geq$ 3, Extent of carotid stenosis >45
Triglycerides, mmol/L	0—TG < 1.7 1—1.7 $\leq$ TG < 2.0 2—TG $\geq$ 2.0
Glucose, mmol/L	0—Glucose $\leq$ 5.5 1—5.5 < Glucose $\leq$ 6.0 2—6.0 < Glucose < 7.0 3—Glucose $\geq$ 7.0
Fibrinogen, g/L	0—Fibrinogen $\leq$ 4.0 1—Fibrinogen > 4.0
hsCRP, mg/L	0—hsCRP < 1.0 1—1.0 $\leq$ hsCRP < 3.0 2–hsCRP $\geq$ 3.0
Adiponectin, µg/mL	0—Adiponectin $\geq$ 8.0 1—Adiponectin < 8.0

CIMT—carotid intima-media thickness; AP—atherosclerosis plaque; hsCRP—high-sensitive C-reactive protein; TG—triglycerides.

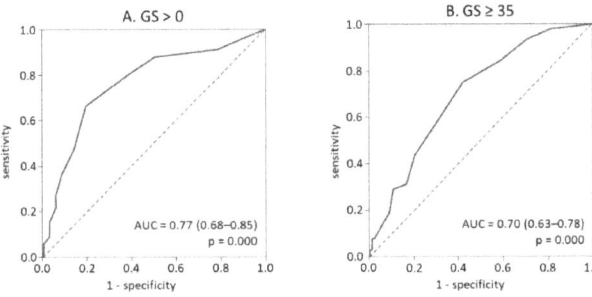

Figure 1. ROC-curve analysis for the prediction of coronary atherosclerosis presence (**A**) or severity (**B**) by i-BIO in the initial cohort.

The i-BIO was validated on an independent (tested) cohort of patients in whom the presence or absence of coronary atherosclerosis was also verified by coronary angiography, and changes in the carotid arteries were detected by duplex scanning. The cohort included 216 patients, their biochemical characteristics are presented in Table 3.

Table 3. Circulating biochemical parameters of the patients from the tested cohort.

Characteristics Means ± SD; Median (Q25–Q75)	GS = 0 (n = 73)	GS > 0 (n = 143)	GS < 35 (n = 144)	GS ≥ 35 (n = 72)
TC, mmol/L	4.5 ± 1.2	4.2 ± 1.1	4.6 ± 1.08	3.8 ± 0.9 [b]
LDL-C, mmol/L	2.6 ± 0.9	2.6 ± 0.9	2.7 ± 0.9	2.2 ± 0.8 [b]
HDL-C, mmol/L	1.2 ± 0.3	1.1 ± 0.3	1.2 ± 0.3	1.0 ± 0.3 [b]
Triglycerides, mmol/L	1.4 (1.0–1.9)	1.3 (1.0–1.8)	1.3 (0.9–1.9)	1.4 (1.1–1.8)
apo AI, g/L	1.57 ± 0.32	1.47 ± 0.29 [a]	1.58 ± 0.29	1.36 ± 0.26 [b]
apo B, g/L	0.86 ± 0.24	0.88 ± 0.23	0.89 ± 0.24	0.84 ± 0.22
hsCRP, mg/L	2.3 (0.9–5.4)	3.0 (1.6–6.3) [a]	2.8 (1.1–4.8)	4.5 (2.1–10.1) [b]
Fibrinogen, g/L	4.30 (3.7–5.2)	4.70 (4.1–5.5) [a]	4.30 (3.8–5.1)	4.90 (4.4–5.7) [b]
Glucose, mmol/L	5.9 ± 1.4	6.6 ± 1.8 [a]	6.1 ± 1.4	6.9 ± 2.0 [b]
Insulin, µU/mL	8.85 (6.1–12.5)	11.0 (7.6–15.9) [a]	9.4 (6.0–13.8)	11.0 (8.2–17,5) [b]
Adiponectin, µg/mL	7.7 (5.9–10.6)	5.1 (5.6–11.2)	8.3 (6.2–11.4)	6.8 (4.7–10.4) [b]
Leptin, ng/mL	19.4 (5.8–57.3)	16.9 (4.8–58.2)	21.4 (5.2–70.7)	10.5 (4.0–37.2) [b]

TC—total cholesterol; LDL-C—low-density lipoprotein cholesterol; HDL-C—high-density lipoprotein cholesterol; hsCRP—high-sensitive C-reactive protein; apo—apolipoprotein; $p < 0.05$: a—between GS = 0 and GS > 0; b—between GS < 35 and GS ≥ 35.

To assess the risk of presence and severity of coronary atherosclerosis in this tested cohort, the same thresholds for i-BIO as for initial cohort were used: i-BIO > 4 or BIO ≥ 9, respectively. Figure 2A demonstrates the results of ROC curve analysis for the feasibility of i-BIO to discriminate between atherosclerosis-free subjects (GS < 0) and patients with coronary atherosclerosis of any severity (GS > 0). At i-BIO > 4, risk of any stage atherosclerosis detection was 3.1 times higher than in subjects having i-BIO ≤ 4: OR = 3.1 (95% CI 1.7–5.7; $p = 0.0002$) with sensitivity of 76.2% and specificity-49.3%.

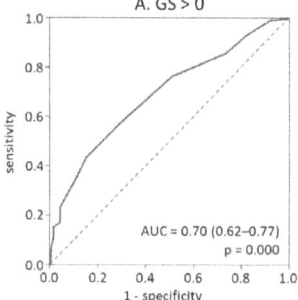
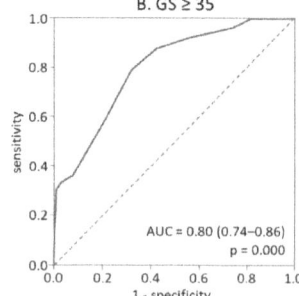

Figure 2. ROC-curve analysis for the prediction of coronary atherosclerosis presence (A) or severity (B) by i-BIO in the tested cohort.

Verified marker i-BIO ≥ 9 allows us to separate patients with multivessel coronary lesions and clinical manifestations (GS ≥ 35) from those who did not have severe atherosclerosis with sensitivity of 50.0% and specificity of 84% (Figure 2B). Risk of severe atherosclerosis at i-BIO $\geq$ 9 was 5.3 times higher than in patients with i-BIO < 9 (OR = 5.3; 95% CI 2.75–10.03; $p = 4 \times 10^{-7}$).

4. Discussion

This study was undertaken to examine a set of clinical and metabolic parameters and their combinations in order to analyze their potential impact on early development of atherosclerotic lesions in coronary arteries to predict the presence and severity of coronary atherosclerosis. We have generated a novel cumulative multi-marker—integrated biomarker, or i-BIO, composed of several imaging and circulating biochemical parameters for non-invasive detection of coronary atherosclerosis and evaluation of its severity. According to the data obtained, i-BIO appeared to be valid and allowed statistically significant separation of both atherosclerosis-free subjects (GS = 0) from patients with any signs of atherosclerosis according to coronary angiography data (GS > 0) and patients without changes on coronary angiography from those with severe atherosclerosis of coronary arteries (GS $\geq$ 35).

Atherosclerosis is a systemic process, and this prompted us to analyze biochemical parameters of function or dysfunction of the major metabolic systems involved into pathogenesis of this disease including serum lipoprotein profile, markers of insulin-dependent glucose utilization, inflammatory and hemostatic markers, and parameters of visceral adipose tissue metabolism.

Biomarkers play an essential role in biomedical research, in daily clinical practice, and in drug development, which should be considered one of the priority areas of translational medicine [27–30]. In this regard, research to find new biomarkers, to evaluate their analytical characteristics, and to confirm their significance seems to be a very relevant task. Moreover, before being introduced into biomedical research any new marker requires verification (validation) either in a prospective study or in cross-sectional studies on independent cohorts.

Now it is becoming increasingly clear that a single-biomarker approach has limited predictive value, while integrated combined biomarkers have a definite advantage over the measurement and analysis of individual parameters and can be used as additional tools to further individual stratification of the patients at risk. The multi-marker approach has been tested in a number of studies [13,16–18,29–31]. In particular, it has been shown that when the initial low correlation between a single marker and the disease or its risk factors increases significantly when they are combined; this approach is very promising [28,32,33]. Several algorithms incorporating multiple markers were used for prediction of coronary heart disease risk [34]. Indeed, integrated biomarkers may add incremental value to other criteria that include traditional risk factors, and should be considered in those patients who require particular management decisions but the physician lacks sufficient information to assess conventional risk factors in these patients. The use of new technologies, including proteomics, metabolomics, lipidomics and advanced structural and functional imaging, enable to detect a number of promising new biomarker candidates [35–37].

Along with this, a certain place is given to the approach used in our study, when combined multi-markers are formed on the basis of generally used in practical healthcare studies and measurements, including non-invasive duplex scanning of carotid arteries and quantification of circulating metabolites included in this biomarker. Another promising approach to analyze a wide set of parameters for new effective scales construction is machine learning, commonly called artificial intelligence [38]. Using machine learning approaches and computational modeling, several studies have been undertaken for the early diagnostics and prediction of coronary artery disease status and progression, for the prediction of atherosclerotic plaque growth [39], or to assess the risk level of diabetes mellitus [40].

In other words, new biomarkers and/or their complexes may well occupy a niche both as auxiliary non-invasive diagnostic tools and as new potential molecular targets. Thus, the study of various combinations of clinical and demographic, imaging, and biochemical/metabolic/genetic parameters available for practical health care, as well as the establishment of integrated biomarkers and assessment of their predictive ability, allowed us to propose multi-marker diagnostic panels for non-invasive (low invasive) personalized detection of coronary atherosclerosis and its severity.

Our study has some limitations. We lack the follow up data for the patients and thus cannot estimate the outcome and evaluate predictive power of the i-BIO for the purpose of calibration and reclassification. However, we verified our data on an independent cohort similar to the initial one; moreover, a follow-up study on the initial cohort is in progress.

5. Conclusions

In conclusion, the novel i-BIO suggested in our study includes imaging characteristics derived from carotid ultrasound dopplerography (CIMT, AP number, and carotid stenosis) and circulating blood tests (serum levels of triglycerides, glucose, fibrinogen, hsCRP, and adiponectin). i-BIO values over 4 points detected patients with any stage of coronary atherosclerosis (GS > 0) with sensitivity of 87.8%, while i-BIO $\geq$ 9 points allows to exclude patients free from severe coronary atherosclerosis (GS < 35) with specificity of 79.8%. Validation of i-BIO on the independent cohort confirmed the feasibility of i-BIO > 4 to separate patients with coronary atherosclerosis of any stage (GS > 0) with sensitivity of 76.2%, and to exclude subjects without atherosclerosis (GS < 35) with specificity of 84.0% with i-BIO $\geq$ 9. Thus, a composite panel of routinely available imaging and blood tests is useful for assessment for coronary atherosclerosis and estimation of its severity.

Author Contributions: Conceptualization, V.A.M. and N.E.G.; methodology, V.A.M., N.E.G. and M.V.Z.; software, E.B.Y.; formal analysis, E.B.Y.; validation, V.A.M. and M.V.Z.; investigation, N.E.G. and M.V.Z.; data curation, V.A.M. and M.V.Z.; writing—original draft preparation, V.A.M.; writing—review and editing, O.M.D.; visualization, V.A.M. and N.E.G.; supervision, V.A.M. and O.M.D.; project administration, O.M.D.; funding acquisition, O.M.D. All authors have read and agreed to the published version of the manuscript.

Funding: This research received no external funding.

Institutional Review Board Statement: This study was performed in accordance with the Declaration of Helsinki and was approved by the Local Ethics Committee (approvals No 07/05-12 and No 09-05/19).

Informed Consent Statement: Written informed consent was signed by each patient before coronary angiography and carotid-ultrasound dopplerography and collecting the blood samples.

Acknowledgments: The authors are grateful to Natalia Gomyranova and Olga Litinskaya for their excellent technical assistance; to Vladimir Kutsenko and Julia Makarova for their help in statistical analysis, and to Oxana Stefanyuk for excellent help during the manuscript preparation.

Conflicts of Interest: The authors declare no conflict of interest.

References

1. Visseren, F.L.J.; Mach, F.; Smulders, Y.M.; Carballo, D.; Koskinas, K.C.; Bäck, M.; Benetos, A.; Biffi, A.; Boavida, J.-M.; Capodanno, D. 2021 ESC Guidelines on cardiovascular disease prevention in clinical practice. *Eur. Heart J.* **2021**, *42*, 3227–3337. [CrossRef] [PubMed]
2. Wang, Y.; Wang, J. Modelling and prediction of global non-communicable diseases. *BMC Public Health* **2020**, *20*, 1–13. [CrossRef] [PubMed]
3. Virani, S.S.; Alonso, A.; Aparicio, H.J.; Benjamin, E.J.; Bittencourt, M.S.; Callaway, C.W.; Carson, A.P.; Chamberlain, A.M.; Cheng, S.; Delling, F.N.; et al. American Heart Association Council on Epidemiology and Prevention Statistics Committee and Stroke Statistics Subcommittee. Heart Disease and Stroke Statistics—2021 Update: A Report from the American Heart Association. *Circulation* **2021**, *143*, e254–e743. [CrossRef]
4. Lloyd-Jones, D.M.; Leip, E.P.; Larson, M.; D'Agostino, R.B.; Beiser, A.; Wilson, P.W.; Wolf, P.A.; Levy, D. Prediction of Lifetime Risk for Cardiovascular Disease by Risk Factor Burden at 50 Years of Age. *Circulation* **2006**, *113*, 791–798. [CrossRef] [PubMed]
5. Hoefer, I.E.; Steffens, S.; Ala-Korpela, M.; Bäck, M.; Badimon, L.; Bochaton-Piallat, M.-L.; Boulanger, C.M.; Caligiuri, G.; Dimmeler, S.; Egido, J.; et al. Novel methodologies for biomarker discovery in atherosclerosis. *Eur. Heart J.* **2015**, *36*, 2635–2642. [CrossRef]

6. Knuuti, J.; Wijns, W.; Saraste, A.; Capodanno, D.; Barbato, E.; Funck-Brentano, C.; Prescott, E.; Storey, R.F.; Deaton, C.; Cuisset, T.; et al. 2019 ESC Guidelines for the diagnosis and management of chronic coronary syndromes: The Task Force for the diagnosis and management of chronic coronary syndromes of the European Society of Cardiology (ESC). *Eur. Heart J.* **2020**, *41*, 407–477. [CrossRef]
7. Patel, M.R.; Peterson, E.D.; Dai, D.; Brennan, J.M.; Redberg, R.F.; Anderson, H.V.; Brindis, R.G.; Douglas, P.S. Low Diagnostic Yield of Elective Coronary Angiography. *N. Engl. J. Med.* **2010**, *362*, 886–895. [CrossRef] [PubMed]
8. Vasan, R.S. Biomarkers of cardiovascular disease: Molecular basis and practical considerations. *Circulation* **2006**, *113*, 2335–2362. [CrossRef]
9. Ghantous, C.M.; Kamareddine, L.; Farhat, R.; Zouein, F.A.; Mondello, S.; Kobeissy, F.; Zeidan, A. Advances in Cardiovascular Biomarker Discovery. *Biomedicines* **2020**, *8*, 552. [CrossRef]
10. Roberts, L.D.; Gerszten, R.E. Toward New Biomarkers of Cardiometabolic Diseases. *Cell Metab.* **2013**, *18*, 43–50. [CrossRef]
11. Gilstrap, L.G.; Wang, T.J. Biomarkers and Cardiovascular Risk Assessment for Primary Prevention: An Update. *Clin. Chem.* **2012**, *58*, 72–82. [CrossRef]
12. Cui, J. Overview of Risk Prediction Models in Cardiovascular Disease Research. *Ann. Epidemiol.* **2009**, *19*, 711–717. [CrossRef] [PubMed]
13. Wang, T.J. Assessing the Role of Circulating, Genetic, and Imaging Biomarkers in Cardiovascular Risk Prediction. *Circulation* **2011**, *123*, 551–565. [CrossRef]
14. Chu, S.H.; Huang, M.; Kelly, R.S.; Benedetti, E.; Siddiqui, J.K.; Zeleznik, O.A.; Pereira, A.; Herrington, D.; Wheelock, C.E.; Krumsiek, J.; et al. Integration of Metabolomic and Other Omics Data in Population-Based Study Designs: An Epidemiological Perspective. *Metabolites* **2019**, *9*, 117. [CrossRef] [PubMed]
15. Helfand, M.; Buckley, D.I.; Freeman, M.; Fu, R.; Rogers, K.; Fleming, C.; Humphrey, L.L. Emerging Risk Factors for Coronary Heart Disease: A Summary of Systematic Reviews Conducted for the U.S. Preventive Services Task Force. *Ann. Intern. Med.* **2009**, *151*, 496–507. [CrossRef] [PubMed]
16. Zethelius, B.; Berglund, L.; Sundstrom, J.; Ingelsson, E.; Basu, S.; Larsson, A.; Venge, P.; Ärnlöv, J. Use of Multiple Biomarkers to Improve the Prediction of Death from Cardiovascular Causes. *N. Engl. J. Med.* **2008**, *358*, 2107–2116. [CrossRef]
17. Blankenberg, S.; Zeller, T.; Saarela, O.; Havulinna, A.S.; Kee, F.; Tunstall-Pedoe, H.; Kuulasmaa, K.; Yarnell, J.; Schnabel, R.B.; Wild, P.S.; et al. Contribution of 30 Biomarkers to 10-Year Cardiovascular Risk Estimation in 2 Population Cohorts: The MONICA, Risk, Genetics, Archiving, and Monograph (MORGAM) biomarker project. *Circulation* **2010**, *121*, 2388–2397. [CrossRef]
18. de Lemos, J.A.; Rohatgi, A. Separating the Contenders from the Pretenders: Competitive high-throughput biomarker screening in large population-based studies. *Circulation* **2010**, *121*, 2381–2383. [CrossRef]
19. Biomarkers Definitions Working (BDW) Group; Atkinson, A.J., Jr.; Colburn, W.A.; DeGruttola, V.G.; DeMets, D.L.; Downing, G.J.; Hoth, D.F.; Oates, J.A.; Peck, C.C.; Spilker, B.A.; et al. Biomarkers and surrogate endpoints: Preferred definitions and conceptual framework. *Clin. Pharmacol. Ther.* **2001**, *69*, 89–95. [CrossRef]
20. Morrow, D.A.; de Lemos, J.A. Benchmarks for the Assessment of Novel Cardiovascular Biomarkers. *Circulation* **2007**, *115*, 949–952. [CrossRef] [PubMed]
21. Gensini, G.G. A more meaningful scoring system for determining the severity of coronary heart disease. *Am. J. Cardiol.* **1983**, *51*, 606. [CrossRef]
22. Gavrilova, N.E.; Metelskaya, V.A.; Perova, N.V.; Yarovaya, E.B.; Boytsov, S.A.; Mazaev, V.P. The comparative analysis of angiographic scores for detection the lesion of coronary arteries. *Russ. J. Cardiol.* **2014**, *19*, 24–29. [CrossRef]
23. Perk, J.; De Backer, G.; Gohlke, H.; Graham, I.; Reiner, Z.; Verschuren, M.; Verschuren, M.; Albus, C.; Benlian, P.; Boysen, G.; et al. European Guidelines on cardiovascular disease prevention in clinical practice (version 2012). The Fifth Joint Task Force of the European Society of Cardiology and Other Societies on Cardiovascular Disease Prevention in Clinical Practice (constituted by representatives of nine societies and by invited experts). *Eur. Heart J.* **2012**, *33*, 1635–1701. [CrossRef] [PubMed]
24. Moore, H.M.; Kelly, A.; Jewell, S.D.; McShane, L.M.; Clark, D.P.; Greenspan, R.; Hainaut, P.; Hayes, D.F.; Kim, P.; Mansfield, E.; et al. Biospecimen Reporting for Improved Study Quality (BRISQ). *Biopreserv. Biobank.* **2011**, *9*, 57–70. [CrossRef] [PubMed]
25. Catapano, A.L.; Graham, I.; De Backer, G.; Wiklund, O.; Chapman, M.J.; Drexel, H.; Hoes, A.W.; Jennings, C.S.; Landmesser, U.; Pedersen, T.R.; et al. 2016 ESC/EAS Guidelines for the Management of Dyslipidaemias. The Task Force for the Management of Dyslipidaemias of the European Society of Cardiology and European Atherosclerosis Society. *Eur. Heart J.* **2016**, *37*, 2999–3058. [CrossRef]
26. Ridker, P.M.; Buring, J.E.; Cook, N.R.; Rifai, N. C-Reactive Protein, the Metabolic Syndrome, and Risk of Incident Cardiovascular Events: An 8-year follow-up of 14719 initially healthy American women. *Circulation* **2003**, *107*, 391–397. [CrossRef]
27. Marcovina, S.M.; Crea, F.; Davignon, J.; Kaski, J.C.; Koenig, W.; Landmesser, U.; Pieri, P.L.; Schulz-Menger, J.; Shaw, L.J.; Sobesky, J. Biochemical and bioimaging markers for risk assessment and diagnosis in major cardiovascular diseases: A road to integration of complementary diagnostic tools. *J. Intern. Med.* **2007**, *261*, 214–234. [CrossRef]
28. Koenig, W. Integrating biomarkers: The new frontier? *Scand. J. Clin. Lab. Investig.* **2010**, *70*, 117–123. [CrossRef]
29. Schnabel, R.B.; Schulz, A.; Messow, C.M.; Lubos, E.; Wild, P.S.; Zeller, T.; Sinning, C.R.; Rupprecht, H.J.; Bickel, C.; Peetz, D.; et al. Multiple marker approach to risk stratification in patients with stable coronary artery disease. *Eur. Heart J.* **2010**, *31*, 3024–3031. [CrossRef]

30. Jackson, C.E.; Haig, C.; Welsh, P.; Dalzell, J.R.; Tsorlalis, I.K.; McConnachie, A.; Preiss, D.; Anker, S.D.; Sattar, N.; Petrie, M.C.; et al. The incremental prognostic and clinical value of multiple novel biomarkers in heart failure. *Eur. J. Hear. Fail.* **2016**, *18*, 1491–1498. [CrossRef]
31. Melander, O.; Newton-Cheh, C.; Almgren, P.; Hedblad, B.; Berglund, G.; Engström, G.; Persson, M.; Smith, J.G.; Magnusson, M.; Christensson, A.; et al. Novel and Conventional Biomarkers for Prediction of Incident Cardiovascular Events in the Community. *JAMA* **2009**, *302*, 49–57. [CrossRef] [PubMed]
32. Tonkin, A.M.; Blankenberg, S.; Kirby, A.; Zeller, T.; Colquhoun, D.M.; Funke-Kaiser, A.; Hague, W.; Hunt, D.; Keech, A.C.; Nestel, P.; et al. for the LIPID Study Investigators. Biomarkers in stable coronary heart disease, their modulation and cardiovascular risk: The LIPID biomarker study. *Int. J. Cardiol.* **2015**, *201*, 499–507. [CrossRef] [PubMed]
33. Siemelink, M.A.; Zeller, T. Biomarkers of Coronary Artery Disease: The Promise of the Transcriptome. *Curr. Cardiol. Rep.* **2014**, *16*, 513. [CrossRef]
34. Hense, H.-W. Observations, predictions and decisions—assessing cardiovascular risk assessment. *Int. J. Epidemiol.* **2004**, *33*, 235–239. [CrossRef]
35. Shah, S.H.; Kraus, W.E.; Newgard, C.B. Metabolomic Profiling for the Identification of Novel Biomarkers and Mechanisms Related to Common Cardiovascular Diseases: Form and function. *Circulation* **2012**, *126*, 1110–1120. [CrossRef]
36. Stegemann, C.; Pechlaner, R.; Willeit, P.; Langley, S.R.; Mangino, M.; Mayr, U.; Menni, C.; Moayyeri, A.; Santer, P.; Rungger, G.; et al. Lipidomics Profiling and Risk of Cardiovascular Disease in the Prospective Population-Based Bruneck Study. *Circulation* **2014**, *129*, 1821–1831. [CrossRef]
37. Wang, N.; Zhu, F.; Chen, L.; Chen, K. Proteomics, metabolomics and metagenomics for type 2 diabetes and its complications. *Life Sci.* **2018**, *212*, 194–202. [CrossRef]
38. Quer, G.; Arnaout, R.; Henne, M.; Arnaout, R. Machine Learning and the Future of Cardiovascular Care: JACC State-of-the-Art Review. *J. Am. Coll. Cardiol.* **2021**, *77*, 300–313. [CrossRef] [PubMed]
39. Pleouras, D.; Rocchiccioli, S.; Pelosi, G.; Michalis, L.K.; Fotiadis, D.I.; Sakellarios, A.I.; Kyriakidis, S.; Kigka, V.; Siogkas, P.; Tsompou, P.; et al. A computational multi-level atherosclerotic plaque growth model for coronary arteries. In Proceedings of the 2019 41st Annual International Conference of the IEEE Engineering in Medicine and Biology Society (EMBC), Berlin, Germany, 23–27 July 2019; Volume 2019, pp. 5010–5013. [CrossRef]
40. Georga, E.I.; Protopappas, V.C.; Mougiakakou, S.G.; Fotiadis, D.I. Short-term vs. long-term analysis of diabetes data: Application of machine learning and data mining techniques. In Proceedings of the 13th IEEE International Conference on BioInformatics and BioEngineering, Chania, Greece, 10–13 November 2013.

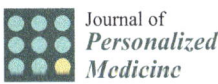

Article

Relationship between Epicardial and Coronary Adipose Tissue and the Expression of Adiponectin, Leptin, and Interleukin 6 in Patients with Coronary Artery Disease

Olga V. Gruzdeva, Yulia A. Dyleva *, Ekaterina V. Belik, Maxim Y. Sinitsky, Aleksandr N. Stasev, Aleksandr N. Kokov, Natalia K. Brel, Evgenia O. Krivkina, Evgenia E. Bychkova, Roman S. Tarasov and Olga L. Barbarash

Federal State Budgetary Scientific Institution "Research Institute for Complex Issues of Cardiovascular Diseases", 650002 Kemerovo, Russia; o_gruzdeva@mail.ru (O.V.G.); sionina.ev@mail.ru (E.V.B.); sinitsky.maxim@gmail.com (M.Y.S.); stasan@kemcardio.ru (A.N.S.); kokoan@kemcardio.ru (A.N.K.); brel.n.k@mail.ru (N.K.B.); kriveo@kemcardio.ru (E.O.K.); eugenia.tarasowa@yandex.ru (E.E.B.); tarars@kemcardio.ru (R.S.T.); barb61@yandex.ru (O.L.B.)
* Correspondence: dyleva87@yandex.ru

Abstract: Adipose tissue (AT) is an endocrine and paracrine organ that synthesizes biologically active adipocytokines, which affect inflammation, fibrosis, and atherogenesis. Epicardial and perivascular fat depots are of great interest to researchers, owing to their potential effects on the myocardium and blood vessels. The aim of the study was to assess the expression and secretion of adipocytokine genes in the AT of patients with coronary artery disease (CAD) and patients with aortic or mitral valve replacement. This study included 84 patients with CAD and 50 patients with aortic or mitral valve replacement. Adipocytes were isolated from subcutaneous, epicardial (EAT), and perivascular AT (PVAT), and were cultured for 24 h. EAT exhibited the lowest level of adiponectin gene expression and secretion, regardless of nosology, and high expression levels of the leptin gene and interleukin-6 (IL-6). However, EAT adipocytes in patients with CAD were characterized by more pronounced changes in comparison with the group with heart defects. High leptin and IL-6 levels resulted in increased pro-inflammatory activity, as observed in both EAT and PVAT adipocytes, especially in individuals with CAD. Therefore, our results revealed the pathogenetic significance of alterations in the adipokine and cytokine status of adipocytes of EAT and PVAT in patients with CAD.

Keywords: adiponectin; leptin; interleukin-6; epicardial adipose tissue; perivascular adipose tissue

1. Introduction

Atherosclerosis-related cardiovascular disease (CVD) remains one of the main causes of death in industrialized countries, despite significant achievements in modern medicine [1]. Moreover, the increasing incidence of obesity is likely to aggravate this problem. Adipose tissue (AT) is universally regarded as an endocrine and paracrine organ that synthesizes biologically active molecules. Adipocytokines are involved in various processes, including inflammation, fibrosis, and atherogenesis [2–4]. It has been shown that local fat depots, such as epicardial (EAT) and perivascular AT (PVAT), are associated with increased cardiovascular events, independent of traditional risk factors [5]. In addition, reports have shown differences in the matrix RNA (mRNA) expression of adipokines in epicardial and subcutaneous AT (SAT) [6]. As different fat depots are characterized by their unique adipocytokinome and secretome, studies on the role of AT adipocytokines at different locations and CVD are relevant.

EAT is of particular interest owing to its close location to the coronary arteries and its possible paracrine action on them [7]. When inflammatory processes are activated, the epicardium becomes a site of impaired adipogenesis, which leads to the secretion of pro-inflammatory adipokines and fibrosis of the atrial and ventricular myocardium. PVAT is also of interest, since its heterogeneity determines the functions of ATs-protective or atherogenic. EAT and PVAT have been shown to be associated with coronary artery disease (CAD) [8]. However, the mechanisms by which adipocytokines affect the pathogenesis of CVD are still not fully understood. Thus, it is necessary to study the expression of adipokine genes in AT in various sites to develop potential therapeutic interventions against pathological activation of AT in CVD.

2. Material and Methods

2.1. Study Inclusion Criteria

Inclusion criteria consisted of the following: CAD, presence of indications for coronary artery bypass grafting (CABG) (based on coronarography data), patient age up to 75 years, and patient consent for participating in the study. Exclusion criteria were as follows: patient age greater than 75 years; presence of type 1 and type 2 diabetes mellitus (DM) as evident in his/her medical history and/or revealed during the hospitalization examination, acute of pervious myocardial infarction (MI), presence of clinically significant comorbidities (anemia, kidney and liver failure, oncological and infectious–inflammatory diseases) in the period of exacerbation, autoimmune diseases, and refusal to participate in the study.

2.2. Study Population

The study included 125 patients with CAD and indications for direct myocardial revascularization by CABG. The study group consisted of 31 women (25%) and 94 men (75%), of an average age of 65.32 (57.35; 69.16) years (Table 1). In the patient history, hypertension, smoking, angina pectoris, and burdened heredity for cardiovascular pathology were recorded more often. In total, 86 patients had a previous history of MI, and 11 people had a history of stroke. The comparison group included 120 patients with heart defects (aortic or mitral valve replacement), consisting of individuals of an average age of 61.22 (55.49; 66.65) years (Table 1) without coronary atherosclerosis (as per coronary angiography). Individuals in group with heart defects were characterized by a low percentage of patients with cardiovascular risk factors.

Table 1. Clinical and anamnestic characteristics of patients with coronary artery disease and heart defects.

Parameter	CAD (n = 125)	Heart Defects (n = 120)	p
Men, n (%)	97 (77.6)	60 (50)	0.011
Body mass index, kg/m^2	28.89 (26.64; 32.12)	26.78 (23.21; 29.01)	0.069
Arterial hypertension, n (%)	118 (94.4)	32 (26.7)	0.001
Hypercholesterolemia, n (%)	31 (24.8)	16 (13.3)	0.025
Smoking, n (%)	90 (72)	10 (8.3)	0.0001
Anamnesis			
Family history of CAD, n (%)	76 (60.8)	42 (35)	0.014
History of myocardial infarction, n (%)	86 (68.8)	0	-
History of stroke, n (%)	11 (8.8)	0	-
Atherosclerosis of other pools, n (%)	21 (16.8)	0	-
No angina, n (%)	8 (6.4)	120 (100)	0.0001
Functional class I angina, n (%)	0	0	-
Functional class II angina, n (%)	51 (40.8)	0	-
Functional class III angina, n (%)	66 (52.8)	0	-
Chronic heart failure NYHA I functional class, n (%)	16 (12.8)	26 (21.7)	0.030

Table 1. Cont.

Parameter	CAD (n = 125)	Heart Defects (n = 120)	p
Chronic heart failure NYHA II functional class, n (%)	11 (8.8)	54 (45)	0.0002
Chronic heart failure NYHA III functional class, n (%)	7 (5.6)	40 (33.3)	0.003
Chronic heart failure NYHA IV functional class, n (%)	0	0	-
Atherosclerosis of the 1st coronary artery, n (%)	10 (8)	0	-
Atherosclerosis of the 2nd coronary artery, n (%)	6 (4.8)	0	-
Atherosclerosis of three or more coronary artery, n (%)	109 (87.2)	0	-
Ejection fraction, %	51.0 (44.13; 56.377)	53.2 (43.41; 58.03)	0.125
Treatment strategy/group of drugs (hospital period)			
Aspirin, n (%)	122 (97.6)	0	-
Clopidogrel, n (%)	21 (16.8)	0	-
Warfarin, n (%)	0	103 (85.8)	-
β-blockers, n (%)	122 (97.6)	111 (92.5)	0.312
Angiotensin-converting enzyme, n (%)	96 (76.8)	95 (79.2)	0.247
Statins, n (%)	125 (100)	98 (81.7)	0.033
Calcium channel Blocker, n (%)	96 (76.8)	90 (75)	0.151
Nitrates, n (%)	11 (8.8)	10 (8.3)	0.417
Diuretics, n (%)	105 (84)	110 (91.7)	0.062

Notes: Hereinafter: CAD, groups of patients with coronary artery disease and indications for direct myocardial revascularization by coronary artery bypass grafting, p, significance level.

All patients were administered standard antianginal and antiplatelet therapies throughout the observation period and in-hospital treatment period (Table 1).

2.3. Measurement of the Area of SAT, EAT, and PVAT

For all patients, the area was measured as abdominal AT, namely, its visceral and subcutaneous components, using multi-spiral computed tomography (MSCT) on a Siemens Somatom 64 computed tomography scanner (Siemens Healthcare, Erlangen, Germany). Scanning was performed at the level of vertebral bodies L4–L5 in the craniocaudal direction. At the level of the intervertebral disc L4–L5, the area of abdominal adipose tissue (AAT) was measured in a semi-automatic mode. Further, the area of visceral adipose tissue (VAT) was determined on the obtained image by highlighting the contour of the peritoneum. The area of SAT was calculated mathematically by subtracting the area of VAT from the area of AAT (Figure 1a).

The determination of EAT thickness was performed by magnetic resonance imaging (MRI) on an Exelart Atlas 1.5-T MR imager (Toshiba, Tokyo, Japan). Thickness measurements of EAT was performed on images oriented along the short axis of the heart. EAT thickness was measured at three points along the anterior wall of the right ventricle, after which the average value was calculated. In addition, the same method was used to measure EAT thickness at the back wall of the left ventricle, followed by the calculation of the mean value (Figure 1b).

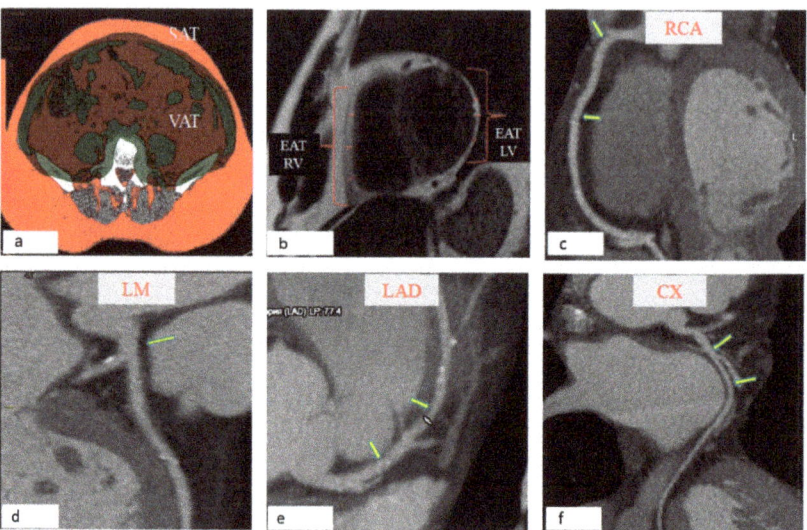

Figure 1. Morphometric assessment of local fat depots. (**a**) Slices centered at the L4–L5 disc spaces were selected. Visceral fat was defined as the fat enclosed by the visceral cavity. Subcutaneous fat was defined as fat outside the visceral cavity, not including that located within the muscular fascia. The total visceral and subcutaneous fat area (cm^2) were automatically calculated using a workstation (Leonardo, Siemens, Germany). (**b**) EAT was defined as the adipose tissue located between the visceral layer of the pericardium and outer surface of the myocardium. EAT was measured on the horizontal long-axis plane in end-diastolic phase. The EAT thickness of the right and left ventricular free wall was recorded by averaging the measurements of 3 different levels. (**c**) The thickness of the PVAT right coronary artery (RCA) was measured at the level of the proximal third of the RCA, for which the orifice of the acute margin artery is the distal end, in the projection of the middle third of the RCA, bounded by the arteries of the acute margin and the posterior interventricular branch of the right coronary artery. (**d**) The thickness of the PVAT of the left coronary artery (LCA) was measured at the level of the left main (LM) coronary artery (Figure 1d). (**e**) The PVAT was assessed at the level of the proximal and middle third of the anterior descending artery (LAD). The proximal third of LAD is a site from the orifice to the origin of the first diagonal artery, while the middle third of the LAD is limited by the orifices of the first and second diagonal arteries. (**f**) The thickness of the PVAT was estimated at the level of the proximal third of the circumflex coronary arteries (CX), which is limited by the ostium of the CX and the branch of the obtuse edge and at the level of the middle third of the CX-a segment from the branch of the obtuse edge to the orifice of the posterior interventricular artery.

Determination of the thickness of the PVAT at different anatomical locations was performed using the MSCT method with the following parameters: 1 mm axial slice thickness, an image matrix of 512 × 512, tube voltage of 120 kV, and a tube current of 100 mA. The MSCT images were acquired using bolus contrast, followed by a quantitative evaluation. The thickness of the PVAT of the right coronary artery (RCA) was measured at the level of the proximal third and in the projection of the middle third of the RCA (Figure 1c). The thickness of the PVAT of the left coronary artery (LCA) was measured at the level of the left main (LM) coronary artery (Figure 1d). The thickness of the PVAT of the anterior descending coronary artery (LAD) was measured at the level of the proximal and middle third of the LAD (Figure 1e). The thickness of the PVAT of the circumflex coronary arteries (CX) was measured at the level of the proximal third of the CX (Figure 1f). The obtained DICOM images were processed on a "Leonardo" multimodal workstation.

2.4. Cell Collection

2.4.1. Obtaining Biopsies of AT from Various Sites

Biopsies of 3–5 g of SAT, EAT, and PVAT samples were obtained during coronary bypass surgery and heart defects (aortic or mitral valve replacement). SAT samples were obtained from the subcutaneous tissue of the lower angle of the mediastinal wound. EAT samples were obtained from the right heart (right atrium and right ventricle), and PVAT samples were obtained from the area of the right coronary artery. The AT samples were placed in Hanks' Balanced Salt Solution (Merck KGaA, St. Louis, MO, USA) containing penicillin (100 U/L), streptomycin (100 mg/mL), and gentamicin (50 µg/mL).

Adipose depots were harvested and fixed overnight in 10% neutral buffered formalin. Sections obtained from paraffin-embedded tissues were stained with hematoxylin and eosin (H&E) using standard protocols (Figure 2).

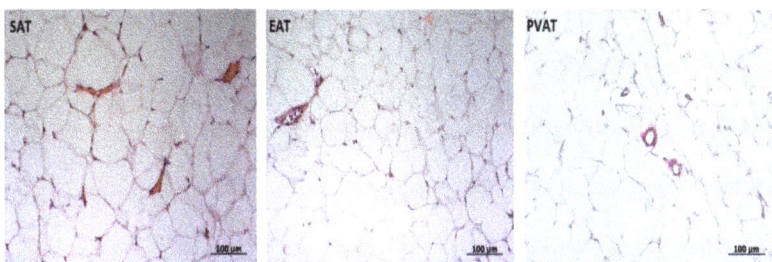

Figure 2. Representative microphotographs of hematoxylin and eosin (upper panels) stained samples of subcutaneous (SAT), epicardial (EAT) and perivascular (PVAT) from patients with coronary artery disease. Scale bar = 100 µm.

2.4.2. Adipocyte Extraction and Culture

Adipocytes were isolated from ATs under sterile conditions in a laminar flow hood (BOV-001-AMS MZMO, Millerovo, Russia) using a previously described method [9]. Adipose tissue samples (3–5 g) were crushed to 1–3 mm^3 fragments and incubated in a collagenase type I solution (0.5 mg/mL) (Thermo Fisher Scientific, Waltham, MA, USA) containing 200 nM adenosine (Merck KGaA, St. Louis, MO, USA) at 37 °C for 30 min. Then, the adipocytes were poured through a Falcon™ 100 µm sterile mesh (Thermo Fisher Scientific, Waltham, MA, USA) and washed with Gibco® M199 culture medium (Thermo Fisher Scientific), 1% 4-(2-hydroxyethyl)-1-piperazineethanesulfonic acid buffer (Thermo Fisher Scientific), 1% l-glutamine with penicillin and streptomycin (Thermo Fisher Scientific), 0.4% amphotericin B (Thermo Fisher Scientific), glucose of 5 mmol/L, 10% fetal bovine serum (Thermo Fisher Scientific). The volume of the liquid containing the cells was adjusted to 5 mL using culture medium, and the cells were centrifuged for 2 min at 200× g. Isolated adipocytes (supernatant) were placed in a separate tube, and the volume was adjusted to 1 mL with culture medium. Adipocytes were counted in a Goryaev's chamber. Cell viability was evaluated according to the method described by Suga et al. [10]. Adipocytes (20 × 10^5) were seeded into a 24-well plate (Greiner Bio One International GmbH, Kremsmünster, Austria), and the volume in each well was adjusted to 1 mL with culture medium. The plates were incubated for 24 h at a temperature of 37 ± 1 °C in an atmosphere of 5% carbon dioxide and 10% oxygen. Subsequently, the adipocytes were carefully extracted from the surface of the culture medium to determine the expression of adipokine and cytokine genes and the culture medium was also extracted from the bottom of the wells for the determination of adipokine and cytokine levels by enzyme-linked immunoassay (ELISA).

2.5. Laboratory Assays

2.5.1. RNA Extraction

Total RNA purification from isolated adipocytes was performed using the commercial RNeasy® Plus Universal Mini Kit (Qiagen, Hilden, Germany), according to the manufacturer's protocol with slight modifications, as described previously [11]. Extracted RNA was stored at −70 °C until use.

The quantity and quality of purified RNA were assessed using a NanoDrop 2000 Spectrophotometer (Thermo Fisher Scientific) by measuring the light absorbance at 280 nm, 260 nm, and 230 nm and calculating the 260/280 (A260/280) and 260/230 (A260/230) ratios. The integrity of the RNA was determined by electrophoresis in agarose gels, followed by visualization using the Gel Doc™ XR + System (Bio-Rad, Hercules, CA, USA).

2.5.2. cDNA Synthesis

Single-stranded cDNA was synthesized using the High-Capacity cDNA Reverse Transcription Kit (Applied Biosystems, Foster City, CA, USA) on a VeritiTM 96-Well Thermal Cycler (Applied Biosystems, Waltham, MA, USA). Reverse transcription was performed using the program settings suggested by the kit's manufacturer. The quantity and quality of synthesized cDNA were assessed using a NanoDrop 2000 Spectrophotometer. Samples were stored at −20 °C.

2.5.3. Real Time Quantitative Polymerase Chain Reaction (qRT-PCR)

Expression of the adiponectin, leptin, leptin receptor and interleukin-6 (IL-6) genes was evaluated by quantitative real-time polymerase chain reaction (qPCR) using TaqManTM Gene Expression Assays (ADIPOQ Hs00605917_m1, LEP Hs00174877_m1, LEPR Hs00174497_m1, IL6 Hs00174131_m1, Applied Biosystems, Waltham, MA, USA) on a ViiA 7 Real-Time PCR System (Applied Biosystems, Waltham, MA, USA). For the negative control, we used 20 µL of the reaction mixture with no cDNA template. Three technical replicates were prepared for each sample and negative control. Results were normalized for three reference genes, *HPRT1* (hypoxanthine phosphoribosyltransferase-1), *GAPDH* (glyceraldehyde-3-phosphatedehydrogenase), and *B2M* (beta-2-microglobulin). To assess the effectiveness of PCR, amplification graphs and standard curves were analyzed using QuantStudioTM Real-Time PCR Software v.1.3 (Applied Biosystems). The expression of the studied genes (normalized quantification ratio, NRQ) was calculated by the Pfaffl method and is represented on a logarithmic (log10) scale as the fold change relative to control samples [12].

2.5.4. ELISA

The concentration of adiponectin, leptin (Human Total Adiponectin/Acro30, DRP300; Human Leptin, DLP00) in the culture medium of adipocytes was determined by ELISA using test systems from R&D Systems, Inc. (Minneapolis, MN, USA) and IL-6 was determined using the test system Interleukin-6 BMS213-2 from eBioscience (Vienna, Austria).

2.6. Statistical Analysis

Statistical analysis was performed using GraphPad Prism 6 (GraphPad Software, La Jolla, CA, USA) and Statistica software, 10.0 (Dell Software, Inc., Round Rock, TX, USA). The Kolmogorov–Smirnov test was used to verify the normal distribution of data. The data were not normally distributed. Therefore, nonparametric methods were used. Data were presented as median (Me) and 25th and 75th quartiles (Q1; Q3). Two independent groups were compared using the Mann–Whitney U test. Three independent groups were compared using the Kruskal–Wallis test by ranks, followed by a pairwise comparison using the nonparametric Mann–Whitney test with the Bonferroni correction. Categorical variables are expressed as percentages and compared using chi-squared test or Fisher's exact test. A p-value of less than 0.05 was considered statistically significant.

To identify the relationship between quantitative indicators and a qualitative trait, the method of stepwise logistic regression analysis and ROC analysis with the construction of the characteristic ROC curve and the calculation of the area under the ROC curve were used. The area under the ROC curve exceeding 0.70 was considered diagnostically significant. Using ROC analysis, the threshold values of the morphometric characteristics of AT of various localization were established.

3. Results

3.1. Visualization of Local Fat Depots (Epicardial, Perivascular, Abdominal) in Patients with Coronary Heart Disease

We observed that the thickness of LV EAT and RV EAT was, on average, 1.2 times higher in patients with CAD than in the group of patients with heart defects (Table 2).

Table 2. Indicators of quantitative assessment of epicardial, perivascular, abdominal fat depots in patients with cardiovascular diseases.

Parameters	CAD 1, (n = 125)	Heart Defects, (n = 120)	p
Thickness EAT LV, mm	3.53 (2.87; 4.36)	2.76 (2.42; 3.21)	$p = 0.022$
Thickness EAT RV, mm	4.58 (4.09; 6.17)	3.65 (3.12; 3.97)	$p = 0.031$
Thickness PVAT p/3 RCA, mm	4.55 (3.53; 5.76)	2.70 (2.41; 3.29)	$p = 0.002$
Thickness PVAT m/3 RCA, mm	4.67 (3.49; 6.13)	2.63 (2.24; 3.29)	$p = 0.003$
Thickness PVAT LCA, mm	3.64 (3.33; 4.46)	2.77 (2.48; 3.12)	$p = 0.027$
Thickness PVAT p/3 anterior descending artery, mm	4.31 (3.51; 4.87)	3.15 (2.56; 3.03)	$p = 0.001$
Thickness PVAT m/3 anterior descending artery, mm	3.71 (3.24; 4.92)	2.62 (2.16; 2.88)	$p = 0.012$
Thickness PVAT p/3 circumflex artery, mm	3.35 (3.12; 4.47)	2.74 (2.34; 2.93)	$p = 0.037$
Thickness PVAT m/3 circumflex artery, mm	3.67 (3.10; 4.99)	2.55 (2.27; 2.83)	$p = 0.002$
Area VAT, cm^2	168.28 (149.21; 198.19)	136.24 (96.28; 142.13)	$p = 0.031$
Area SAT, cm^2	264.51 (190.15; 311.46)	277.36 (197.12; 344.31)	$p = 0.418$

Notes. The data presented are the medians (25th quartiles and 75th quartiles). EAT, epicardial adipose tissue, LV, left ventricle, RV, right ventricle, PVAT, perivascular adipose tissue, p/3, proximal third, RCA, right coronary artery, m/3, middle third, LCA, left coronary artery, VAT, visceral adipose tissue, SAT, subcutaneous adipose tissue.

In a comparative analysis of the quantitative parameters of PVAT in the study groups of patients with CAD, we observed that the thickness of PVAT of the proximal and middle third of the RCA was higher by 60% and 75%, respectively, than in patients with heart defects. In patients with CAD, the thickness of the PVAT at the level of the trunk of the left coronary artery (LCA) and the thickness at the level of the proximal and middle third of the RCA were 24%, 30%, and 31% higher, respectively, in comparison with that of group patients with heart defects. There was also an increase in the thickness of the PVAT at the level of the proximal and middle third of the circumflex artery in patients with CAD by 21% and 30%, respectively, than that of group patients with heart defects. Upon assessing the abdominal fat depot in patients with CAD, we observed that the VAT area exceeded the parameters of patients with heart defects by 1.2 times (Table 2).

The next step was to identify the relationship between the morphometric parameters of AT and the presence of atherosclerosis in the coronary arteries using logistic regression.

The results are presented in Table 3. We observed that the parameter with the closest association with the presence of atherosclerosis in the coronary arteries is the thickness of the EAT LV, the thickness of the PVAT of the LCA trunk, the proximal third of the anterior descending artery, the proximal third of the circumflex artery, and the area of the VAT.

Table 3. Area under the ROC curve and 95% confidence interval for atherosclerotic coronary artery disease.

Parameters	AUC	p	95% Confidence Interval (CI)	
Thickness EAT LV, mm	0.871	$p < 0.012$	0.693	0.983
Thickness EAT RV, mm	0.611	$p < 0.025$	0.552	0.739
Thickness PVAT p/3 RCA, mm	0.706	$p < 0.031$	0.708	0.979
Thickness PVAT m/3 RCA, mm	0.649	$p < 0.037$	0.523	0.729
Thickness PVAT LCA, mm	0.793	$p < 0.022$	0.642	0.937
Thickness PVAT p/3 anterior descending artery, mm	0.832	$p < 0.014$	0.704	0.956
Thickness PVAT m/3 anterior descending artery, mm	0.626	$p < 0.033$	0.686	0.769
Thickness PVAT p/3 circumflex artery, mm	0.771	$p < 0.019$	0.631	0.847
Thickness PVAT m/3 circumflex artery, mm	0.611	$p < 0.041$	0.556	0.718
Area VAT, cm^2	0.809	$p < 0.026$	0.694	0.963
Area SAT, cm^2	0.598	$p < 0.035$	0.386	0.627

EAT, epicardial adipose tissue; LV, left ventricle; RV, right ventricle; PVAT, perivascular adipose tissue; p/3, proximal third, RCA, right coronary artery; m/3, middle third, LCA, left coronary artery; VAT, visceral adipose tissue; SAT, subcutaneous adipose tissue; AUG, area under the ROC curve.

Threshold values were set for quantitative indicators of fat storage most associated with coronary atherosclerosis. Thus, for the thickness of the EAT LV, this parameter was 3.3 mm (sensitivity = 87.4, specificity = 88.9) for the thickness of the PVAT LCA was 3.4 mm (sensitivity = 86.4, specificity = 87.2), p/3 anterior descending artery was 3.7 mm (sensitivity = 88.3, specificity = 87.5), and p/3 circumflex artery was 3.35 mm (sensitivity = 86.4, specificity = 88.1)). The critical level of the VAT area was 106.1 cm^2 (sensitivity = 90.9, specificity = 89.2).

3.2. Adiponectin Gene Expression and Concentration of Adiponectin in the Daily Adipocyte Culture of Various Fat Depots

Adipocytes in the EAT expressed the lowest amount of *ADIPOQ* relative to adipocytes in different locations in both groups (Figure 3a).

In patients with CAD, *ADIPOQ* expression in the EAT was significantly lower than in the culture of SAT and PVAT (1.2 times ($p = 0.038$) and 1.5 times ($p = 0.027$), respectively). Similarly, in group patients with aortic or mitral valve replacement, *ADIPOQ* expression in EAT adipocytes was lower compared to adipocytes in the SAT and PVAT (1.4 times ($p = 0.001$) and 1.5 times ($p = 0.002$), respectively). Moreover, in Group 2, the mRNA level of *ADIPOQ* in EAT adipocytes was higher than that of patients with CAD by 1.2 times ($p = 0.031$). High mRNA levels of *ADIPOQ* were observed in the culture of PVAT. Further, *ADIPOQ* expression in cultures of SAT and PVAT adipocytes was not statistically different between patients with CAD and heart defects (Figure 1).

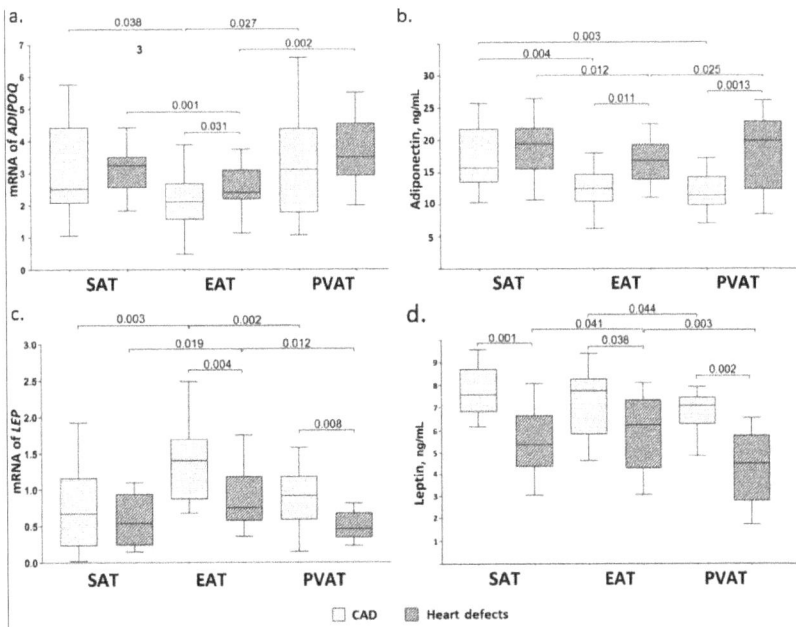

Figure 3. Adipokine gene expression and secretion in various fat depots in the daily culture of adipocytes derived from patients with CAD and patients with heart defects (aortic or mitral valve replacement). (**a**) Adiponectin gene expression (**b**) Adiponectin concentration (**c**) Leptin gene expression (**d**) Leptin concentration Notes: *ADIPOQ*-gene of adiponectin, *LEP*-gene of leptin, CAD-patients with coronary artery disease and those with indications of direct myocardial revascularization by coronary artery bypass grafting, Heart defects patients with aortic or mitral valve replacement, p-significant differences as compared to subcutaneous adipocytes, ($p \leq 0.05$).

The concentration of adiponectin in the daily culture of EAT adipocytes was lower than that of SAT in both groups (1.3 times ($p = 0.004$) and 1.13 times ($p = 0.012$), respectively) (Figure 3b).

Moreover, adiponectin levels in group with heart defects were 1.4 times higher than in group patients with CAD individuals ($p = 0.011$). The lowest level of adiponectin secretion was detected in PVAT adipocytes of patients with CAD than that of adipocyte cultures at different locations. By contrast, in patients heart defects, adiponectin levels in the PVAT exceeded that of fat depots at different locations by 1.8 times ($p = 0.001$). Adiponectin concentrations in cultures of SAT adipocytes were not statistically different between groups patients with CAD and heart defects (Figure 3b).

3.3. Leptin Gene Expression and Concentration of Leptin in the Daily Adipocyte Culture of Various Fat Depots

High levels of *LEP* expression were observed in the culture of EAT adipocytes in patients of both groups compared with adipocytes at a different location (Figure 3c). In group patients with CAD, *LEP* expression was 1.9 times higher than in group with heart defects ($p = 0.004$). Thus, mRNA levels of the *LEP* gene in EAT adipocytes exceeded that of the SAT and PVAT adipocytes by 2.1 ($p = 0.003$) and 1.5 times ($p = 0.002$), respectively, among patients with CAD, and by 1.4 ($p = 0.019$) and 1.6 times ($p = 0.012$), respectively, in patients with heart defects. Moreover, in group patients with heart defects, the lowest mRNA level of the *LEP* was detected in the PVAT culture, which was two times ($p = 0.008$) lower than that in patients with CAD. However, *LEP* expression in SAT adipocyte cultures did not show a statistically significant difference, independent of nosology (Figure 3c).

Leptin concentration was also the highest in the culture of EAT adipocytes in both groups, whereas among patients with CAD, it exceeded that group of heart defects by 1.2 times ($p = 0.038$) (Figure 3d). However, statistically significant differences compared with SAT were only found in individuals of patients with heart defects (1.2 times, $p = 0.041$). The lowest leptin concentration was observed in PVAT adipocytes compared to adipocyte cultures of other locations, and statistically significant differences were found relative to EAT adipocytes. Leptin levels in the PVAT were 1.1 times ($p = 0.044$) lower than that of the EAT in group patients with CAD and 1.5 times ($p = 0.003$) lower than that of group with heart defects. Further, leptin concentration in the PVAT adipocyte supernatant of patients with CAD was 1.5 times higher than that of comparison group ($p = 0.002$). There were no statistically significant differences in leptin concentration in the culture of SAT adipocytes between groups (Figure 3d).

3.4. IL-6 Gene Expression and Concentration of IL-6 in the Daily Adipocyte Culture of Various Fat Depots

Upon measuring pro-inflammatory *IL6* expression in a 24 h culture of adipocytes at various locations, maximum levels were observed in the EAT relative to the SAT and PVAT in group patients with CAD (2.1 times with $p = 0.0012$ and 1.4 times with $p = 0.0024$, respectively) and comparison group relative to the PVAT (1.9 times with $p = 0.0002$). Moreover, mRNA level of the *IL6* in the EAT of patients with CAD exceeded that of group patients with heart defects by 1.4 times ($p = 0.0013$) (Table 4). Further, *IL6* expression in PVAT adipocytes in group patients with CAD was 1.9 times ($p = 0.0001$) higher than that of patients with heart defects. Subcutaneous adipocytes in both groups did not show differences in IL-6 gene expression.

Table 4. Gene expression IL-6 and IL-6 concentration in adipocyte cultures of various fat depots in patients with coronary artery disease and patients with aortic or mitral valve replacement.

Parameter	Subcutaneous Adipocytes		Epicardial Adipocytes		Perivascular Adipocytes			*p*
	CAD	Heart Defects	CAD	Heart Defects	CAD	Heart Defects		
	1	2	3	4	5	6		
IL6 expression, Delta Ct	0.037 (0.025; 0.051)	0.053 (0.034; 0.061)	0.077 (0.062; 0.081)	0.056 (0.049; 0.075)	0.048 (0.037; 0.057)	0.029 (0.021; 0.032)	0.012	$P_{1-3} = 0.003$ $P_{3-5} = 0.011$ $P_{2-6} = 0.0001$ $P_{4-6} = 0.0001$
	$P_{1-2} = 0.124$		$P_{3-4} = 0.002$		$P_{5-6} = 0.0002$			
IL-6, pg/mL	12.37 (9.12; 16.27)	13.92 (10.01; 16.26)	29.35 (25.18; 37.16)	21.55 (17.77; 23.34)	18.12 (15.61; 21.06)	11.64 (8.79; 14.17)	0.011	$P_{1-3} = 0.0001$ $P_{3-5} = 0.0002$ $P_{2-4} = 0.022$ $P_{4-6} = 0.001$
	$P_{1-2} = 0.071$		$P_{3-4} = 0.022$		$P_{5-6} = 0.025$			

The data presented are the medians (25th quartiles, 75th quartiles). *IL6*, interleukin-6 gene, IL-6, interleukin-6.

The concentration of IL-6 in the EAT adipocyte culture was higher compared to SFU and PVAT, regardless of nosology (Table 4). Thus, in patients with CAD, the concentration of IL-6 in the EAT was 2.5 and 1.8 times higher than that in the SAT and PVAT, respectively. In Group 2, the EAT was 1.5 times and 1.8 times higher than that in the SAT and PVAT, respectively. Moreover, the concentration of IL-6 in the EAT and PVAT in patients with CAD exceeded the level of patients with heart defects by 1.4 times ($p = 0.022$ and $p = 0.018$, respectively). IL-6 secretion in SAT adipocytes did not differ between groups.

3.5. Relationship between Gene Expression and Secretion of Adipocytokines in AT with Indicators of Morphometric Characteristics of Local Fat Depots of the Heart and Blood Vessels in Patients with CAD

Patients with CAD were divided into groups in accordance with the threshold values of the size of fat depots to identify the factors most associated with the expression and secretion of adipocytokines and morphometric characteristics of AT of ectopic localization. For example, the number of patients in whom the values of the thickness of the EAT LV,

PVAT LCA, p/3 anterior descending artery, p/3 circumflex artery, and the area of the VAT exceeded the threshold values amounted to 60 (48%).

Among all the studied indicators of adipocytokine status, the expression of *ADIPOQ* in the EAT and PVAT, *LEP* in the EAT, *IL6* in the EAT and PVAT, the concentration of adiponectin in the EAT, and leptin in the EAT and PVAT were most associated with an increase in the size of local fat depots (Table 5).

Table 5. Association of the level of expression and secretion of adipocytokines from local fat depots with an increase in morphometric parameters of adipose tissues in patients with CAD.

Parameters	Odds Ratio (OR)	95% Confidence Interval (CI)		p
ADIPOQ expression in EAT	0.47	0.39	0.53	$p = 0.013$
ADIPOQ expression in PVAT	0.63	0.55	0.71	$p = 0.002$
LEP expression in EAT	1.54	1.44	1.60	$p = 0.022$
IL6 expression in EAT	1.51	1.43	1.59	$p = 0.002$
IL6 expression in PVAT	1.41	1.35	1.50	$p = 0.002$
Adiponectin concentration in EAT	0.55	0.46	0.61	$p = 0.001$
Leptin concentration in EAT	2.52	2.46	2.60	$p = 0.014$
Leptin concentration in PVAT	2.34	2.25	2.40	$p = 0.001$
IL-6 concentration in EAT	1.49	1.40	1.58	$p = 0.002$

4. Discussion

Recently, AT of the heart and blood vessels has been gaining attention as a new modifiable risk factor for the development and progression of CVD [13,14]. At the same time, it is well known that AT performs a number of key functions necessary for maintaining tissue and cellular myocardial homeostasis [15]. The dualism of the physiological and pathological effects of AT a given site is not fully understood, although it has been noted that an unfavorable course of CVD is associated with AT dysfunction in the heart and blood vessels. Further, fat deposits around the heart and blood vessels can play an important role in the pathogenesis of CVD owing to their anatomical proximity to vascular structures and the myocardium. It has been proven that the paracrine effect of PVAT on the vascular wall consists of the secretion of adipocytokines involved in vasoconstriction and vasodilation [16]. Moreover, adipocytes secrete adipokines and proinflammatory cytokines' the level of the secretion is known to correlate with obesity [17].

One of the objectives of this study was a comparative assessment of the morphometric parameters of EAT in patients with coronary and non-coronary heart disease. The results obtained indicate that patients with CAD exhibited higher values of EAT thickness along the anterior wall of the RV, which indicates an uneven distribution of EAT along the heart surfaces. These features are presumably anatomically and physiologically determined. It has previously been shown that the left and right ventricles contain the same absolute amount of fat on their epicardial surfaces [18]. However, taking into account the obvious differences in the mass of the myocardium of the respective ventricles, the proportion of AT in the left ventricle was less than in the right one. At the same time, the maximum EAT thickness was observed in patients with CAD. According to Iantorno et al., an increase in the linear indicators of EAT was observed in patients with CAD and immunodeficiency in comparison with persons with no signs of CAD [(13.9 ± 3.1 mm) and (10.7 ± 3.3) mm, respectively ($p = 0.001$)] [19]. Similar results were obtained by Picard et al., who reported that the thickness of EAT in patients with CAD was 2.74 ± 2.4 mm, whereas it was (2.08 ± 2.1) mm ($p = 0.0001$) in healthy individuals [20]. An increase in the size of EAT in patients with CAD may be due to a low level of AT oxygenation due to impaired blood supply to the myocardium in coronary heart disease (AT of the heart is in general circulation with the myocardium). Previous studies have found an inverse relationship between adipocyte size and AT blood flow [21].

Statin therapy plays an important role in the primary and secondary prevention of cardiovascular disease. In addition to inhibiting β-hydroxy β-methylglutaryl-CoA reductase, statins can interfere with various processes such as signaling, differentiation, and cell proliferation. The modulation of EAT by statins may be one of the most important pleiotropic effects of this class of drugs. One study has also suggested a potential anti-inflammatory effect of statins on VAT, [22]. However, there is little evidence of an effect on VAT in the cardiac region.

Indeed, there are positive results from studies conducted for different durations. In the study by Alexopoulos, statin therapy for 12 months resulted in a decrease in EAT compared with placebo [23]. In a relatively recent study, intensive statin therapy for patients with CAD when used for 3 to 72 months also indicates a direct effect on EAT thickness (assessed by ECHO-CT) and inflammatory status [24].

In the experimental study by Ishihara, treatment of 3T3-L1 preadipocytes with different concentrations of pitavastatin and the daily administration of the drug to female mice showed that statins significantly reduce (by 16.8%) the number of hypertrophied adipocytes, the total mass of which remained unchanged [25]. Later, in another pilot study, it was similarly demonstrated that low concentrations of statins (10 mg/kg atorvastatin and 3 mg/kg rosuvastatin for 48 days) consistently reduce AT mass and adipocyte size in mice on a high-fat diet [26].

Thus, statins are undoubtedly potential drugs capable of directly affecting the AT of the heart and modulating the functional activity and size of adipocytes; however, for the manifestation of these effects, their long-term use from several months to 1 year is required. In our study, patients took statins for 5 days before CABG and, therefore, before receiving VT biopsies. Additionally, the measurement of the morphometric parameters of fat depots was carried out in the period from 1 to 4 days before the operation; therefore, we assume that statin therapy in our case could not significantly affect the results of the study.

This study also showed that there was an increase in the thickness of the PVAT at the level of the proximal and middle third of the RCA, the proximal and middle thirds of the LAD and CX, as well as the trunk of the LCA in patients with CAD, compared with patients with heart defects. Thus, there is a significant predominance of PVAT in the basin of the RCA. The data obtained are consistent with the results of the study by Demircelk et al. The average thickness of the PVAT was significantly higher in patients with signs of obstructive atherosclerotic lesions in comparison with those with no signs of CAD and minor signs of coronary atherosclerosis [27].

An increase in the PVAT indices in patients with CAD may be due to mechanisms similar to that operating in the EAT. A decrease in oxygen supply against the background of atherosclerotic lesions of the coronary arteries can affect the pericoronary AT, causing hypoxia, and leading to an increase in the size of adipocytes. In addition, studies conducted in recent decades have shown the participation of adventitia and the surrounding PVAT in the development of atherosclerosis in the coronary arteries [28].

The identified associations may be associated with an increase in the secretory activity of cardiac and vascular AT in patients with CAD. Previously, it was shown that the adipocytes of EAT and PVAT are characterized by impaired differentiation and disproportionate adipocytokine secretion, manifested by a decrease in adiponectin levels and an increase in leptin and IL-6 levels in comparison with adipocytes of SAT and perirenal adipocytes [29]. According to our results, adiponectin gene expression levels in the culture of EAT adipocytes was the lowest in patients of both groups. In addition, the level of adiponectin in the EAT and PVAT is associated with an increase in the size of local fat depots around the heart and blood vessels. The data obtained in our study is consistent with the study of Bambacea et al. [6]. and Iacobellis at al [30]. In a study by Eiras at al., a reduced mRNA level of the *ADIPOQ* detected in the EAT relative to the SAT in patients without CAD [31]. However, other authors have shown no differences between patients with CAD and patients with aortic or mitral valve replacement. For example, Iglesias et al. showed that adiponectin gene expression in the EAT was lower than in the SAT, but there were no statistically significant differences between patients after CABG and with valve replacement [32]. The authors explain this by gender characteristics, as mRNA level of the *ADIPOQ* in the EAT were higher in women. PVAT is also actively involved in atherogenesis, and it synthesizes proinflammatory molecules that are involved in the formation of unstable plaques that are prone to rupture and atherothrombosis and promote the progression of CAD [8,33]. Due to this close interaction, the PVAT is the first fat depot that recognizes and reacts to emerging changes in homeostasis through the synthesis and production of adipocytokines [34]. Adiponectin plays a crucial role, as its protective and anti-inflammatory properties are known. Our results demonstrate that PVAT had the highest level of adiponectin gene expression. Moreover, adiponectin was higher in group patients with heart defects. Similar data were demonstrated by Cybularz et al. [35]. Reduced adiponectin gene expression in combination with high expression of the leptin gene may be associated with the activation of key atherogenic pathways, contributing to the progression of CAD [36].

Based on the literature, it can be assumed that the levels of adipocytokine mRNA in the AT are not always a complete reflection of their concentration [37]. In this study, PVAT adipocytes of patients with CAD were characterized by the highest level of adiponectin gene expression, yet they exhibited the lowest concentration in the culture supernatants compared to adipocyte cultures at other locations. One of the reasons for this difference may be the low expression of adiponectin receptors in these fat depots. In a study by Guo at al., which assessed the role of adiponectin and its receptors in vivo, the authors found that angiotensin II (Ang II)-induced hypertension led to a significant decrease in the expression of both adiponectin and its AdipoR1 and AdipoR2 receptors in perivascular adipocytes and vascular cells [38]. Nacci et al. investigated the effect of infliximab on adiponectin gene expression in PVAT and showed a decrease in the level of adiponectin mRNA, AdipoR1, and AdipoR2 in mice with type 1 DM. Taken together, the findings suggest that the PVAT is a site of adiponectin/AdipoR dysregulation, and secondly, it is most susceptible to proinflammatory signals [39].

Another reason may be the long-term processes of post-translational modification and oligomerization of adiponectin. The observed high level of adiponectin in PVAT is due to the longer processes of "maturation" of adiponectin in CAD, which occur in the endoplasmic reticulum (ER) of adipocytes and are controlled by special proteins/chaperones in the ER such as Ero1-Lα. It is assumed that part of the synthesized adiponectin undergoes decay or proteolysis, and the delayed release of adiponectin is due to disruption of protein-chaperones that regulate adiponectin secretion from the cell [40]. In addition, Bauchea et al. showed that adiponectin was to be able to suppress its own production and expression of its AdipoR2 receptor in transgenic mice [41]. Further, Kadowaki et al. demonstrated a decrease in the number of adiponectin receptors in metabolic syndrome and obesity [42].

Leptin, the most studied adipokine marker of obesity, participates in the regulation of atherogenesis, thrombogenesis, and vascular revascularization. Further, it stimulates inflammatory processes, oxidative stress, and vascular smooth muscle cell hypertrophy. Leptin plays a role in the pathogenesis of hypertension, CAD, and type 2 DM and the development of their complications [43]. According to our data, a higher expression of the leptin gene was observed in the culture of EAT adipocytes compared to the SAT in patients. Furthermore, in patients with CAD, *LEP* expression was the highest in PVAT adipocytes. An increase in the level of *LEP* expression in EFT is associated with an increase in the size of fat depots in the heart and around the coronary vessels. This data is consistent with the data provided by other groups [44]. Polyakova et al. showed that in men, regardless of the presence of coronary heart disease, the *LEP* expression in the EAT was significantly higher than the SAT [45]. Furthermore, the authors explain the observed differences by the predominance of men among patients with CAD, and the incidence of more severe atherosclerotic lesions of the coronary arteries in male patients [46]. However, Iglesias et al.

showed that *LEP* expression in the EAT was lower than the SAT from 46 patients who were undergoing heart surgery, coronary artery bypass surgery, or aortic or mitral valve replacement. Moreover, leptin mRNA expression in EAT was higher in women than men [32]. Increased leptin gene expression in the EAT culture of patients can have a negative effect on both adipocytes and cardiomyocytes by activating inflammatory and atherosclerotic processes [47].

Thus, the "protective" potential of AT depends on its localization. EFT adipocytes of CAD patients are characterized by changes in the adipocytokine system: low level of adiponectin gene expression against a high level of leptin gene expression and secretion compared to adipocytes at other locations.

IL-6 has been shown to produce various types of cells. However, adipocytes are also able to secrete proinflammatory IL-6 [48]. Approximately 30% of the IL-6 in the body is synthesized by AT, and its production is increased in overweight individuals. IL-6 is involved in the regulation of the energy balance of fat and muscle tissues, triggering regenerative mechanisms of immune protection and regulation of fat intake into AT. In addition, IL-6 is able to limit the inflammatory response by inhibiting the synthesis of a number of proinflammatory cytokines, including tumor necrosis factor-α (TNF-α) [49]. In vitro studies have shown that isolated visceral fat synthesizes more IL-6 than subcutaneous fat, and increased IL-6 production has been observed in adipocyte hypertrophy. plasma levels of IL-6 correlate with the area of epicardial and abdominal visceral AT in patients with coronary artery atherosclerosis, suggesting a potential effect of these fat depots on the development of atherosclerosis through paracrine rather than systemic effects [14].

We found that *IL6* expression in the daily culture of EAT adipocytes was the highest in comparison to the SAT and PVAT in both patients with CAD and those with aortic or mitral valve replacement. Moreover, the level of *IL6* mRNA in the EAT and PVAT in individuals with CAD was higher than in patients with heart defects. These identified features are consistent other studies. Shibasaki at al. found that *IL6* expression in the EAT was significantly higher than that in the SAT [50]. Moreover, *IL6* and *LEP* expression in the EAT was higher in patients with CAD, and *ADIPOQ* expression were comparable in both groups. In the SAT, *IL6* and *LEP* expression levels were moderately higher in patients with CAD compared to those without CAD. However, there were no differences in plasma cytokine levels between the two groups. [50].

Increased *IL6* expression and secretion in EAT and PVAT adipocytes can contribute to the high level of *LEP* expression and content observed in these types of AT. It is known that leptin has a stimulating effect on immune cells and is able to regulate the production of pro- and anti-inflammatory cytokines. [51]. In addition, some studies have noted homology in the structure of leptin and IL-6 receptors, also suggesting an interaction between leptin and circulating factors, through which cytokines inhibit binding of the leptin receptor to block its signaling activity in cell culture [52].

Experimental in vitro findings demonstrated that secretory products of adipocytes increase the secretion of inflammatory cytokines by macrophages and other immune cells, and pro-inflammatory cytokines, in particular IL-6, increase the transcription of leptin, which was confirmed by in vivo studies. Pro-inflammatory stimuli such as TNF-α and IL-6 itself can enhance IL-6 production in vitro. The content of IL-6 in AT is hundred times higher than in the plasma, suggesting important auto and paracrine regulatory functions in this tissue [53].

5. Conclusions

In conclusion, increased production of leptin and IL-6 and decreased production of cardioprotective adiponectin led to activation of immune cells and inflammation. This manifested primarily in EAT and PVAT adipocytes, especially in individuals with CAD, which creates favorable conditions for the development and progression of atherosclerosis. Moreover, leptin is able to affect the vascular wall and activate platelet aggregation, increasing the risk of thrombosis. Established changes in the content of the studied adipocytokines in epicardial adipocytes is a prognostically unfavorable sign in this category of patients. Therefore, the study of EAT revealed the pathogenetic significance of changes in the adipokine and cytokine status of adipocytes in patients with CAD.

Author Contributions: Conceptualization, O.V.G.; data curation, O.V.G., O.L.B.; formal analysis Y.A.D., E.V.B., E.E.B.; investigation Y.A.D., E.V.B., M.Y.S., N.K.B., E.E.B., E.O.K.; methodology, O.V.G., Y.A.D., A.N.K., R.S.T.; administration, O.L.B.; resources, A.N.S.; supervision, O.L.B.; validation, O.V.G.; writing—original draft preparation, O.V.G., Y.A.D., E.V.B.; writing—review and editing, O.V.G., Y.A.D. All authors have read and agreed to the published version of the manuscript.

Funding: This research is conducted within the fundamental research project No. 0546-2015-0012 "Multivessel coronary artery disease, polyvascular disease and comorbid conditions. The diagnosis and risk management in a large industrial region of Siberia" (Principal Investigator-director of the NII KPSSZ, M.D., Ph.D., Prof., Barbarash O.L.).

Institutional Review Board Statement: The study was performed at the Federal State Budgetary Institution's Research Institute for Complex Issues of Cardiovascular Diseases. The study protocol No. 1 from 4.02.2020 was approved by the Local Ethics Committee of the Federal State Budgetary Institution Research Institute for Complex Issues of Cardiovascular Diseases and was developed according to the World Medical Association's Declaration of Helsinki on Ethical Principles for Medical Research Involving Human Subjects, 2000 edition, and the "GCP Principles in the Russian Federation", approved by the Russian Ministry of Health.

Informed Consent Statement: Informed consent was obtained from all subjects involved in the study.

Conflicts of Interest: The authors declare no conflict of interest.

References

1. Nakamura, K.; Fuster, J.J.; Walsh, K. Adipokines: A link between obesity and cardiovascular disease. *J. Cardiol.* **2014**, *63*, 250–259. [CrossRef]
2. Tanaka, K.; Fukuda, D.; Sata, M. Roles of epicardial adipose tissue in the pathogenesis of coronary atherosclerosis—An update on recent findings. *Circ. J.* **2020**, *85*, 2–8. [CrossRef]
3. Bambace, C.; Sepe, A.; Zoico, E.; Telesca, M.; Olioso, D.; Venturi, S.; Rossi, A.; Corzato, F.; Faccioli, S.; Cominacini, L.; et al. Inflammatory profile in subcutaneous and epicardial adipose tissue in men with and without diabetes. *Heart Vessels* **2014**, *29*, 42–48. [CrossRef]
4. Anthony, S.R.; Guarnieri, A.R.; Gozdiff, A.; Helsley, R.N.; Owens, A.P., III; Tranter, M. Mechanisms linking adipose tissue inflammation to cardiac hypertrophy and fibrosis. *Clin. Sci.* **2019**, *133*, 2329–2344. [CrossRef]
5. Mahabadi, A.A.; Berg, M.H.; Lehmann, N.; Kalsch, H.; Bauer, M.; Kara, K.; Dragano, N.; Moebus, S.; Jockel, K.H.; Erbel, R.; et al. Association of epicardial fat with cardiovascular risk factors and incident myocardial infarction in the general population. *J. Am. Coll. Cardiol.* **2013**, *61*, 1388–1395. [CrossRef]
6. Bambacea, C.; Telescab, M.; Zoicoa, E.; Sepe, A.; Olioso, D.; Rossi, A.; Corzato, F.; Di Francesco, V.; Mazzucco, A.; Santini, F.; et al. Adiponectin gene expression and adipocyte diameter: A comparison between epicardial and subcutaneous AT in men. *Cardiovasc. Pathol.* **2011**, *20*, e153–e156. [CrossRef]
7. Lehr, S.; Hartwig, S.; Lamers, D.; Famulla, S.; Muller, S.; Hanisch, F.G.; Cuvelier, C.; Ruige, J.; Eckardt, K.; Ouwens, D.M.; et al. Identification and validation of novel adipokines released from primary human adipocytes. *Mol. Cell Proteom.* **2012**, *11*, M111.010504. [CrossRef]
8. Verhagen, S.N.; Visseren, F.L. Perivascular AT as a cause of atherosclerosis. *Atherosclerosis* **2011**, *214*, 3–10. [CrossRef]
9. Gruzdeva, O.V.; Dyleva, Y.A.; Antonova, L.V.; Matveeva, V.G.; Uchasova, E.G.; Fanaskova, E.V.; Karetnikova, V.N.; Ivanov, S.V.; Barbarash, O.L. Adipokine and cytokine profiles of epicardial and subcutaneous at in patients with coronary heart disease. *Bull. Exp. Biol. Med.* **2017**, *163*, 608–611. [CrossRef]
10. Suga, H.; Matsumoto, D.; Inoue, K.; Shigeura, T.; Eto, H.; Aoi, N.; Kato, H.; Abe, H.; Yoshimura, K. Numerical Measurement of Viable and Nonviable Adipocytes and Other Cellular Components in Aspirated Fat Tissue. *Plast. Reconstr. Surg.* **2008**, *122*, 103–114. [CrossRef]
11. Sinitsky, M.Y.; Dyleva, Y.A.; Uchasova, E.G.; Belik, E.V.; Yuzhalin, A.E.; Gruzdeva, O.V.; Matveeva, V.G.; Ponasenko, A.V. Adipokine gene expression in adipocytes isolated from different fat depots of coronary artery disease patients. *Arch. Physiol. Biochem.* **2019**, 1–9. [CrossRef]
12. Pfaffl, M.W. A new mathematical model for relative quantification in real-time RT-PCR. *Nucleic Acids Res.* **2001**, *29*, e45. [CrossRef]
13. Mookadam, F.; Goel, R.; Alharthi, M.S.; Jiamsripong, P.; Cha, S. Epicardial fat and its association with cardiovascular risk: A cross-sectional observational study. *Heart Views* **2010**, *11*, 103.

14. Chu, C.Y.; Lee, W.H.; Hsu, P.C.; Lee, M.K.; Lee, H.H.; Chiu, C.A.; Lin, T.H.; Lee, C.S.; Yen, H.W.; Voon, W.C.; et al. Association of Increased Epicardial Adipose Tissue Thickness With Adverse Cardiovascular Outcomes in Patients With Atrial Fibrillation. *Medicine* **2016**, *95*, e2874. [CrossRef]
15. Guglielmi, V.; Sbraccia, P. Epicardial adipose tissue: At the heart of the obesity complications. *Acta Diabetol.* **2017**, *54*, 805–812. [CrossRef]
16. Ben-Zvi, D.; Savion, N.; Kolodgie, F.; Simon, A.; Fisch, S.; Schafer, K.; Bachner-Hinenzon, N.; Cao, X.; Gertler, A.; Solomon, G.; et al. Local application of leptin antagonist attenuates angiotensin ii-induced ascending aortic aneurysm and cardiac remodeling. *J. Am. Heart Assoc.* **2016**, *5*, e003474. [CrossRef]
17. Trayhurn, P.; Wood, I.S. Signalling role of AT: Adipokines and inflammation in obesity. *Biochem. Soc. Trans.* **2005**, *33*, 1078–1081. [CrossRef]
18. Corradi, D.; Maestri, R.; Callegari, S.; Pastori, P.; Goldoni, M.; Luong, T.V.; Bordi, C. The ventricular epicardial fat is related to the myocardial mass in normal, ischemic and hypertrophic hearts. *Cardiovasc. Pathol.* **2004**, *13*, 313–316. [CrossRef]
19. Iantorno, M.; Soleimanifard, S.; Schar, M.; Brown, T.T.; Bonanno, G.; Barditch-Crovo, P.; Mathews, L.; Lai, S.; Gerstenblith, G.; Weiss, R.G.; et al. Regional coronary endothelial dysfunction is related to the degree of local epicardial fat in people with HIV. *Atherosclerosis* **2018**, *278*, 7–14. [CrossRef]
20. Picard, F.A.; Gueret, P.; Laissy, J.P.; Champagne, S.; Leclercq, F.; Carrie, D.; Juliard, J.M.; Henry, P.; Niarra, R.; Chatellier, G.; et al. Epicardial adipose tissue thickness correlates with the presence and severity of angiographic coronary artery disease in stable patients with chest pain. *PLoS ONE* **2014**, *9*, e110005. [CrossRef]
21. Trayhurn, P. Hypoxia and adipose tissue function and dysfunction in obesity. *Physiol. Rev.* **2013**, *93*, 1–21. [CrossRef] [PubMed]
22. Labuzek, K.; Bułdak, L.; Dułwa-Bułdak, A.; Bielecka, A.; Krysiak, R.; Madej, A.; Okopien, B. Atorvastatin and fenofibric acid differentially affect the release of adipokines in the visceral and subcutaneous cultures of adipocytes that were obtained from patients with and without mixed dyslipidemia. *Pharmacol. Rep.* **2011**, *63*, 1124–1136. [CrossRef]
23. Alexopoulos, N.; Melek, B.H.; Arepalli, C.D.; Hartlage, G.R.; Chen, Z.; Kim, S.; Raggi, E.S.P. Effect of intensive versus moderate lipid-lowering therapy on epicardial adipose tissue in hyperlipidemic post-menopausal women: A substudy of the BELLES Trial (Beyond endorsed lipid lowering with EBT scanning). *JACC* **2013**, *61*, 1956–1961. [CrossRef]
24. Parisi, V.; Petraglia, L.; D'Esposito, V.; Cabaro, S.; Rengo, G.; Caruso, A.; Grimaldi, M.G.; Baldascino, F.; De Bellis, A.; Vitale, D.; et al. Statin therapy modulates thickness and inflammatory profile of human epicardial adipose tissue. *Int. J. Cardiol.* **2019**, *274*, 326–330. [CrossRef]
25. Ishihara, Y.; Ohmori, K.; Mizukawa, M.; Hasan, A.U.; Noma, T.; Kohno, M. Beneficial direct adipotropic actions of pitavastatin in vitro and their manifestations in obese mice. *Atherosclerosis* **2010**, *212*, 131–138. [CrossRef]
26. Lee, S.; Lee, Y.; Kim, J.; An, J.; Kim, K.; Lee, H.; Kong, H.; Song, Y.; Kim, K. Atorvastatin and rosuvastatin improve physiological parameters and alleviate immune dysfunction in metabolic disorders. *Biochem. Biophys. Res. Commun.* **2016**, *478*, 1242–1247. [CrossRef]
27. Demircelik, M.B.; Yilmaz, O.C.; Gurel, O.M.; Selcoki, Y. Epicardial adipose tissue and pericoronary fat thickness measured with 64-multidetector computed tomography: Potential predictors of the severity of coronary artery disease. *Clinics* **2014**, *69*, 388–392. [CrossRef]
28. Kolodgie, F.D.; Virmani, R.; Cornhill, J.F.; Herderick, E.E.; Smialek, J. Increase in atherosclerosis and adventitial mast cells in cocaine abusers: An alternative mechanism of cocaine-associated coronary vasospasm and thrombosis. *J. Am. Coll. Cardiol.* **1991**, *17*, 1553–1560. [CrossRef]
29. Omar, A.; Chatterjee, T.K.; Tang, Y.; Hui, D.Y.; Weintraub, N.L. Proinflammatory phenotype of perivascular adipocytes. *Arterioscler. Thromb. Vasc. Biol.* **2014**, *34*, 1631–1636. [CrossRef]
30. Iacobellis, G.; Pistilli, D.; Gucciardo, M.; Leonetti, F.; Miraldi, F.; Brancaccio, G.; Gallo, P.; di Gioia, C.R.T. Adiponectin expression in human epicardial AT in vivo is lower in patients with coronary artery disease. *Cytokine* **2005**, *29*, 251–255. [CrossRef] [PubMed]
31. Eiras, S.; Teijeira-Fernández, E.; Shamagian, L.G.; Fernandez, A.L.; Vazquez-Boquete, A.; Gonzalez-Juanatey, J.R. Extension of coronary artery disease is associated with increased IL-6 and decreased adiponectin gene expression in epicardial AT. *Cytokine* **2008**, *43*, 174–180. [CrossRef]
32. Iglesias, M.J.; Eiras, S.; Pineiro, R.; Lopez-Otero, D.; Gallego, R.; Fernandez, Á.L.; Lago, F.; González-Juanatey, J.R. Gender differences in adiponectin and leptin expression in epicardial and subcutaneous Adipose Tissue. findings in patients undergoing cardiac surgery. *Rev. Esp. Cardiol.* **2006**, *59*, 1252–1260. [CrossRef]
33. Lee, H.Y.; Despres, J.P.; Koh, K.K. Perivascular AT in the pathogenesis of cardiovascular disease. *Atherosclerosis* **2013**, *230*, 177–184. [CrossRef]
34. Withers, S.B.; Bussey, C.E.; Saxton, S.N.; Melrose, H.M.; Watkins, A.E.; Heagerty, A.M. Mechanisms of adiponectin-associated perivascular function in vascular disease. *Arterioscler. Thromb. Vasc. Biol.* **2014**, *34*, 1637–1642. [CrossRef]
35. Cybularz, M.; Langbein, H.; Zatschler, B.; Brunssen, C.; Deussen, A.; Matschke, K.; Morawietz, H. Endothelial function and gene expression in perivascular adipose tissue from internal mammary arteries of obese patients with coronary arterydisease. *Atheroscler. Suppl.* **2017**, *30*, 149–158. [CrossRef]
36. Payne, G.A.; Kohr, M.C.; Tune, J.D. Epicardial perivascular AT as a therapeutic target in obesity-related coronary artery disease. *Br. J. Pharmacol.* **2012**, *165*, 659–669. [CrossRef]

37. Mazurek, T.; Zhang, L.F.; Zalewski, A.; Mannion, J.D.; Diehl, J.T.; Arafat, H.; Sarov-Blat, L.; O'Brien, S.; Keiper, E.A.; Johnson, A.G.; et al. Human epicardial adipose tissue is a source of inflammatory mediators. *Circulation* **2003**, *108*, 2460–2466. [CrossRef]
38. Guo, R.; Han, M.; Song, J.; Liu, J.; Sun, Y. Adiponectin and its receptors are involved in hypertensive vascular injury. *Mol. Med. Rep.* **2018**, *17*, 209–215. [CrossRef] [PubMed]
39. Nacci, C.; Leo, V.; De Benedictis, L.; Potenza, M.A.; Sgarra, L.; De Salvia, M.A.; Quon, M.J.; Montagnani, M. Infliximab therapy restores adiponectin expression in perivascularAT and improves endothelial nitric oxide-mediatedvasodilation in mice with type 1 diabetes. *Vasc. Pharmacol.* **2016**, *87*, 83–91. [CrossRef] [PubMed]
40. Tao, L.; Gao, E.; Jiao, X.; Yuan, Y.; Li, S.; Christopher, T.A.; Lopez, B.L.; Koch, W.; Chan, L.; Goldstein, B.J.; et al. Adiponectin cardioprotection after myocardial ischemia/reperfusion involves the reduction of oxidative/nitrative stress. *Circulation* **2007**, *115*, 1408–14016. [CrossRef] [PubMed]
41. Bauche, I.B.; El Mkadem, S.A.; Rezsohazy, R.; Funahashi, T.; Maeda, N.; Miranda, L.M.; Brichard, S.M. Adiponectin downregulates its own production and the expression of its AdipoR2 receptor in transgenic mice. *Biochem. Biophys. Res. Commun.* **2006**, *345*, 1414–1424. [CrossRef] [PubMed]
42. Kadowaki, T. Adiponectin and adiponectin receptors in insulin resistance, diabetes, and the metabolic syndrome. *J. Clin. Investig.* **2006**, *116*, 1784–1792. [CrossRef]
43. Hasty, A.H.; Shimano, H.; Osuga, J.; Namatame, I.; Takahashi, A.; Yahagi, N.; Perrey, S.; Iizuka, Y.; Tamura, Y.; Amemiya-Kudo, M.; et al. Severe hypercholesterolemia, hypertriglyceridemia, and atherosclerosis in mice lacking both leptin and the low density lipoprotein receptor. *J. Biol. Chem.* **2001**, *276*, 37402–37408. [CrossRef] [PubMed]
44. Gormez, S.; Demirkan, A.; Atalar, F.; Caynak, B.; Erdim, R.; Sozer, V.; Gunay, D.; Akpinar, B.; Ozbek, U.; Buyukdevrim, A.S. Adipose tissue gene expression of adiponectin, tumor necrosis factor alpha and leptin in metabolic syndrome patients with coronary artery disease. *Intern. Med.* **2011**, *50*, 805–910. [CrossRef] [PubMed]
45. Polyakova, E.A.; Kolodina, D.A.; Miroshnikova, V.V.; Razgildina, N.D.; Bogdanova, E.O.; Lyapina, E.N.; Belyaeva, O.D.; Pchelina, S.N.; Berkovich, O.A.; Baranova, E.I. Subcutaneous and epicardial adipose tissue leptin gene expression in coronary artery disease patient. *Transl. Med.* **2019**, *6*, 25–35. (In Russian) [CrossRef]
46. Bokeriya, L.A.; Aronov, D.M. Russian clinical guidelines. Coronary artery bypass grafting in patients with ischemic heart disease: Rehabilitation and secondary prevention. *Cardiosomatics* **2016**, *7*, 5–71. [CrossRef]
47. Drosos, I.; Chalikias, G.; Pavlaki, M.; Kareli, D.; Epitropou, G.; Bougioukas, G.; Mikroulis, D.; Konstantinou, F.; Giatromanolaki, A.; Ritis, K.; et al. Differences between perivascular AT surrounding the heart and the internal mammary artery: Possible role for the leptin-inflammation-fibrosis-hypoxia axis. *Clin. Res. Cardiol.* **2016**, *105*, 887–900. [CrossRef]
48. Gotsman, I.; Stabholz, A.; Planer, D.; Pugatsch, T.; Lapidus, L.; Novikov, Y.; Masrawa, S.; Soskolne, A.; Lotan, C. Serum cytokine tumor necrosis factor-alpha and interleukin-6 associated with the severity of coronary artery disease: Indicators of an active inflammatory burden? *Isr. Med. Assoc. J.* **2008**, *10*, 494–498.
49. Dandona, P.; Aljada, A.; Chaudhuri, A.; Mohanty, P.; Garg, R. Metabolic syndrome: A comprehensive perspective based on interaction between obesity, diabetes, and inflammation. *Circulation* **2005**, *111*, 1448–1454. [CrossRef]
50. Shibasaki, I.; Nishikimi, T.; Mochizuki, Y.; Yamada, Y.; Yoshitatsu, M.; Inoue, Y.; Kuwata, T.; Ogawa, H.; Tsuchiya, G.; Ishimitsu, T.; et al. Greater expression of inflammatory cytokines, adrenomedullin, and natriuretic peptide receptor-C in epicardial AT in coronary artery disease. *Regul. Pept.* **2010**, *165*, 210–217. [CrossRef]
51. Yang, R.; Barouch, L.A. Leptin signaling and obesity. *Circ. Res.* **2007**, *101*, 545–559. [CrossRef] [PubMed]
52. Fujimaki, S.; Kanda, T.; Fujita, K.; Tamura, J.; Kobayashi, I. The significance of measuring plasma leptin in acute myocardial infarction. *J. Int. Med. Res.* **2001**, *29*, 13–108. [CrossRef] [PubMed]
53. Hoene, M.; Weigert, C. The role of interleukin-6 in insulin resistence, body fat distribution and energy balance. *Obes. Rev.* **2008**, *9*, 20–29. [PubMed]

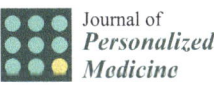

Article

The Determinants of the 13-Year Risk of Incident Atrial Fibrillation in a Russian Population Cohort of Middle and Elderly Age

Marina Shapkina [1,*], Andrey Ryabikov [1,2], Ekaterina Mazdorova [1], Anastasia Titarenko [1], Ekaterina Avdeeva [1], Elena Mazurenko [1], Lilia Shcherbakova [1], Hynek Pikhart [3], Martin Bobak [3] and Sofia Malyutina [1]

1. Institute of Internal and Preventive Medicine—Branch of Federal State Budgeted Research Institution, "Federal Research Center, Institute of Cytology and Genetics, Siberian Branch of the Russian Academy of Sciences", 630090 Novosibirsk, Russia; a_ryabikov@hotmail.com (A.R.); mazdorova@mail.ru (E.M.); titav@inbox.ru (A.T.); avdeeva_08@inbox.ru (E.A.); poltorackayaes@gmail.com (E.M.); 9584792@mail.ru (L.S.); smalyutina@hotmail.com (S.M.)
2. Federal State Budget Educational Institution of Higher Education, Novosibirsk State Medical University of the Ministry of Health of the Russian Federation, 630091 Novosibirsk, Russia
3. Institute of Epidemiology and Health Care, University College London, London WC1E6BT, UK; h.pikhart@ucl.ac.uk (H.P.); m.bobak@ucl.ac.uk (M.B.)
* Correspondence: shapkina7331@gmail.com; Tel.: +7(965)-990-73-31

Citation: Shapkina, M.; Ryabikov, A.; Mazdorova, E.; Titarenko, A.; Avdeeva, E.; Mazurenko, E.; Shcherbakova, L.; Pikhart, H.; Bobak, M.; Malyutina, S. The Determinants of the 13-Year Risk of Incident Atrial Fibrillation in a Russian Population Cohort of Middle and Elderly Age. *J. Pers. Med.* **2022**, *12*, 122. https://doi.org/10.3390/jpm12010122

Academic Editor: Amelia Filippelli

Received: 11 December 2021
Accepted: 12 January 2022
Published: 17 January 2022

Publisher's Note: MDPI stays neutral with regard to jurisdictional claims in published maps and institutional affiliations.

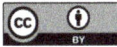

Copyright: © 2022 by the authors. Licensee MDPI, Basel, Switzerland. This article is an open access article distributed under the terms and conditions of the Creative Commons Attribution (CC BY) license (https://creativecommons.org/licenses/by/4.0/).

Abstract: Atrial fibrillation (AF) is the most common arrhythmia and a predictor of the complications of atherosclerotic cardiovascular diseases (ASCVDs), particularly thromboembolic events and the progression of heart failure. We analyzed the determinants of the 13-year risk of incident AF in a Russian population cohort of middle and elderly age. A random population sample (n = 9360, age 45–69 years) was examined at baseline in 2003–2005 and reexamined in 2006–2008 and 2015–2017 in Novosibirsk (the HAPIEE study). Incident AF was being registered during the average follow-up of 13 years. The final analysis included 3871 participants free from baseline AF and cardiovascular disease (CVD) who participated in all three data collections. In a multivariable-adjusted Cox regression model, the 13-year risk of AF was positively associated with the male sex (hazard ratio (HR) = 2.20; 95% confidence interval (CI) 1.26–3.87); age (HR = 1.10 per year; 95% CI 1.07–1.14); body mass index (BMI), (HR = 1.11 per unit; 95% CI 1.07–1.15); systolic blood pressure (SBP), (HR = 1.02 per 1 mmHg; 95% CI 1.01–1.02), and it was negatively associated with total cholesterol (TC), (HR = 0.79 per 1 mmol/L; 95% CI 0.66–0.94). In women, the risk of AF was more strongly associated with hypertension (HT) and was also negatively related to total cholesterol (TC) level (HR = 0.74 per 1 mmol/L; 95% CI 0.56–0.96). No independent association was found with mean alcohol intake per drinking occasion. These results in a Russian cohort have an implication for the prediction of AF and ASCVD complications in the general population.

Keywords: HAPIEE study; atrial fibrillation; atherosclerosis; arterial hypertension; obesity; diabetes mellitus; aging; determinants; prevalence; Russian population cohort; Cox regression analysis

1. Introduction

With the worldwide increase in life expectancy, aging-related conditions are becoming increasingly important. Atrial fibrillation (AF) is the most common arrhythmia, worldwide burden, and an important predictor of the complications of atherosclerotic cardiovascular diseases (ASCVDs), particularly thromboembolic events and progression of heart failure [1–4]. The prevalence of AF is increasing, and it is expected to become an epidemic in the coming decades, as the population is aging [2,5–9], and will reach up to 14–17 million AF patients by 2030 in the European Union [10].

AF is most prevalent in multimorbid patients with ASCVDs (such as coronary artery disease and stroke), hypertension, heart failure, valvular heart disease, obesity, diabetes mellitus, or chronic kidney disease [5,11–16]. About 20–30% of patients with ischemic stroke have AF diagnosed before, during, or after the initial event [17–19]. Cognitive impairment [20–22], decreased quality of life [23,24], and depressed mood [25] are common in patients with AF. In addition, AF increased the risk of dementia in those without stroke (RR: 1.67; 95% confidence interval (CI): 1.17, 2.38) [26].

The prognostic importance of AF underlined the development and regular update of guidelines for the management of AF [2,3], but the asymptomatic and paroxysmal course often allows only a retrospective verification of AF as a mechanism of complications that have already arisen. Consequently, preclinical assessment of AF risk and the identification of patterns of AF predictors is a priority.

For this report, we investigated the determinants of the 13-year risk of incident AF in a Russian population cohort of the middle and elderly age.

2. Materials and Methods

Study Population

A random population sample (n = 9360, age 45–69 years) was examined at baseline in 2003–2005 in Novosibirsk within the Russian arm of the HAPIEE (Health, Alcohol and Psychosocial Factors in Eastern Europe) study [27]. The average follow-up period was 12.8 years (standard deviation (SD) = 0.78, median = 12.7) in men and 12.9 years (SD = 0.77, median = 12.9) in women (until 31 December 2017). During the follow-up, two reexaminations of the cohort were being conducted in 2005–2008 (2nd, n = 6031, age 47–72 years) and 2015–2017 (3rd, n = 3898, age 55–84 years).

The analysis included respondents with available rest electrocardiogram (ECG) at the survey: 9255 participants at baseline examination and 3878 on the 3rd reexamination.

The design of this study is a prospective cohort study.

The study was approved by the Ethics Committee (Protocol No. 1 from 14 March 2002 and Protocol No. 12 from 8 December 2020) of the IIPM—Branch of IC&G SB RAS (Institute of Internal and Preventive Medicine – Branch of Federal State Budgeted Research Institution, "Federal Research Center, Institute of Cytology and Genetics, Siberian Branch of the Russan Academy of Sciences"). All study participants signed the patient informed consent form.

The research protocol of examinations throughout all stages (waves) included a standard epidemiological assessment of cardiovascular diseases (CVDs) and their risk factors and health parameters. Details of the study protocol have been described elsewhere [27]. In this analysis, we included the following instrumental and laboratory parameters: body mass index (BMI), blood pressure (BP), heart rate, resting ECG, levels of total cholesterol (TC), triglycerides (TGs), high-density lipoprotein cholesterol (HDLC), gamma-glutamyl transpeptidase (GGTP), and glucose in blood serum were measured enzymatically. Low-density lipoprotein cholesterol (LDLC) was calculated using the Friedewald formula.

To assess fasting plasma glucose (FPG), we converted the fasting serum glucose level using the formula of the European Association for the Study of Diabetes (EASD), 2007 [28]:

FPG (mmol/L) = $-0.137 + 1.047 \times$ Glucose of serum (mmol/L).

The resting ECG was recorded in 12 standard leads using electrocardiograph Cardiax (IMED Ltd., Budapest, Hungary), the timeframe for resting ECG was 30 s (including two records for 6 leads each, record at inspiration and record "for rhythm"). ECG changes were assessed manually by Minnesota Code (MC) [29] by two readers (S.M., M.S.). For repeatability of ECG, we conducted a double-blind assessment of ECG in a random sample (100 records), the mean agreement coefficient Kappa was 0.85.

HT was established at levels of systolic (SBP) or diastolic (DBP) blood pressure $\geq$ 140/90 mm Hg according to European Society of Cardiology (ESC) Guidelines, 2018 [30], and/or under antihypertensive treatment during the last 2 weeks.

Diabetes mellitus (DM) was defined in the presence of a history of diabetes with glucose-lowering treatment and/or by fasting plasma glucose level of $\geq$7 mmol/L [31].

The presence of coronary artery disease (CHD) was determined according to epidemiological criteria based on (1) survey data (positive response to the Rose questionnaire for angina pectoris and/or "ischemic" ECG changes (1, 4, 5 MC classes) or (2) medical history of myocardial infarction, or acute coronary syndrome, or coronary artery bypass grafting, or percutaneous transluminal coronary angioplasty confirmed by hospitalization.

The presence of stroke was established on the basis of a medical history of stroke or a transient ischemic attack confirmed by hospitalization. The history of chronic heart disease (CHD) and/or stroke was determined as the presence of CVD.

A person who smoked at least one cigarette a day was classified as a smoker. Smoking status was categorized as current smoker, former smoker, and never smoked.

The amount of alcohol consumed was converted to pure ethanol (g). The alcohol consumption in the present study was analyzed by the mean dose per occasion. Marital status was dichotomized as married (or cohabiting) and single (never been married, divorced, or widower/widow). The level of education was dichotomized as high education and education less than high.

The new-onset AF revealed at the reexamination during the follow-up was registered as an endpoint (permanent type) and was defined by Minnesota Code (MC 8-3-1, 8-3-2; 6-8 with "fibrillation" for atria).

Firstly, for the sake of the cross-sectional estimates of the AF prevalence, we included all subjects that have adequate resting ECG at the baseline examination (n = 9255) and 3rd examination (n = 3878).

Secondly, for cohort analysis of the incident AF, we excluded individuals with prevalent AF (n = 146) and CVD at baseline (n = 1888), non-responders in any of the follow-up examinations (n = 2759), those with technically inadequate ECGs at any wave (n = 105), or missing baseline data on the factors analyzed (n = 592). Finally, the data on 3871 persons (1775 men and 2096 women) aged 45–69 years at baseline were analyzed for the risk of incident AF. The analysis in the CVD-free population was applied in correspondence with a similar approach in other cohort studies of the AF risk [32–35].

Thirdly, for the sensitivity analysis, we repeated calculations based on a cohort without exclusion of the baseline CVD.

Statistical analysis was performed using the Statistical Package for Social Sciences (SPSS) version 13.0 for Windows (IBM, Armonk, NY, USA). First, we used ANOVA and nonparametric tests, to compare continuous variables between those who developed AF and their counterparts, and cross-tabulation to compare categorical variables. Second, we used Cox regression (age- and multivariable-adjusted models) to analyze predictors of AF.

Model 1 was age- and sex adjusted in total population and age adjusted in analysis split by sex; model 2 was adjusted for age, sex, BMI, SBP, TC, TG, smoking, alcohol consumption (mean dose per occasion, g) based on the risk factors preselected in model 1; model 3 was adjusted for age, sex, BMI, TC, HT, DM, smoking, alcohol consumption, level of education, and marital status. Hypothesis testing was considered statistically significant at p-value < 0.05.

3. Results

In cross-sectional analysis, the prevalence of AF in the cohort population increased from 1.6% (n = 146/9255) at the age of 45–69 years (1.1% in women and 2.1% in men) to 4.2% (n = 164/3878) at the age of 55–84 years (3.0% in women and 6.1% in men) over the 13-year follow-up period (Figure 1).

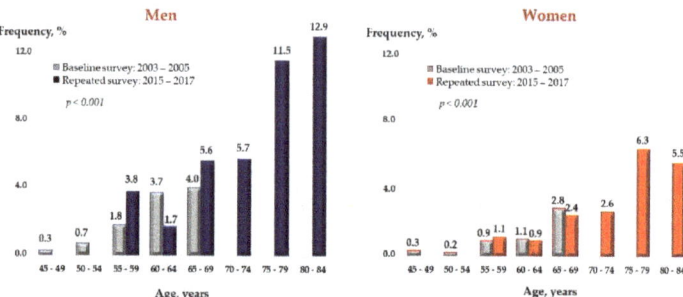

Figure 1. Prevalence of AF 2003–2017 by age groups in 2003–2005 and 2015–2017. The HAPIEE study, Russian population cohort. AF, atrial fibrillation.

Among participants free from baseline AF and CVD, 122 new cases of AF were identified, accounting for 3.2% ($n = 122/3871$), 2.6% in women, and 3.8% in men.

The baseline characteristics of participants with incident AF occurred during the follow-up, and those without AF are presented in Table 1. Both men and women with incident AF were older and had stronger expressed cardiometabolic risk factors than their counterparts (higher values of BMI, SBP, and DBP), and higher HT prevalence (among women). There was no difference between groups in blood lipid profile or carbohydrate metabolism parameters. In addition, there was no significant difference in behavioral factors (smoking and alcohol consumption) and in socioeconomic status (educational level and marital status).

Table 1. Sex-specific characteristics of baseline sample depending on incident AF. The HAPIEE study, Russian population cohort free from baseline AF and CVD, $n = 3871$.

Risk Factors	Men, Mean (SD)/n (%)			Women, Mean (SD)/n (%)		
	iAF(−) n = 1707	iAF(+) n = 68	p^1	iAF(−) n = 2042	iAF(+) n = 54	p^2
Age, years	57.6 (6.99)	60.6 (6.30)	<0.001	57.2 (6.95)	61.4 (5.76)	<0.001
Heart rate, b/min	71.1 (12.48)	70.7 (12.16)	0.807	71.2 (10.33)	68.7 (10.7)	0.078
BMI, kg/m^2	26.0 (4.13)	28.0 (4.25)	<0.001	29.5 (5.42)	32.5 (5.70)	<0.001
SBP, mmHg	142.3 (22.98)	151.0 (24.89)	0.002	141.5 (24.89)	158.9 (27.46)	<0.001
DBP, mmHg	89.8 (13.18)	93.1 (13.29)	0.045	89.0 (13.01)	96.1 (15.40)	<0.001
HT	1002 (58.7%)	45 (66.2%)	0.134	1272 (62.3%)	46 (85.2%)	<0.001
DM	152 (9.0%)	8 (12.1%)	0.253	175 (8.7%)	2 (3.8%)	0.160
TC, mmol/L	5.9 (1.21)	5.9 (1.21)	0.585	6.5 (1.26)	6.2 (1.12)	0.077
LDLC, mmol/L	3.8 (1.08)	3.7 (1.01)	0.690	4.2 (1.13)	3.9 (0.98)	0.060
HDLC, mmol/L	1.5 (0.38)	1.5 (0.30)	0.230	1.6 (0.34)	1.6 (0.37)	0.521
TG, mmol/L	1.4 (0.75)	1.5 (0.69)	0.514	1.5 (0.82)	1.4 (0.76)	0.403
GGTP, U/L	38.3 (45.03)	35.1 (20.01)	0.566	28.1 (30.40)	28.7 (17.15)	0.891
Glucose, mmol/L	5.9 (1.49)	5.9 (0.87)	0.916	5.9 (1.39)	5.6 (0.61)	0.193
Alcohol per occasion, g	55.4 (45.89)	62.5 (48.11)	0.216	22.0 (16.83)	20.4 (12.89)	0.482
Smoking status:						
Never smoked	458 (26.8)	21 (30.9)		1756 (86.0)	49.0 (90.7)	
Former smoker	390 (22.9)	20 (29.4)	0.215	87 (4.3)	1 (1.9)	0.559
Current smoker	858 (50.3)	27 (39.7)		199 (9.7)	4 (7.4)	
The level of education:						
Higher	575 (33.7)	26 (38.2)	0.257	615 (30.1)	13 (24.1)	0.212
Other	1132 (66.3)	42 (61.8)		1427 (69.9)	41 (75.9)	
Marital status:						
Married	1495 (87.6)	62 (91.2)	0.250	1255 (61.5)	27.0 (50.0)	0.060
Single	212 (12.4)	6 (8.8)		787 (38.5)	27,0 (50.0)	

[1] p-value between groups depending on incident AF in men; [2] p-value between groups depending on incident AF in women; iAF(+) or iAF(−)—a presence or an absence incident AF, respectively. AF, Atrial fibrillation; CVD, cardiovascular disease; SD, standard deviation; iAF, incident AF; BMI, body mass index; SBP, systolic blood pressure; DBP, diastolic blood pressure; HT, hypertension; DM, diabetes mellitus; TC, total cholesterol; LDLC, low-density lipoprotein cholesterol; HDLC, high-density lipoprotein cholesterol; TG, triglycerides; GGTP, gamma-glutamyl transpeptidase.

In the series of age- and sex-adjusted Cox regression of model 1, 18 risk factors were tested. The 13-year risk of incident AF was positively associated with male sex, BMI, SBP, DBP, or presence of HT, and it was negatively associated with TC and LDLC levels (Supplementary Table S1). According to the results of age-adjusted model 1, the following covariates were included for further analysis: age, sex, BMI, SBP, TC, TG, smoking, alcohol consumption (mean dose per occasion, g) in model 2; age, sex, BMI, TC, HT, DM, smoking, alcohol consumption (mean dose per occasion, g), education, and marital status in model 3.

Men in our studied population sample had a 2.2-fold increased risk of AF (95% CI 1.17–3.47), compared with women, regardless of other factors. Thus, further analysis of the contribution of the studied risk factors to the 13-year risk of AF was performed with stratification by sex.

In men (Table 2, Figure 2), in age-adjusted models, the risk of incident AF was positively associated with the value of BMI, SBP, and alcohol intake. After controlling by biological and behavioral factors, the risk of incident AF was positively associated with age (HR = 1.09; 95% CI 1.04–1.13), BMI (HR = 1.10; 95% CI 1.04–1.17), and value of SBP (HR = 1.01; 95% CI 1.001–1.021) in model 2. Some associations attenuated after additional adjustment for HT, DM, education, and marital status in model 3, and AF remained to be associated with age (HR = 1.10; 95%CI 1.06–1.14) and value of BMI (HR=1.11; 95% CI 1.04–1.17), regardless of other factors.

Table 2. Associations between risk factors and 13-risk of incident AF in men free from baseline AF and CVD. Cox regression analysis, age- and multivariable-adjusted models.

Risk Factors	Model 1 HR (95% CI)	Model 2 HR (95% CI)	Model 3 HR (95% CI)
Age, per 1 years	1.09 (1.05–1.13)	1.09 (1.04–1.13)	1.10 (1.06–1.14)
Heart rate, per 1 b/min	1.01 (0.99-1.03)	1.00 (0.98–1.03)	1.01 (0.99–1.03)
BMI, per 1 kg/m^2	1.11 (1.05–1.17)	1.10 (1.04–1.17)	1.11 (1.04–1.17)
SBP, per 1 mmHg	1.01 (1.00–1.02)	1.01 (1.00–1.02)	
TC, per 1 mmol/L	0.90 (0.73–1.11)	0.83 (0.66–1.04)	0.84 (0.67–1.05)
LDLC, per 1 mmol/L	0.88 (0.70–1.11)		
TG, per 1 mmol/L	1.13 (0.85–1.51)		0.97 (0.67–1.40)
Glucose, per 1 mmol/L	1.01 (0.84–1.21)		
GGTP, per 1 U/L	1.00 (1.00–1.01)		
HT, yes vs. no	1.35 (0.81–2.25)		1.13 (0.66–1.93)
DM, yes vs. no	1.44 (0.69–3.01)		1.15 (0.53–2.48)
Alcohol, per 20 g	1.10 (1.00–1.22)	1.08 (0.98–1.20)	1.00 (1.00–1.01)
Smoking status:			
- Former smoker vs. Never	1.24 (0.67–2.23)	1.16 (0.63–2.15)	1.15 (0.61–2.15)
- Current smoker vs. Never	1.12 (0.63–2.01)	1.30 (0.70–2.40)	1.28 (0.69–2.38)
Level of education:			
- Other vs. higher	1.06 (0.65–1.74)		1.05 (0.63–1.75)
Marital status:			
- Single vs. married	0.79 (0.34–1.82)		0.68 (0.27–1.72)

HR, hazard ratio; CI, confidence interval; model 1 adjusted for age; model 2: adjusted for age, BMI, SBP, TC, TG, smoking, alcohol consumption; model 3 adjusted for age, BMI, TC, HT, DM, smoking, alcohol consumption, education, and marital status.

In women (Table 3, Figure 3), in age-adjusted models, the risk of incident AF was positively associated with the value of BMI (HR = 1.10; 95% CI 1.05–1.15), SBP (HR = 1.02; 95% CI 1.01–1.03), or the presence of HT (HR = 2.79; 95% CI 1.30–5.99), and negatively related to TC (HR = 0.70; 95% CI 0.55–0.89) and LDLC (HR = 0.68; 95% CI 0.52–0.88). These relationships remained significant in models 2 and 3 independent of biological, behavioral, and social factors, except for the value of LDLC.

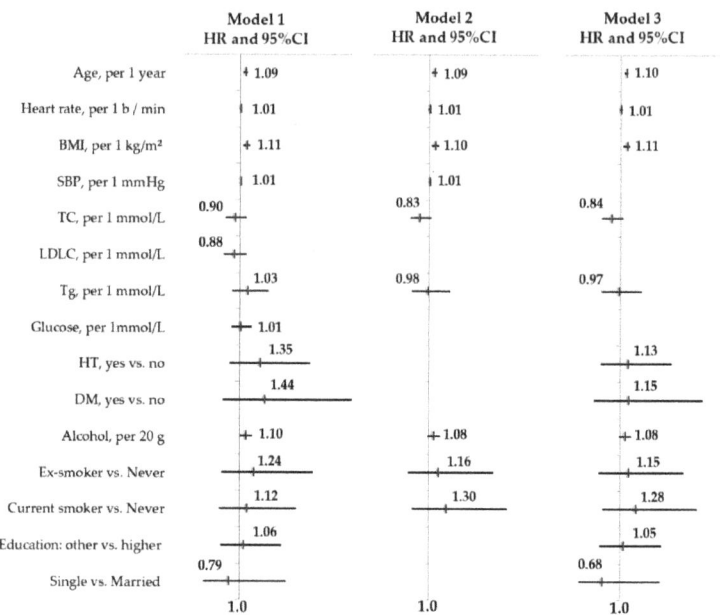

Figure 2. Determinants of 13-year risk of incident AF in men free from baseline AF and CVD. Cox regression analysis, age- and multivariable-adjusted models. The HAPIEE study, Russian population cohort, n = 1775. AF, atrial fibrillation; CVD, cardiovascular disease; BMI, body mass index; SBP, systolic blood pressure; TC, total cholesterol; LDLC, low-density lipoprotein cholesterol; TG, triglycerides; HT, hypertension; DM, diabetes mellitus; HR, hazard ratio; CI, confidence interval.

Table 3. Associations between risk factors and 13-risk of incident AF in women free from baseline AF and CVD. Cox regression analysis, age- and multivariable-adjusted models.

Risk Factors	Model 1 HR (95% CI)	Model 2 HR (95% CI)	Model 3 HR (95% CI)
Age, per 1 years	1.10 (1.06–1.15)	1.09 (1.06–1.12)	1.10 (1.07–1.14)
Heart rate, per 1 b/min	0.98 (0.95–1.00)	0.98 (0.95–1.00)	0.98 (0.95–1.00)
BMI, per 1 kg/m^2	1.10 (1.05–1.15)	1.09 (1.04–1.14)	1.09 (1.04–1.14)
SBP, per 1 mmHg	1.02 (1.01–1.03)	1.02 (1.01–1.03)	
TC, per 1 mmol/L	0.70 (0.55–0.89)	0.74 (0.57–0.96)	0.70 (0.54–0.89)
LDLC, per 1 mmol/L	0.68 (0.52–0.88)		
TG, per 1 mmol/L	0.74 (0.47–1.15)		0.76 (0.45–1.28)
Glucose, per 1 mmol/L	0.74 (0.52–1.05)		
GGT, per 1 U/L	1.01 (1.00–1.01)		
HT, yes vs. no	2.79 (1.30–5.98)		2.37 (1.07–5.25)
DM, yes vs. no	0.39 (0.09–1.60)		0.37 (0.09–1.53)
Alcohol, per 20 g	1.06 (0.67–1.49)	0.89 (0.60–1.32)	0.90 (0.63–1.35)
Smoking status:			
- Former smoker vs. Never	0.79 (0.11–5.79)	1.06 (0.14–7.93)	0.95 (0.13–7.11)
- Current smoker vs. Never	1.59 (0.55–4.64)	2.04 (0.68–6.15)	2.10 (0.70–6.27)
Level of education:			
- Other vs. Higher	1.36 (0.73–2.54)		1.32 (0.67–2.58)
Marital status:			
- Single vs. Married	1.41 (0.82–2.42)		1.40 (0.81–2.44)

HR, hazard ratio; CI, confidence interval; model 1 adjusted for age; model 2 adjusted for age, BMI, SBP, TC, TG, smoking, alcohol consumption; model 3 adjusted for age, BMI, TC, HT, DM, smoking, alcohol consumption, education, and marital status.

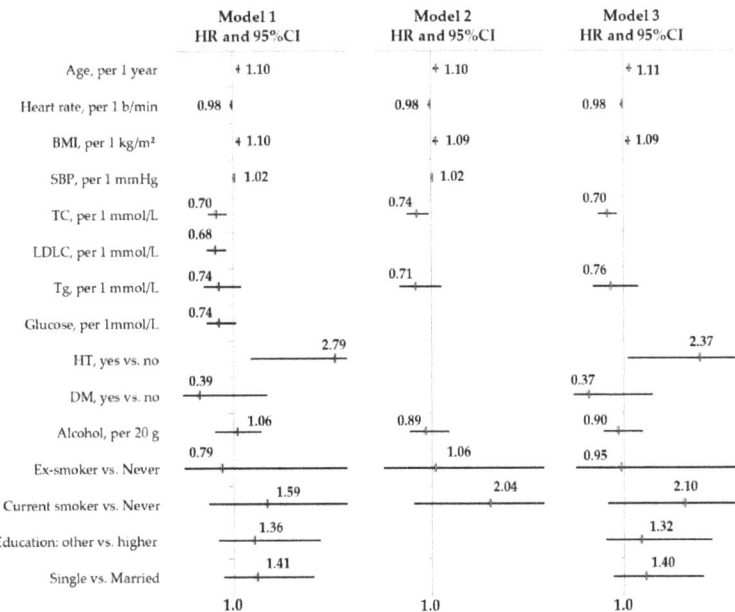

Figure 3. Determinants of 13-year risk of incident AF in women free from baseline AF and CVD. Cox regression analysis, age- and multivariable-adjusted models. The HAPIEE study, Russian population cohort, n = 2096.

In sensitivity analysis among all subjects, regardless of the prevalent CVD, the presence of baseline CVD was associated with AF risk (HR = 2.25 per year; 95% CI 1.59–3.17). The HRs for associations between primarily revealed determinants and AF slightly attenuated but remained significant; we did not find additional associations between other studied risk factors and AF.

4. Discussion

In this Russian population-based cohort, the baseline prevalence of AF was 1.6% at the age of 45–69 years and about 4% at the age of 55–84 years. The frequency of AF increased from 0.3% in the younger age group (45–50 years) up to 13% in men and 6% in women in the older age group (80–84 years). Our results were close to the findings from the North American and European population studies. In the prospective analyses, among the persons free from baseline CVD, the 13-year risk of incident AF was positively associated with male sex, SBP, or the presence of hypertension, and BMI value independent of other factors. In the total cohort, the risk of incident AF was also associated with the prevalent CVD.

AF is an age- and sex-specific condition. In the AnTicoagulation and Risk Factors In Atrial Fibrillation (ATRIA) study (USA), the prevalence of AF was 0.1% among adults younger than 55 years and 9.0% for those aged 80 years and older [5]. The overall prevalence of AF in the Rotterdam study was 5.5%, rising from 0.7% in the age group of 55–59 years to 17.8% in those aged 85 years and above [36].

The profile of AF determinants and the strength of their effects were similar to other studies worldwide. For example, the 38-year follow-up data from the Framingham study (FHS) showed that men were 1.5-fold more likely to develop AF than women, adjusted for age and predisposing conditions [13]. In our study, over a 13-year follow-up period, being male had an approximately twofold increased risk of incident AF, independent of other risk factors.

The FHS data also demonstrated that age is the strongest risk factor for AF when compared with other factors, including male sex, BMI, diabetes, smoking, alcohol intake, SBP, heart failure, and myocardial infarction [37]. In our study, age also strongly contributed to the risk of incident AF and increased the risk of AF by 10% each year.

With regard to elevated BP, in the studied Russian population sample, those with incident AF during follow-up had higher baseline SBP and DBP, compared with those free from this condition, and this relationship was stronger among women. In women, the presence of HT was a powerful predictor of AF and independently associated with the risk of AF, increasing by 2.3 times, compared with normotensives. The value of SBP was positively associated with the risk of AF in both sexes. The Cohorts for Heart and Aging Research in Genomic Epidemiology model for atrial fibrillation (CHARGE-AF) consortium also found that both systolic and diastolic BP were predictors of AF risk [38]. In the FHS, the adjusted risk for AF was slightly weaker and amounted to 1.4- and 1.5-fold risk for women and men with HT, respectively [13].

Long-term (13-year) trajectories of systolic blood pressure and hypertension in the Tromsø study were also associated with an increased incidence of AF. However, this association was stronger in women with baseline elevated systolic blood pressure and doubled the risk of AF incidence, regardless of the dynamics of SBP during the follow-up period [39].

Elevated BMI is both an independent risk factor for AF and a predisposing for the development of HT, DM, and CVD. In our population cohort, those who developed AF during the 13-year follow-up period had higher baseline BMI values ($p < 0.001$); an increase in BMI by 1 kg/m^2 increased the risk of AF by 10% in both, men and women, independent of other factors. The association between the value of BMI and increased risk of developing AF was reported in numerous population studies [40–42]. For example, in the Danish Diet, Cancer, and Health Study, the adjusted hazard ratio for AF per unit of increase in the body mass index was 1.08 (95% CI: 1.05–1.11) in men and 1.06 (95% CI: 1.03–1.09) in women [36]. A dose–response relationship was observed, with each one-unit increase in BMI associated with a 3–4.7% increase in AF risk [40,43,44].

The blood lipid fractions have a complex relationship with AF. In our analysis, LDLC and TC values were negatively related to the 13-year risk of incident AF in age-adjusted models; for TC, this association remained significant after controlling for other risk factors and was mainly confer to women. In a combined analysis of data from the Multi-Ethnic Study of Atherosclerosis (MESA) and the FHS, on the contrary, a high level of HDLC was inversely associated with AF risk (HR 0.64, 95% CI 0.48–0.87 in those with levels ≥60 mg/dL versus <40 mg/dL), whereas high TG value was associated with a higher risk of AF (HR = 1.60, 95% CI 1.25–2.05 in those with levels ≥200 mg/dL versus <150 mg/dL). TC and LDLC were not related to the risk of AF in the referred analysis [45]. In contrast, the data on the Atherosclerosis Risk in Communities (ARIC) study showed that the high levels of LDLC and TC were associated with a lower risk of AF, whereas HDLC and TG were not related to AF risk [46]. A similar inverse association between LDLC and the risk of AF was found in the Women's Health Study [47]. The mechanisms of this inverse association between atherogenic lipids and AF are not fully understood and might be related to the complex relationship between the cholesterol and the stabilizing effect on myocardial membranes and ion channel function [48–50], along with its role in chronic inflammation and oxidative stress [51]. In addition, AF is an age-associated condition, and blood lipid levels generally decrease in patients of the age of over 60. Additionally, subclinical hyperthyroidism with reduced lipid levels may be an independent risk factor for AF [52].

In general, the identified cluster of AF predictors, such as obesity, hypertension, age, and male sex, make it possible to consider AF as an atherosclerotic cardiovascular condition. Some differences in AF determinants or coefficients between studies might be due to various study designs and approaches in the diagnosis of AF, as well as racial characteristics, morbidity, and risk factors profile, socio-economic characteristics, medical care, and lifestyle in the studied populations.

Study Limitations

The present study has some limitations. The incident AF cases in the analysis were limited to permanent AF form recorded by resting ECG in repeated examination and did not include the cases of paroxysmal AF that occurred during the follow-up, including the fatal ones. This might lead to underestimation of risk coefficients but is unlikely to change the identified determinants of AF.

We did not find associations between incident AF and behavioral factors, which can also be related to the fact that we included only cases of permanent AF.

To overcome this shortage, at the next stage of analysis, we plan to update the completeness of AF endpoints by ascertainment of paroxysmal and persistent AF cases, both fatal and non-fatal, during the 13-year follow-up from CVD and mortality registers. Upon data completeness, we plan further post hoc analyses.

Another limitation might be related to the approach that only respondents free from baseline AF and CVD were included in the analysis of AF determinants. This is a common practice in the cohort studies for cardiovascular outcomes including the risk of AF (for example, Framingham Heart study [32], Renfrew/Paisley study [33], nation-wide cohort study of Swedish [34], REasons for Geographic And Racial Differences in Stroke (REGARDS) study [35]), and the using of this approach allows us to compare results. Moreover, to assess the overall burden of AF, we additionally performed a sensitivity analysis of the determinants of the risk of incident AF among all respondents, regardless of the presence of CVD. As expected, baseline CVD was associated with the AF risk; the HRs for associations between primarily revealed determinants and AF slightly attenuated but remained significant. Additionally, we did not find additional associations between the studied risk factors and AF. Thus, the final results practically did not change (Supplementary Table S2).

The last limitation relates to non-response or attrition bias where persons more prone to AF risk due to CVD, arrhythmia, or other health problems did not attend the examination. However, we addressed the cohort free from baseline CVD and AF, and this issue has no impact on the baseline results. Non-response for reexamination limited the number of incident AF cases registered, but it is unlikely that individuals with chronic conditions as permanent AF would be systematically more prone to not attending the examination. Moreover, in separate analyses, we observed that non-responders have better health than responders (personal communication with D. Denissova [53]).

At the same time, according to our knowledge, this is the first cohort study in Russia that explored the risk of AF and identified the predictors and individual risk coefficients for incident AF at the population level.

5. Conclusions

In this Russian population-based cohort of middle-aged and older individuals, the prevalence of AF registered by resting ECG increased from 1.6% to 4.2% with the age from 45–69 to 55–84 years. The incidence rate of new-onset AF cases among persons free from baseline CVD was 3.2%. The 13-year risk of incident AF was positively associated with male sex, age, BMI, SBP, or the presence of hypertension, and was negatively associated with total cholesterol level. In women, the 13-year risk of incident AF was more strongly associated with HT and inversely associated with total cholesterol levels.

The present study was limited by the consideration of largely permanent AF based on the resting ECG and did not include the cases of paroxysmal AF during the follow-up. Further studies are needed to cover the overall burden of AF at longitudinal follow-up in a population setting.

At the same time, the findings in this Russian cohort are generally consistent with the data obtained in the European and North American population studies. The findings of individual risk of AF in the Russian cohort have implications for the prediction of AF and ASCVD complications.

Supplementary Materials: The following are available online at https://www.mdpi.com/article/10.3390/jpm12010122/s1, Table S1: Associations between risk factors and 13-risk of incident AF. Cox regression analysis, age- and multivariable-adjusted models (The HAPIEE study, Russian population cohort free from baseline CVD, n = 3871), Table S2: Associations between risk factors and 13-risk of incident AF. Cox regression analysis, age- and multivariable-adjusted models (The HAPIEE study, Russian population cohort, n = 5759).

Author Contributions: Conceptualization, S.M. and M.S.; methodology, S.M., M.S. and L.S.; software, L.S. and S.M.; validation, M.S., S.M., L.S. and H.P.; formal analysis, M.S. and S.M.; investigation, M.S., A.R., E.M. (Ekaterina Mazdorova), A.T., E.A. and E.M. (Elena Mazurenko); resources, S.M., M.B. and H.P.; data curation, S.M., L.S., M.B. and H.P.; writing—original draft preparation, M.S. and S.M.; writing—review and editing, A.R., M.B., H.P. and L.S.; visualization, S.M., M.S. and A.R.; supervision, M.S.; project administration, S.M. and M.B.; funding acquisition, M.B., S.M. and M.S. All authors have read and agreed to the published version of the manuscript.

Funding: This research was supported by RFBR grant #20-313-90015, RSF grant #20-15-00371, The HAPIEE study was funded by the Wellcome Trust (WT064947, WT081081) and the US National Institute of Aging (1RO1AG23522).

Institutional Review Board Statement: The study was conducted according to the guidelines of the Declaration of Helsinki and approved by the Ethics Committee of IIPM—Branch of IC&G SB RAS (Institute of Internal and Preventive Medicine—Branch of Federal State Budgeted Research Institution, "Federal Research Center, Institute of Cytology and Genetics, Siberian Branch of the Russian Academy of Sciences") Protocol No. 1 from 14 March 2002 and Protocol No. 12 from 08 December 2020. The study did not involve humans or animals.

Informed Consent Statement: Informed consent was obtained from all subjects involved in the study.

Data Availability Statement: The data presented in this study are available in tabulated form on request. The data are not publicly available due to ethical restrictions and project regulations.

Acknowledgments: The authors acknowledge M. Holmes, D. Stefler, J. Hubacek, for valuable advice on manuscript planning and discussion, and Eu. Verevkin for help in data management. M. Shapkina, A. Ryabikov, E. Mazdorova, A. Titarenko, E. Avdeeva, E. Mazurenko, L. Scherbakova, and S. Malyutina were supported by the Russian Academy of Science, State Assignment (AAAA-A17-117112850280-2).

Conflicts of Interest: The authors declare no conflict of interest.

References

1. Gillis, A.M. Atrial Fibrillation and Ventricular Arrhythmias. *Circulation* **2017**, *135*, 593–608. [CrossRef]
2. Kirchhof, P.; Benussi, S.; Kotecha, D.; Ahlsson, A.; Atar, D.; Casadei, B.; Castella, M.; Diener, H.-C.; Heidbuchel, H.; Hendriks, J.; et al. 2016 ESC Guidelines for the management of atrial fibrillation developed in collaboration with EACTS. *Eur. J. Cardio.-Thorac. Surg.* **2016**, *50*, e1–e88. [CrossRef]
3. Hindricks, G.; Potpara, T.; Dagres, N.; Arbelo, E.; Bax, J.J.; Blomström-Lundqvist, C.; Boriani, G.; Castella, M.; Dan, G.-A.; Dilaveris, P.E.; et al. 2020 ESC Guidelines for the diagnosis and management of atrial fibrillation developed in collaboration with the European Association for Cardio-Thoracic Surgery (EACTS): The Task Force for the diagnosis and management of atrial fibrillation of the European Society of Cardiology (ESC) Developed with the special contribution of the European Heart Rhythm Association (EHRA) of the ESC. *Eur. Heart J.* **2021**, *42*, 373–498. [CrossRef]
4. Timmis, A.; Townsend, N.; Gale, C.; Grobbee, R.; Maniadakis, N.; Flather, M.; Wilkins, E.; Wright, L.; Vos, R.; Bax, J.; et al. European Society of Cardiology: Cardiovascular Disease Statistics 2017. *Eur. Heart J.* **2017**, *39*, 508–579. [CrossRef]
5. Ball, J.; Carrington, M.J.; Mcmurray, J.; Stewart, S. Atrial fibrillation: Profile and burden of an evolving epidemic in the 21st century. *Int. J. Cardiol.* **2013**, *167*, 1807–1824. [CrossRef] [PubMed]
6. Go, A.S.; Hylek, E.M.; Phillips, K.A.; Chang, Y.; Henault, L.E.; Selby, J.V.; Singer, D.E. Prevalence of Diagnosed Atrial Fibrillation in Adults. *JAMA* **2001**, *285*, 2370–2375. [CrossRef] [PubMed]
7. Miyasaka, Y.; Barnes, M.E.; Gersh, B.J.; Cha, S.S.; Bailey, K.R.; Abhayaratna, W.P.; Seward, J.B.; Tsang, T.S. Secular Trends in Incidence of Atrial Fibrillation in Olmsted County, Minnesota, 1980 to 2000, and Implications on the Projections for Future Prevalence. *Circulation* **2006**, *114*, 119–125. [CrossRef]

8. Naccarelli, G.V.; Varker, H.; Lin, J.; Schulman, K.L. Increasing Prevalence of Atrial Fibrillation and Flutter in the United States. *Am. J. Cardiol.* **2009**, *104*, 1534–1539. [CrossRef] [PubMed]
9. Krijthe, B.P.; Kunst, A.; Benjamin, E.; Lip, G.Y.; Franco, O.; Hofman, A.; Witteman, J.C.; Stricker, B.H.; Heeringa, J. Projections on the number of individuals with atrial fibrillation in the European Union, from 2000 to 2060. *Eur. Heart J.* **2013**, *34*, 2746–2751. [CrossRef]
10. Chugh, S.S.; Havmoeller, R.; Narayanan, K.; Singh, D.; Rienstra, M.; Benjamin, E.J.; Gillum, R.F.; Kim, Y.-H.; McAnulty, J.H., Jr.; Zheng, Z.-J.; et al. Worldwide Epidemiology of Atrial Fibrillation: A Global Burden of Disease 2010 Study. *Circulation* **2014**, *129*, 837–847. [CrossRef]
11. Zoni-Berisso, M.; Lercari, F.; Carazza, T.; Domenicucci, S. Epidemiology of atrial fibrillation: European perspective. *Clin. Epidemiol.* **2014**, *6*, 213–220. [CrossRef]
12. McManus, D.D.; Rienstra, M.; Benjamin, E. An Update on the Prognosis of Patients With Atrial Fibrillation. *Circulation* **2012**, *126*, e143–e146. [CrossRef]
13. Kannel, W.; Wolf, P.; Benjamin, E.; Levy, D. Prevalence, incidence, prognosis, and predisposing conditions for atrial fibrillation: Population-based estimates. *Am. J. Cardiol.* **1998**, *82*, 2N–9N. [CrossRef]
14. Nguyen, T.N.; Hilmer, S.N.; Cumming, R.G. Review of epidemiology and management of atrial fibrillation in developing countries. *Int. J. Cardiol.* **2013**, *167*, 2412–2420. [CrossRef]
15. Oldgren, J.; Healey, J.S.; Ezekowitz, M.; Commerford, P.; Avezum, A.; Pais, P.; Zhu, J.; Jansky, P.; Sigamani, A.; Morillo, C.A.; et al. Variations in Cause and Management of Atrial Fibrillation in a Prospective Registry of 15 400 Emergency Department Patients in 46 Countries. *Circulation* **2014**, *129*, 1568–1576. [CrossRef] [PubMed]
16. Chiang, C.-E.; Naditch-Brûlé, L.; Murin, J.; Goethals, M.; Inoue, H.; O'Neill, J.; Silva-Cardoso, J.; Zharinov, O.; Gamra, H.; Alam, S.; et al. Distribution and Risk Profile of Paroxysmal, Persistent, and Permanent Atrial Fibrillation in Routine Clinical Practice. *Circ. Arrhythmia Electrophysiol.* **2012**, *5*, 632–639. [CrossRef]
17. Kishore, A.; Vail, A.; Majid, A.; Dawson, J.; Lees, K.R.; Tyrrell, P.J.; Smith, C. Detection of Atrial Fibrillation After Ischemic Stroke or Transient Ischemic Attack. *Stroke* **2014**, *45*, 520–526. [CrossRef]
18. Henriksson, K.M.; Farahmand, B.; Åsberg, S.; Edvardsson, N.; Terént, A. Comparison of Cardiovascular Risk Factors and Survival in Patients with Ischemic or Hemorrhagic Stroke. *Int. J. Stroke* **2011**, *7*, 276–281. [CrossRef] [PubMed]
19. Grond, M.; Jauss, M.; Hamann, G.; Stark, E.; Veltkamp, R.; Nabavi, D.; Horn, M.; Weimar, C.; Köhrmann, M.; Wachter, R.; et al. Improved Detection of Silent Atrial Fibrillation Using 72-Hour Holter ECG in Patients With Ischemic Stroke. *Stroke* **2013**, *44*, 3357–3364. [CrossRef]
20. Ott, A.; Breteler, M.M.; de Bruyne, M.C.; van Harskamp, F.; Grobbee, D.E.; Hofman, A. Atrial Fibrillation and Dementia in a Population-Based Study. *Stroke* **1997**, *28*, 316–321. [CrossRef]
21. Knecht, S.; Oelschläger, C.; Duning, T.; Lohmann, H.; Albers, J.; Stehling, C.; Heindel, W.; Breithardt, G.; Berger, K.; Ringelstein, E.B.; et al. Atrial fibrillation in stroke-free patients is associated with memory impairment and hippocampal atrophy. *Eur. Hear. J.* **2008**, *29*, 2125–2132. [CrossRef]
22. Ball, J.; Carrington, M.J.; Stewart, S.; On Behalf of the SAFETY Investigators. Mild Cognitive Impairment in high-risk patients with chronic atrial fibrillation: A forgotten component of clinical management? *Heart* **2013**, *99*, 542–547. [CrossRef]
23. Marzona, I.; O'Donnell, M.; Teo, K.; Gao, P.; Anderson, C.; Bosch, J.; Yusuf, S. Increased risk of cognitive and functional decline in patients with atrial fibrillation: Results of the ONTARGET and TRANSCEND studies. *Can. Med. Assoc. J.* **2012**, *184*, E329–E336. [CrossRef] [PubMed]
24. Thrall, G.; Lane, D.; Carroll, D.; Lip, G.Y. Quality of Life in Patients with Atrial Fibrillation: A Systematic Review. *Am. J. Med.* **2006**, *119*, 448.e1–448.e19. [CrossRef]
25. Rothe, A.V.E.; Hutt, F.; Baumert, J.; Breithardt, G.; Goette, A.; Kirchhof, P.; Ladwig, K.-H. Depressed mood amplifies heart-related symptoms in persistent and paroxysmal atrial fibrillation patients: A longitudinal analysis—Data from the German Competence Network on Atrial Fibrillation. *Europace* **2015**, *17*, 1354–1362. [CrossRef] [PubMed]
26. Santangeli, P.; Di Biase, L.; Bai, R.; Mohanty, S.; Pump, A.; Brantes, M.C.; Horton, R.; Burkhardt, J.D.; Lakkireddy, D.; Reddy, Y.M.; et al. Atrial fibrillation and the risk of incident dementia: A meta-analysis. *Heart Rhythm* **2012**, *9*, 1761–1768.e2. [CrossRef]
27. Peasey, A.; Bobak, M.; Kubinova, R.; Malyutina, S.; Pajak, A.; Tamosiunas, A.; Pikhart, H.; Nicholson, A.; Marmot, M. Determinants of cardiovascular disease and other non-communicable diseases in Central and Eastern Europe: Rationale and design of the HAPIEE study. *BMC Public Health* **2006**, *6*, 255. [CrossRef] [PubMed]
28. Rydén, L.; Standl, E.; Bartnik, M.; Berghe, G.V.D.; Betteridge, J.; De Boer, M.-J.; Cosentino, F.; Jonsson, B.; Laakso, M.; Malmberg, K.; et al. Guidelines on diabetes, pre-diabetes, and cardiovascular diseases: Executive summary: The Task Force on Diabetes and Cardiovascular Diseases of the European Society of Cardiology (ESC) and of the European Association for the Study of Diabetes (EASD). *Eur. Hear. J.* **2006**, *28*, 88–136. [CrossRef]
29. Rose, G.A.; Blackburn, H.; Gillum, R.F. *Cardiovascular Survey Methods*, 2nd ed.; WHO: Geneva, Switzerland, 1984; p. 223. ISBN 9242400564.
30. Williams, B.; Mancia, G.; Spiering, W.; Agabiti Rosei, E.; Azizi, M.; Burnier, M.; Clement, D.L.; Coca, A.; De Simone, G.; Dominiczak, A.; et al. 2018 ESC/ESH Guidelines for the management of arterial hypertension: The Task Force for the management of arterial

hypertension of the European Society of Cardiology (ESC) and the European Society of Hypertension (ESH). *Eur. Heart J.* **2018**, *39*, 3021–3104. [CrossRef] [PubMed]
31. Rydén, L.; Grant, P.J.; Anker, S.D.; Berne, C.; Cosentino, F.; Danchin, N.; Deaton, C.; Escaned, J.; Hammes, H.-P.; Huikuri, H.; et al. ESC Guidelines on diabetes, pre-diabetes, and cardiovascular diseases developed in collaboration with the EASD. *Eur. Heart J.* **2013**, *34*, 3035–3087. [CrossRef]
32. Kim, E.-J.; Yin, X.; Fontes, J.D.; Magnani, J.W.; Lubitz, S.A.; McManus, D.D.; Seshadri, S.; Vasan, R.S.; Ellinor, P.T.; Larson, M.G.; et al. Atrial fibrillation without comorbidities: Prevalence, incidence and prognosis (from the Framingham Heart Study). *Am. Heart J.* **2016**, *177*, 138–144. [CrossRef]
33. Stewart, S.; Hart, C.L.; Hole, D.J.; McMurray, J.J. A population-based study of the long-term risks associated with atrial fibrillation: 20-year follow-up of the Renfrew/Paisley study. *Am. J. Med.* **2002**, *113*, 359–364. [CrossRef]
34. Andersson, T.; Magnuson, A.; Bryngelsson, I.-L.; Frøbert, O.; Henriksson, K.M.; Edvardsson, N.; Poçi, D. Gender-related differences in risk of cardiovascular morbidity and all-cause mortality in patients hospitalized with incident atrial fibrillation without concomitant diseases: A nationwide cohort study of 9519 patients. *Int. J. Cardiol.* **2014**, *177*, 91–99. [CrossRef]
35. Singleton, M.J.; Ahmad, M.I.; Kamel, H.; O'Neal, W.T.; Judd, S.E.; Howard, V.J.; Howard, G.; Soliman, E.Z.; Bhave, P.D. Association of Atrial Fibrillation Without Cardiovascular Comorbidities and Stroke Risk: From the REGARDS Study. *J. Am. Hear. Assoc.* **2020**, *9*, e016380. [CrossRef]
36. Heeringa, J.; Van Der Kuip, D.A.M.; Hofman, A.; Kors, J.A.; Van Herpen, G.; Stricker, B.H.C.; Stijnen, T.; Lip, G.Y.H.; Witteman, J.C.M. Prevalence, incidence and lifetime risk of atrial fibrillation: The Rotterdam study. *Eur. Heart J.* **2006**, *27*, 949–953. [CrossRef]
37. Schnabel, R.B.; Yin, X.; Gona, P.; Larson, M.G.; Beiser, A.; McManus, D.D.; Newton-Cheh, C.; Lubitz, S.A.; Magnani, J.W.; Ellinor, P.; et al. 50 year trends in atrial fibrillation prevalence, incidence, risk factors, and mortality in the Framingham Heart Study: A cohort study. *Lancet* **2015**, *386*, 154–162. [CrossRef]
38. Alonso, A.; Krijthe, B.P.; Aspelund, T.; Stepas, K.A.; Pencina, M.J.; Moser, C.B.; Sinner, M.F.; Sotoodehnia, N.; Fontes, J.D.; Janssens, A.C.; et al. Simple Risk Model Predicts Incidence of Atrial Fibrillation in a Racially and Geographically Diverse Population: The CHARGE-AF Consortium. *J. Am. Hear. Assoc.* **2013**, *2*, e000102. [CrossRef] [PubMed]
39. Sharashova, E.; Wilsgaard, T.; Ball, J.; Morseth, B.; Gerdts, E.; Hopstock, L.A.; Mathiesen, E.B.; Schirmer, H.; Løchen, M.-L. Long-term blood pressure trajectories and incident atrial fibrillation in women and men: The Tromsø Study. *Eur. Heart J.* **2019**, *41*, 1554–1562. [CrossRef]
40. Wang, T.J.; Parise, H.; Levy, D.; D'Agostino, R.B., Sr.; Wolf, P.A.; Vasan, R.S.; Benjamin, E.J. Obesity and the Risk of New-Onset Atrial Fibrillation. *JAMA* **2004**, *292*, 2471–2477. [CrossRef] [PubMed]
41. Frost, L.; Hune, L.J.; Vestergaard, P. Overweight and obesity as risk factors for atrial fibrillation or flutter: The Danish Diet, Cancer, and Health Study. *Am. J. Med.* **2005**, *118*, 489–495. [CrossRef]
42. Murphy, N.F.; Macintyre, K.; Stewart, S.; Hart, C.L.; Hole, D.; McMurray, J.J.V. Long-term cardiovascular consequences of obesity: 20-year follow-up of more than 15 000 middle-aged men and women (the Renfrew–Paisley study). *Eur. Heart J.* **2005**, *27*, 96–106. [CrossRef] [PubMed]
43. Tedrow, U.B.; Conen, D.; Ridker, P.M.; Cook, N.R.; Koplan, B.A.; Manson, J.E.; Buring, J.E.; Albert, C. The Long- and Short-Term Impact of Elevated Body Mass Index on the Risk of New Atrial Fibrillation: The WHS (Women's Health Study). *J. Am. Coll. Cardiol.* **2010**, *55*, 2319–2327. [CrossRef]
44. Gami, A.S.; Hodge, D.O.; Herges, R.M.; Olson, E.J.; Nykodym, J.; Kara, T.; Somers, V.K. Obstructive Sleep Apnea, Obesity, and the Risk of Incident Atrial Fibrillation. *J. Am. Coll. Cardiol.* **2007**, *49*, 565–571. [CrossRef]
45. Alonso, A.; Yin, X.; Roetker, N.S.; Magnani, J.W.; Kronmal, R.A.; Ellinor, P.; Chen, L.; Lubitz, S.A.; McClelland, R.L.; McManus, D.D.; et al. Blood Lipids and the Incidence of Atrial Fibrillation: The Multi-Ethnic Study of Atherosclerosis and the Framingham Heart Study. *J. Am. Hear. Assoc.* **2014**, *3*, e001211. [CrossRef]
46. Lopez, F.L.; Agarwal, S.K.; MacLehose, R.F.; Soliman, E.Z.; Sharrett, A.R.; Huxley, R.; Konety, S.; Ballantyne, C.M.; Alonso, A. Blood Lipid Levels, Lipid-Lowering Medications, and the Incidence of Atrial Fibrillation. *Circ. Arrhythmia Electrophysiol.* **2012**, *5*, 155–162. [CrossRef]
47. Mora, S.; Akinkuolie, A.O.; Sandhu, R.K.; Conen, D.; Albert, C.M. Paradoxical Association of Lipoprotein Measures With Incident Atrial Fibrillation. *Circ. Arrhythmia Electrophysiol.* **2014**, *7*, 612–619. [CrossRef]
48. Goonasekara, C.L.; Balse, E.; Hatem, S.; Steele, D.F.; Fedida, D. Cholesterol and cardiac arrhythmias. *Expert Rev. Cardiovasc. Ther.* **2010**, *8*, 965–979. [CrossRef]
49. Levitan, I.; Christian, A.E.; Tulenko, T.N.; Rothblat, G.H. Membrane Cholesterol Content Modulates Activation of Volume-Regulated Anion Current in Bovine Endothelial Cells. *J. Gen. Physiol.* **2000**, *115*, 405–416. [CrossRef]
50. Abi-Char, J.; Maguy, A.; Coulombe, A.; Balse, E.; Ratajczak, P.; Samuel, J.-L.; Nattel, S.; Hatem, S.N. Membrane cholesterol modulates Kv1.5 potassium channel distribution and function in rat cardiomyocytes. *J. Physiol.* **2007**, *582*, 1205–1217. [CrossRef] [PubMed]
51. Patel, P.; Dokainish, H.; Tsai, P.; Lakkis, N. Update on the Association of Inflammation and Atrial Fibrillation. *J. Cardiovasc. Electrophysiol.* **2010**, *21*, 1064–1070. [CrossRef] [PubMed]
52. Rizos, C. Effects of Thyroid Dysfunction on Lipid Profile. *Open Cardiovasc. Med. J.* **2011**, *5*, 76–84. [CrossRef] [PubMed]
53. Denissova, D.; (Dr., Chief Researcher, the Laboratory of Preventive Medicine, Institute of Internal and Preventive Medicine—Branch of Federal State Budgeted Research Institution, "Federal Research Center, Institute of Cytology and Genetics, Siberian Branch of the Russian Academy of Sciences", Novosibirsk, Russia). Personal communication, 2015.

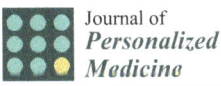

Article

The Relationship between Epigenetic Age and Myocardial Infarction/Acute Coronary Syndrome in a Population-Based Nested Case-Control Study

Sofia Malyutina [1,*], Olga Chervova [2], Taavi Tillmann [3], Vladimir Maximov [1], Andrew Ryabikov [1], Valery Gafarov [1], Jaroslav A. Hubacek [4], Hynek Pikhart [5], Stephan Beck [2] and Martin Bobak [5]

1. Research Institute of Internal and Preventive Medicine-Branch of Institute of Cytology and Genetics SB RAS, 630089 Novosibirsk, Russia; medik11@mail.ru (V.M.); a_ryabikov@hotmail.com (A.R.); valery.gafarov@gmail.com (V.G.)
2. UCL Cancer Institute, University College London, London WC1E 6BT, UK; o.chervova@ucl.ac.uk (O.C.); s.beck@ucl.ac.uk (S.B.)
3. Institute for Global Health, University College London, London WC1E 6BT, UK; t.tillmann@ucl.ac.uk
4. Experimental Medicine Centre, Institute for Clinical and Experimental Medicine, 14021 Prague, Czech Republic; jahb@ikem.cz
5. Institute of Epidemiology and Health Care, University College London, London WC1E 6BT, UK; h.pikhart@ucl.ac.uk (H.P.); m.bobak@ucl.ac.uk (M.B.)
* Correspondence: smalyutina@hotmail.com; Tel.: +7-913-929-33-63

Abstract: We investigated the relationship between 'epigenetic age' (EA) derived from DNA methylation (DNAm) and myocardial infarction (MI)/acute coronary syndrome (ACS). A random population sample was examined in 2003/2005 (n = 9360, 45–69, the HAPIEE project) and followed up for 15 years. From this cohort, incident MI/ACS (cases, n = 129) and age- and sex-stratified controls (n = 177) were selected for a nested case-control study. Baseline EA (Horvath's, Hannum's, PhenoAge, Skin and Blood) and the differences between EA and chronological age (CA) were calculated (ΔAHr, ΔAHn, ΔAPh, ΔASB). EAs by Horvath's, Hannum's and Skin and Blood were close to CA (median absolute difference, MAD, of 1.08, −1.91 and −2.03 years); PhenoAge had MAD of −9.29 years vs. CA. The adjusted odds ratios (ORs) of MI/ACS per 1–year increments of ΔAHr, ΔAHn, ΔASB and ΔAPh were 1.01 (95% CI 0.95–1.07), 1.01 (95% CI 0.95–1.08), 1.02 (95% CI 0.97–1.06) and 1.01 (0.93–1.09), respectively. When classified into tertiles, only the highest tertile of ΔAPh showed a suggestion of increased risk of MI/ACS with OR 2.09 (1.11–3.94) independent of age and 1.84 (0.99–3.52) in the age- and sex-adjusted model. Metabolic modulation may be the likely mechanism of this association. In conclusion, this case-control study nested in a prospective population-based cohort did not find strong associations between accelerated epigenetic age markers and risk of MI/ACS. Larger cohort studies are needed to re-examine this important research question.

Keywords: DNA methylation; epigenetic age; myocardial infarction; acute coronary syndrome; population; nested case-control; HAPIEE project

Citation: Malyutina, S.; Chervova, O.; Tillmann, T.; Maximov, V.; Ryabikov, A.; Gafarov, V.; Hubacek, J.A.; Pikhart, H.; Beck, S.; Bobak, M. The Relationship between Epigenetic Age and Myocardial Infarction/Acute Coronary Syndrome in a Population-Based Nested Case-Control Study. *J. Pers. Med.* 2022, 12, 110. https://doi.org/10.3390/jpm12010110

Academic Editors: Yuliya I. Ragino and José Braganca

Received: 16 November 2021
Accepted: 10 January 2022
Published: 14 January 2022

Publisher's Note: MDPI stays neutral with regard to jurisdictional claims in published maps and institutional affiliations.

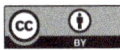

Copyright: © 2022 by the authors. Licensee MDPI, Basel, Switzerland. This article is an open access article distributed under the terms and conditions of the Creative Commons Attribution (CC BY) license (https://creativecommons.org/licenses/by/4.0/).

1. Introduction

Increasing life expectancy worldwide is accompanied by an aging population. Currently, there are at least 900 million people over 60 years old in the world and, according to the United Nations estimates, the world's population is expected to reach 8.6 billion people by 2030, of which more than 1.4 billion will be over the age of 60 [1].

Cardiovascular diseases (CVDs), particularly atherosclerotic CVDs such as coronary heart disease (CHD) and cerebrovascular diseases, are the leading cause of mortality and morbidity, being responsible for about 30% of global deaths [2], and aging is a major risk factor. In the multidimensional process of decline in health status during aging, molecular markers of 'biological age' are regarded as determinants of the rate of aging.

Epigenetic modifications such as DNA methylation (DNAm) have been shown to be the most accurate molecular readout of aging but their possible functional role remains poorly understood [3,4]. Altered epigenetic patterns may therefore be important causes and/or signals of this aging process.

Epigenetic modifications are mitotically (and in some cases meiotically) heritable. They can change gene and genome function independently of changes in the nucleotide sequence of the DNA [5]. The epigenetic phenomenon of DNAm involves the addition or removal of a methyl group to the 5' cytosines, most commonly in the context of CpG dinucleotides; areas of relatively high CpG density are referred to as CpG islands which are often associated with a gene promoter [6]. DNAm can be measured quantitatively, and it is increasingly used in human studies [7].

It has been repeatedly shown that DNAm levels at specific sites in the genome are strongly associated with age and that, in some cases, it has been used to accurately predict chronological age [6,8–10]. These sites underline the concept of 'epigenetic clocks' and several DNAm-based estimators of chronological age, referred to as 'epigenetic age', have been constructed [11]. Hannum's Blood-based clock is based on 71 CpG sites [9], Horvath's Pan-Tissue clock is based on 353 CpG sites [12], Levine's PhenoAge clock is based on 513 CpG sites capturing age-related and functional phenotype modifications [13] and Horvath's Skin and Blood clock is based on 391 CpGs for human fibroblasts and other cell types [14]. Further to these, over 30 epigenetic clocks have been published [15], including those recently developed on the base of the Illumina Methylation EPIC 850 BeadChip (850 K) [16].

In our study, we chose to use Horvath's and Hannum's clocks because they are among the most popular first-generation clocks and are featured (and continue to be used) in many studies of associations between age and phenotypes. The Skin and Blood clock was chosen as an example of a specialized second-generation clock which is known in the research community as the most accurate chronological age predictor reported to date. PhenoAge, which is another second-generation clock, was also chosen based on its popularity among age–trait association studies, including mortality.

We would like to note that second-generation clocks (PhenoAge, GrimAge [17], etc.) are less precise in terms of chronological age prediction in comparison to first-generation or specialized epigenetic clocks. This is because those clocks were designed to incorporate other phenotypes (or comorbidities) and were not primarily aimed at reflecting chronological age. In our experience, PhenoAge is usually well below the chronological age in the vast majority of moderately healthy individuals, which is supported by several publications, including [13,18].

A number of studies have shown an association between epigenetic age and risk of mortality, as summarized in various meta-analyses [19–24]. Both positive and negative correlations have been made on the relationship between epigenetic age and CVD and, specifically, CHD [15,21,24,25], however, these studies are limited, heterogeneous in design and the findings remain largely inconclusive.

In Russia, the proportion of the elderly population is growing, but life expectancy at birth remains on average 8 years lower than in Western Europe [26,27], although the causes of this gap remain unclear [28–30]. This points toward the need to understand all aspects of aging in the Russian population. There have been no longitudinal studies of the relationship between epigenetic measures of age and CVD and chronic diseases in the Russian population. For these reasons, the current analysis is relevant both locally and across the world at large.

Objective of our study was to investigate the relationship between epigenetic age (EA) and myocardial infarction (MI)/acute coronary syndrome (ACS) in a population-based nested case-control study.

2. Methods

2.1. Study Population and Design

A random population sample was examined in the Russian arm of the HAPIEE study at baseline in 2003/05 ($n = 9360$, age 45–69) and re-examined in 2006–2008 and 2015–2017 The cohort was followed up until 31.12.2019 for an average of 15.9 (SD 0.64, median 15.9) years for fatal and non-fatal cardiovascular events and all-cause mortality.

Data on fatal and non-fatal coronary heart disease (CHD) (ICD-10: I20–I25) events were collected at the Research Institute of Internal and Preventive Medicine (IIPM) using a Register of Myocardial Infarction originally established in the WHO MONICA project by combining 'hot pursuit' and 'cold pursuit' methods and using medical records and hospital discharge reports. The data on all-cause and cause-specific mortality were collected at the IIPM using various sources, including the Population Registration Bureau (ZAGS) and the Novosibirsk Office of the State Statistical Bureau (Rosstat), and information received at repeated waves of the study (this includes the address bureau, as well as contacts with relatives of deceased study participants).

2.2. Sample Selection Process

During a 15-year follow-up period, 1475 events of myocardial infarction (MI) or acute coronary syndrome (ACS) were ascertained in 9360 unique persons including serial events in some individuals. Using a nested case-control study design, we applied the following exclusion criteria for selecting MI/ACS cases in this study: prevalent baseline CVD (MI, ACS, stroke), data not available for DNA analysis. Exclusion criteria for selection in the control group of this study were the same, with additional exclusion of controls with baseline cancer or those who died before the end of follow-up. We then randomly selected participants with incident MI/ACS (cases) and age- and sex-frequency matched controls. Assuming that a small proportion of DNA samples would be unavailable or rejected by quality control, we selected initially 161 cases and 243 controls. Among them, 139 cases and 187 controls were available and appropriate for DNAm profiling. After DNAm quality control (procedures are described below), 129 cases and 177 controls were included in the analysis. DNAm profiles of 88 subjects available from the earlier pilot study [31] were included in the sampling algorithm and were included in the 'expanded control group' ($n = 265$) for additional analyses. The general characteristics of expanded controls are summarized in Table S2.

2.3. Ethics

All study participants provided informed consent and study protocols were approved by the ethical committee of the Research Institute of Internal and Preventive Medicine. The study was conducted in accordance with the relevant ethical guidelines and regulations.

2.4. Data Collection

Baseline data collection in the HAPIEE study was conducted using a comprehensive questionnaire, medical examination and the collection of venous blood samples. The protocol included assessment of history of cardiovascular and other chronic diseases, lifestyle habits and health, socio-economic circumstances, objective measurement of blood pressure (BP), anthropometric parameters and physical performance. The details of the protocol are reported elsewhere [32].

The lifestyle habits, health and socio-economic circumstances were assessed by structured interview. A person who smoked at least one cigarette a day was classified as a smoker. Smoking status was categorized as current smoker, former smoker and never smoked.

The level of education was categorized into 4 categories (high, secondary, vocational and primary or less than primary education). For the current analysis, marital status was dichotomized as married (or cohabiting) and single (never been married, divorced or widower/widow).

The height and weight were measured with accuracy to 1 mm and 100 g, respectively; body mass index (BMI) was calculated as kg/m^2. Blood pressure (BP) was measured three times (Omron M-5 tonometer) on the right arm in a sitting position after a 5 min rest period with a 2 min interval between measurements. The average of three BP measurements was calculated.

Blood samples were drawn following at least 8 h of fasting. Serum was stored at minus 80 °C and analyses for lipids and glucose were conducted within one month after sample collection. The levels of total cholesterol (TC), triglycerides (TG), high-density lipoprotein cholesterol (HDLC) and glucose in blood serum were measured enzymatically by a KoneLab Prime 30i autoanalyzer (Thermo Fisher Scientific Inc., Waltham, MA, USA) using kits from Thermo Fisher Scientific (Thermo Fisher Scientific Inc., Waltham, MA, USA). Low-density lipoprotein cholesterol (LDLC) was calculated using the Friedewald formula.

Genomic DNA was isolated from whole blood cells by phenol-chloroform extraction and stored at minus 70 °C until further laboratory analysis.

2.5. DNAm Profiling

Whole blood DNAm profiling was performed using Illumina Infinium Methylation EPIC BeadChip arrays following the manufacturer's recommended protocol (Illumina Inc, San Diego, CA, USA). The arrays were scanned using the iScan Microarray Scanner with an autoloader (Illumina Inc, San Diego, CA, USA) to produce the raw signal intensity files (.idat files) in accordance with standard operating procedures.

2.6. Data Preprocessing and Quality Control (QC)

All the data preprocessing and QC procedures were performed using R version 4.1.0 (R Foundation for Statistical Computing, Vienna, Austria) and dedicated R libraries minfi [33], ChAMP [34] and ENmix [35], following the steps described in [36]. In particular, our QC checks included array control probes' metrics as described in Illumina Bead Control Reporter guidelines, detection p-values and bead count numbers. In addition, we inspected the concordance of the reported sex with one inferred from DNAm data, and for the samples with available repeated DNAm profiling at a different time point, we performed sample matching using the data from 59 EPIC array SNP control probes. In our analysis, we only used data from the samples with less than 1% CpGs with detection p-values above the threshold 0.01, and probes (CpGs) with bead count numbers of at least 3 and p-values below 0.01 across at least 99% of samples.

2.7. DNAm Age Calculation

Baseline EA was calculated using Horvath's [12], Hannum's [9], PhenoAge [13] and Skin and Blood DNAm clocks [14]. The missing probes required for the DNAm age calculation were imputed using the kNN method [37,38], implemented in the ENmix R library. Following the definition in [12], we calculated age acceleration as a difference between EA and chronological age (CA) for each clock. Corresponding age accelerations for Horvath's, Hannum's, PhenoAge and Skin and Blood clocks were denoted as ∆AHr, ∆AHn, ∆APh and ∆ASB, respectively.

2.8. Statistical Analysis

Statistical analysis was conducted using SPSS (v19.0, Inc., Chicago, IL, USA) and R (v4.1.0) software packages (R Foundation for Statistical Computing, Vienna, Austria). The dataset includes 129 MI/ACS cases and 177 controls.

First, descriptive analysis compared chronological age (CA), EA and general characteristics of case and control groups using ANOVA and cross-tabulation techniques.

Second, logistic regression was used to estimate odds ratios of MI/ACS per 1–year increment of EA as a continuous variable. The dependent variable was cases of incident MI/ACS. Model 1 was adjusted for baseline age; Model 2 was adjusted for age and sex; Model 3a was adjusted for age, sex and smoking; Model 4 was adjusted for age, sex, smoking, systolic blood pressure (SBP), total cholesterol (TC), body mass index (BMI) and education level.

Finally, we classified subjects into tertiles of the difference between EA and CA for the four EA measures (ΔAHr, ΔAHn, ΔAPh, ΔASB), and logistic regression was used to estimate odds ratios of MI/ACS by EA tertile using cases of incident MI/ACS as the dependent variable. For the independent variable (difference between EA and CA), the reference category consisted of the tertile of participants with the smallest EA–CA difference. The tertile cutpoints were ΔAHr (−1.38; 3.26), ΔAHn (−3.95; 0.13), ΔAPh (−11.50; −6.21), ΔASB (−3.52; −0.31). Age-adjusted and multivariable-adjusted models were estimated with the same covariates as above.

3. Results

3.1. Cases and Controls Have Significant Differences in Basic Phenotype Characteristics

After the quality control procedures, the analytical sample consisted of 129 cases and 177 controls. The general characteristics of case and control participants are summarized in Table 1.

Table 1. Distribution of baseline covariates among cases of incident MI/ACS and control (the Russian arm of the HAPIEE study).

Covariates	Cases (Incident MI/ACS)	Controls	p-Value [a]
Observed	129	177	
Age at baseline, years (mean, SD)	59.8 (6.87)	54.5 (6.45)	<0.001
Females (%)	62 (48.1)	73 (58.8)	0.064
Systolic blood pressure, mmHg (mean, SD)	151.6 (26.93)	133.2 (21.87)	<0.001
Diastolic blood pressure, mmHg (mean, SD)	92.3 (14.36)	86.0 (12.69)	<0.001
Body mass index, kg/sqm (mean, SD)	28.8 (5.73)	27.50 (4.90)	0.031
Waist/hip ratio, unit (mean, SD)	0.90 (0.077)	0.87 (0.087)	0.002
Total cholesterol mmol/L (mean, SD)	6.61 (1.27)	6.42 (1.28)	0.204
LDL cholesterol, mmol/L (mean, SD)	4.32 (1.14)	4.15 (1.13)	0.207
Glucose, plasma, mmol/L mean, SD)	6.41 (2.29)	5.77 (0.85)	0.001
Hypertension (%)	96 (74.4)	80 (45.2)	<0.001
HT treatment (among HT), (%)	46 (47.9)	46 (27.5)	0.006
Diabetes mellitus type 2 (%)	24 (18.9)	10 (5.8)	<0.001
DM2 treatment (among DM2), (%)	8 (33.3)	3.(30.0)	0.850
Frequency of drinking (%)			
Non-drinkers	24 (18.6)	15 (8.5)	
<1/month	55 (42.6)	76 (42.9)	0.050
1–3/month	25 (19.4)	35 (19.8)	
1–4/week	22 (17.1)	48 (27.1)	
5+/week	3 (2.3)	3 (1.7)	
Smoking (%)			
Never smoked	75 (58.1)	105 (59.3)	0.066
Former smoking	10 (7.8)	27 (15.3)	
Present smoker	44 (34.1)	56 (31.6)	
Married (%)	96 (74.4)	135 (76.3)	0.405
University education (%)	27 (20.9)	56 (31.6)	<0.001
Difference EA–chronological age by four measures:			
ΔAHr, year	0.055 (5.35)	1.663 (5.09)	0.008
ΔAHn, year	−2.702 (5.36)	−1.161 (4.82)	0.009
ΔAPh, year	−8.945 (6.43)	−8.762 (6.38)	0.806
ΔASB, year	−2.551 (4.06)	−1.550 (3.58)	0.023

SD—standard deviation; EA—epigenetic age; CVD—cardiovascular disease. [a]—ANOVA or chi-square test.

The individuals with incident cases of MI/ACS were slightly older, as expected, they had higher BP, anthropometric measures (body mass index, BMI, and waist/hip ratio, WHR) and levels of plasma glucose, more frequently had hypertension (HT) and type 2 diabetes (DM2) and were less educated compared to controls.

DNAm ages calculated by Horvath's, Hannum's and Skin and Blood clocks were similar to participants' CA; the corresponding median absolute differences (MADs) were 1.08, −1.91 and −2.03 years (Figure 1). Means (SD) were 0.98 (5.25), −1.81 (5.10) and −1.97

(3.81) for ΔAHr, ΔAHn and ΔASB, respectively. As expected, PhenoAge's predictions were less precise with MAD = −9.29 and ΔAPh mean (SD) −8.84 (6.39). Scatterplots of chronological vs. epigenetic age by Horvath's, Hannum's, PhenoAge and Skin and Blood clocks are presented in Figure 2 and Figure S1 (Supplementary Material). The correlation coefficients between CA and EA were between 0.688, $p < 0.001$ (for PhenoAge) and 0.856, $p < 0.001$ (for Skin and Blood age), Figure S2 (Supplementary Material). Sex-specific distribution of the epigenetic age acceleration for all four clocks is shown on Supplementary Figure S3.

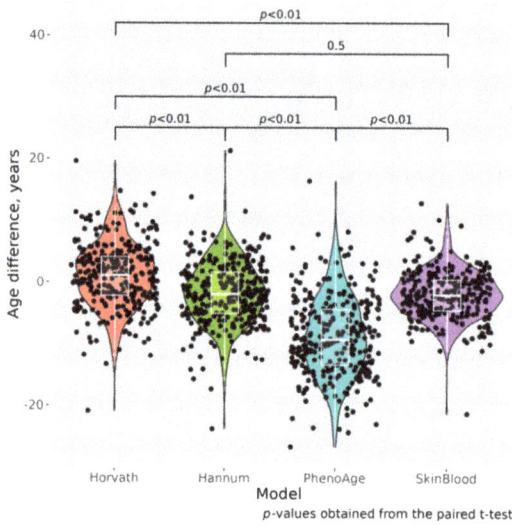

Figure 1. Boxplots of differences between chronological and epigenetic age (cases and controls, $n = 306$).

The mean ΔAHr, ΔAHn and ΔASB were significantly lower in MI/ACS cases compared to controls, 0.055 (5.35) vs. 1.66 (5.09), $p = 0.008$, −2.70 (5.36) vs. −1.16 (4.82), $p = 0.009$ and −2.55 (4.06) vs. −1.55 (3.58), $p = 0.023$, correspondingly (Table 1). ΔAPh was similar in cases and controls. Sex-specific distribution of the epigenetic age acceleration for all four clocks is shown on Supplementary Figure S3.

3.2. Association between Age Acceleration and Risk of MI/ACS

Odds ratios of MI/ACS per 1-year increment of EA measures, modeled as a continuous variable, are presented in Table 2. ORs of MI/ACS per 1-year increment of EA measures were 1.016 (95% CI 0.96–1.07) for ΔAHr; 1.023 (95% CI 0.95–1.08) for ΔAHn; 1.032 (95% CI 0.99–1.07) for ΔAPh; and 1.002 (95% CI 0.94–1.07) for ΔASB in age-adjusted models (Table 2). In multivariable analyses (fully adjusted Model 4), the ORs were 1.009 (95% CI 0.95–1.07), 1.012 (95% CI 0.95–1.08), 1.017 (95% CI 0.97–1.06) and 1.009 (95% CI 0.93–1.09), respectively, and were not statistically significant.

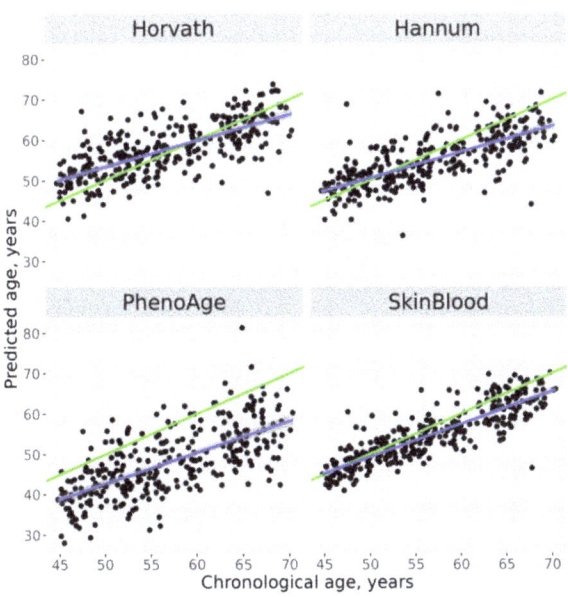

Figure 2. Scatterplots of chronological vs. epigenetic age by Horvath's, Hannum's, PhenoAge and Skin and Blood clocks. Diagonal green line corresponds to the predicted age equal to the chronological age, blue straight line corresponds to the linear regression.

Table 2. Relationship between MI/ACS and epigenetic age acceleration, per 1-year increment of the difference between baseline EA and CA (cases, $n = 129$ and controls, $n = 177$).

Measure of Epigenetic Age	n, Case/Control	Model 1 OR (95% CI)	Model 2 OR (95% CI)	Model 3 OR (95% CI)	Model 4 OR (95% CI)
ΔAHr, per 1 year	129/177	1.016 (0.96–1.07)	1.003 (0.87–1.36)	1.008 (0.95–1.06)	1.009 (0.95–1.07)
p-value for trends		0.563	0.911	0.785	0.763
ΔAHn, per 1 year	129/177	1.023 (0.95–1.08)	1.001 (0.95–1.06)	1.006 (0.95–1.07)	1.012 (0.95–1.08)
p-value for trends		0.418	0.961	0.842	0.708
ΔAPh, per 1 year	129/177	1.032 (0.99–1.07)	1.021 (0.98–1.06)	1.017 (0.98–1.06)	1.017 (0.97–1.06)
p-value for trends		0.126	0.310	0.430	0.459
ΔASB, per 1 year	129/177	1.002 (0.94–1.07)	0.991 (0.93–1.06)	0.997 (0.93–1.07)	1.009 (0.93–1.09)
p-value for trends		0.962	0.802	0.927	0.825

ΔAHr—difference between EA by Horvath's and chronological age; ΔAHn—difference between EA by Hannum's and chronological age; ΔAPh—difference between phenotypic EA and chronological age; ΔASB—difference between Skin and Blood EA and chronological age; OR—odds ratio; CI—confidence interval; Model 1: age-adjusted; Model 2: adjusted for age and sex; Model 3: adjusted for age, sex and smoking; Model 4: adjusted for age, sex, smoking, SBP, TC, BMI and education.

The results are presented separately for men and women in Table S1. The relationships between EAA and MI/ACS were of the same directions compared to pooled results and were not statistically significant.

Odds ratios of MI/ACS by tertiles of EA measures are presented in Table 3. After controlling for age, the risk of MI/ACS was modestly higher in ΔAHr tertile 3 vs. tertile 1: OR = 1.26 (95% CI 0.65–2.44). Similarly, the risk of MI/ACS was higher in tertile 3 of ΔAHn compared with the lowest tertile, the OR was 1.57 (95% CI 0.79–3.14). In multivariable models adjusted for age, sex, smoking, SBP, BMI, total cholesterol and education, the ORs were 1.24 (95% CI 0.60–2.56) and 1.36 (95% CI 0.63–2.96), respectively. However, as the lower margin of 95% confidence intervals was always less than 1.00, it is possible that these results arose by chance alone.

Table 3. Relationship between MI/ACS and epigenetic age acceleration by tertiles of the difference between baseline EA and CA (cases, n = 129 and controls, n = 177).

Measure of Epigenetic Age	n, Case/Control	Tertiles	Absolute Difference T1-T2	Model 1 OR (95% CI)	Model 2 OR (95% CI)	Model 3 OR (95% CI)	Model 4 OR (95% CI)
ΔAHr, year	129/177	T1 (ref)	T2-T3	1.0	1.0	1.0	1.0
		T2	5.64	0.89 (0.49–1.63)	0.83 (0.45–1.53)	0.83 (0.44–1.54)	0.91 (0.47–1.77)
		T3	5.48	1.26 (0.65–2.44)	1.14 (0.59–2.22)	1.21 (0.61–2.40)	1.24 (0.60–2.56)
		p-value for trends		0.510	0.738	0.624	0.593
ΔAHn, year	129/177	T1 (ref)		1.0	1.0	1.0	1.0
		T2	5.35	1.28 (0.68–2.39)	1.20 (0.63–2.24)	1.26 (0.66–2.40)	1.22 (0.61–2.44)
		T3	5.40	1.57 (0.79–3.14)	1.26 (0.61–2.60)	1.36 (0.65–2.85)	1.36 (0.63–2.96)
		p-value for trends		0.198	0.526	0.408	0.437
ΔAPh, year	129/177	T1 (ref)		1.0	1.0	1.0	1.0
		T2	6.49	1.19 (0.64–2.21)	1.18 (0.63–2.20)	1.21 (0.65–2.28)	1.17 (0.61–2.27)
		T3	7.40	2.09 (1.11–3.94)	1.84 (0.99–3.52)	1.78 (0.92–3.43)	1.64 (0.82–3.31)
		p-value for trends		0.022	0.065	0.088	0.171
ΔASB, year	129/177	T1 (ref)		1.0	1.0	1.0	1.0
		T2	3.94	0.88 (0.47–1.62)	0.80 (0.43–1.51)	0.84 (0.45–1.58)	0.99 (0.50–1.94)
		T3	4.06	1.13 (0.60–2.11)	1.00 (0.53–1.89)	1.09 (0.57–2.09)	1.18 (0.60–2.37)
		p-value for trends		0.699	0.948	0.738	0.637

ΔAHr—difference between EA by Horvath's and chronological age; ΔAHn—difference between EA by Hannum's and chronological age; ΔAPh—difference between phenotypic EA and chronological age; ΔASB—difference between Skin and Blood EA and chronological age; OR—odds ratio; CI—confidence interval; Model 1: age-adjusted; Model 2: adjusted for age and sex; Model 3: adjusted for age, sex and smoking; Model 4: adjusted for age, sex, smoking, SBP, TC, BMI and education.

The risk of MI/ACS increased in tertile 3 vs. tertile 1 of ΔAPh, with OR = 2.09 (95% CI 1.11–3.94), p = 0.022 independent of age, and a statistically not significant OR of 1.8 (CI 95% 0.99-3.52), p = 0.065 was found in the sex- and age-adjusted Model 2 (Table 2). This association was partly explained (or mediated) by smoking and metabolic factors (blood pressure, body mass index, total and LDL cholesterol). The relationships between tertiles of ΔAHn and MI/ACS were also positive but statistically not significant. The second tertile of ΔAHr was negatively related to MI/ACS in any type of adjustment. There was no association found between tertiles of baseline ΔASB and the risk of MI/ACS.

For internal validation, we also assessed the association between MI/ACS and EA measures in case and expanded control groups (Tables S2–S4). The results were similar but somewhat weaker for continuous epigenetic age acceleration (EAA) and for EAA by tertiles than in the original case-control groups. In the expanded sample, the age-adjusted OR of MI/ACS per 1-year increment of EAA was 1.014 (95% CI 0.98–1.05) for ΔAPh. The risk of MI/ACS was higher in the top tertile 3 vs. tertile 1 for ΔAPh, with OR = 1.42 (95% CI 0.85–2.42), but statistically not significant in the age-adjusted model and with further adjustment. For ΔAHn, the relationships with MI/ACS were of a similar direction but weaker still; ΔAHr and ΔASB were not associated with the risk of MI/ACS.

4. Discussion

In this nested case-control study in Novosibirsk (Russia), we selected CVD-free participants with incident MI/ACS (cases) and age- and sex-frequency matched controls from a population-based cohort (HAPIEE); participants were followed up over 15 years. Epigenetic ages derived from DNAm with Horvath's, Hannum's and Skin and Blood clocks were close to the chronological ages, but PhenoAge's predictions were less close to CA. From the EA indices tested in this study, the relationship between incident MI/ACS and 1–year increments of the difference between baseline EA and CA assessed by the PhenoAge clock was positive but statistically not significant. The relationships between the risk of MI/ACS and acceleration of EA assessed by ΔAHr, ΔAHn and ΔASB were of the same direction but were weaker and also statistically not significant.

When EAA was classified into tertiles, the risk of MI/ACS modestly increased in tertile 3 vs. tertile 1 of EAA assessed by the PhenoAge clock only in the minimally adjusted model independent of age and was borderline in the age- and sex-adjusted model. This association appeared to be explained (or mediated) by smoking and metabolic factors. We did not find significant associations between EAA tertiles of other studied DNAm clocks and MI/ACS in our sample.

Age is one of the strongest risk factors for many human diseases, including CVD and, specifically, CHD [16,24]. Given the significance of biological aging, a variety of estimators of biological age were constructed. DNAm-based estimators (epigenetic age) precisely predict chronological age and their positive deviation from chronological age is considered as 'accelerated biological aging' (EAA).

In our dataset, EAA was higher in the control group than in MI/ACS cases. That could be explained by the differences in chronological ages in case and control group subjects. Indeed, it is known that EAA is non-linear and tends to decrease with age [10], and in our sample, the chronological age at the time of blood draw in the control subjects is lower than that of the cases. To address the potential interaction between chronological age at baseline and EAA, an analysis stratified by age group would be needed; unfortunately, our study was not large enough to do so.

Evidence is growing on the association between epigenetic age and risk of all-cause mortality and some cause-specific mortality [13,19–24]. In a recent meta-analysis, Fransquet et al. (2019) (41,607 subjects) defined that each 5–year increase in epigenetic age acceleration (EAA) was associated with 8% and 15% increased risk of all-cause mortality (by Hannum's and Horvath's, correspondingly) [24]. Another meta-analysis of Marioni et al. (2015) [22], based on four large cohorts (two Lothian Birth Cohorts, Framingham Heart Study and Normative Aging Study), revealed a pooled effect of 16% and 9% increases in total mortality risk by 5–year higher EAA (by Hannum's and Horvath's, respectively).

EAA has been extensively investigated in relation to age-dependent diseases, health, lifestyle and environmental factors, with inconsistent results [15,21,25,39–42]. In our study, the relationship between MI/ACS and PhenoAge acceleration by 1–year was positive but statistically not significant. We found modestly increased risk of incident MI/ACS in the top vs. the lowest tertile of baseline difference between EA and CA confined to the PhenoAge clock in the minimally adjusted model. The direction of association for PhenoAge is broadly in line with associations between EA acceleration and MI or CHD risk reported in a meta-analysis of five cohorts [13], in the NAS and KORA F4 cohorts [43] and in comparative analysis between GrimAge and other EA estimators [17]. For instance, in the meta-analysis of the NAS cohort ($n = 737$ white men) and KORA F4 cohort ($n = 1725$) with follow-up ranging from 8.5–14 years, the HR of MI was 1.15 per 1 SD of PhenoAge acceleration [43]. In a meta-analysis of five cohorts (WHI (two cohorts), FHS, NAS, JHS), a 1–year increase in PhenoAge was associated with CHD risk with $\beta=0.016$ to 0.073 [13]. A recent systematic review based on 156 publications and a meta-analysis of 57 factors by Oblack et al. [15] obtained similar effects, with HR for CVD risk ranging from 1.011 to 1.083 per year assessed by four epigenetic clocks (Horvath's, Hannum's, PhenoAge and GrimAge).

We observed ORs of MI/ACS ranging from 1.009–1.012 per 1 year of EAA and from 1.2–1.3 in the top tertile vs. the lowest tertile of EAA by Horvath's and Hannum's clocks; these coefficients were not statistically significant but close to those previously reported in the ARIC study [44], a German ESTHER case cohort [20] and cumulative data from a recent meta-analysis [15]. For example, in the ARIC study of a sub-cohort of black participants ($n = 2543$) followed for 21 years, the HR of fatal CHD was 1.17 and 1.22 per 5–year increment of Hannum's and Horvath's EAA independent of other factors; the HR for MI modestly increased by 1.12 for Hannum's EAA [44]. In the ESTHER case cohort study ($n = 1864$), the HR of CVD mortality was 1.19 for a 5–year increment of Horvath's

EAA independent of other factors and similar but weaker for Hannum's EAA measure [20]. On the other hand, for example, Horvath et al. (2016) [25] did not report an association between EAA and incident CHD in the Women's Health Initiative dataset.

The OR in our analysis for EAA by PhenoAge tertile was substantially attenuated after controlling for metabolic factors (BMI, SBP, TC) and education. The residual associations, although still of meaningful magnitude, had wide confidence intervals, and they may have arisen by chance alone on account of our relatively small sample size. This is in contrast to some of the larger aforementioned studies that have reported associations in multivariable-adjusted models.

The impact of metabolic risk factors to mediate the relationship between epigenetic age and risk of atherosclerotic CVD and acute coronary outcomes is well supported. Original studies and comprehensive reviews consistently demonstrate that BMI is strongly correlated with epigenetic age, independent of other covariates [15,21,39,45]. Obesity is a known risk factor for many age-related diseases; it is associated with oxidative stress and a pro-inflammatory state that enhances white blood cell turnover and is considered as pro-aging [39]. The exact mechanisms linking DNA methylation profiles and CVD are not entirely clear, but DNAm is considered as a key player in the genetic regulation of genes related to cardiac homeostasis [46]. In the last decade, several DNAm studies (including EWASs) have linked CHD and atherosclerosis to differentially methylated sites related to genes most commonly involved to the pathways of obesity, adiposity, lipid and carbohydrate metabolism, inflammation, macrophage activity, smooth muscle cell proliferation and renin–angiotensin regulation [45,47–51].

The diversity across previous studies in the relationship between EA and CVD/CHD regarding the presence and magnitude of association might be related to the heterogeneity of the studied outcomes and study design, age, ethnic and sex composition and volume of the sample, population-specific characteristics of morbidity, risk factor profiles and environmental exposure, covariates and multiple statistical testing, as well as the exact DNAm platform and EA clocks used in the analysis.

5. Study Limitations and Advantages

The study has several limitations, particularly the relatively small sample size. In this nested case-control study, we randomly selected cases of incident fatal and non-fatal MI and ACS among all new-onset CHD events occurring in a large population cohort (9360) during a 15-year follow-up; the cases and controls were frequency matched by age and sex. This makes it more likely that we obtained a representative sample of typical acute coronary disease for this population, but the study was under-powered to study relatively small effects. The sample size was determined by the numbers of eligible events with DNA samples and by the cost of the lab analyses. In post hoc power calculations (with 160 cases and 240 controls), the estimated statistical power of the analysis to detect a difference between cases and controls in delta (epigenetic age–chronological age) of 1.5 and 2 years was 80% > 90%, respectively. For internal validation, we repeated the analysis using another (expanded) control group which did not significantly alter the results. However, further enlarging of the MI/ACS sample would certainly improve the statistical power to detect significant associations for EAA metrics.

For practical reasons, we used frequency matching of cases and controls by 5–year age groups and sex instead of an individual matching procedure. After exclusions by quality control, the distribution of age groups between cases and controls slightly changed but the statistical adjustment would take this into account. Sex distribution remained practically uniform (50–60%) between cases and controls. We also conducted internal validation using an expanded control sample with age–sex distribution closer to cases (mean age 59.8 years in cases vs. 57.5 years in expanded controls); the use of an expanded sample did not significantly alter the results.

To protect against misclassification which could not be excluded for CHD as a potentially heterogonous outcome, we focused on the most strictly defined categories of

CHD (MI and ACS) ascertained from the data of 'MI Register' using standardized and internationally validated criteria. To ensure completeness of registration, we additionally used overlapping sources of case ascertainment and both hot-pursuit and cold-pursuit approaches were combined by MI Register.

Another potential limitation relates to the arguable differences in DNAm between sexes [50]. To overcome this limitation, the sampling procedure kept the sex distribution uniform among cases and controls (nearly 50–60%), and we adjusted the estimates by sex (Model 2). Finally, in the sensitivity analysis split by sex we received ORs of the same directions and similar values compared to pooled results and they were insignificant (data are shown in Supplement Material, Table S1).

Our study also has several strengths. First, it is the first population-based prospective nested case-control study exploring the relationship between epigenetic age and risk of incident MI/ACS in the Russian population as well as in the Eastern European population.

Second, we used the latest platform, Illumina Epic 850 BeadChip, for DNA methylation analysis, applied standardized multistep quality control and included longitudinal analysis at a different time point. We only used high-quality data from samples with less than 1% CpGs with detection p-values above the threshold 0.01, and CpGs with bead count numbers of at least 3 and p-values below 0.01 across at least 99% of samples.

Third, we used four estimators of epigenetic age (Horvath's, Hannum's, PhenoAge and Skin and Blood clocks) with established precision in estimating chronological age, age-related diseases and mortality [16] and constructed with a variety of approaches (blood-based, pan-tissue or phenotype-based).

Finally, our data provide the first evidence of the magnitude and potential consequences of EAA in the Russian population.

6. Conclusions

In this case-control study nested in a prospective population-based cohort, we did not find strong associations between accelerated epigenetic age markers and risk of MI/ACS. There was a modest association between acceleration of epigenetic age and increased risk of MI/ACS confined only to the highest tertile of the PhenoAge clock, which appeared to be partly modulated by smoking and metabolic factors. However, this isolated positive finding may have been a false positive result and needs to be interpreted with caution. If confirmed in larger studies, however, epigenetic age acceleration may prove to be a useful predictor of the risk of acute coronary events in older age, with a potential for practical implications for CVD prevention.

Supplementary Materials: The following are available online at https://www.mdpi.com/article/10.3390/jpm12010110/s1, Figure S1: Boxplots showing age distribution in case and control groups for A—all samples, B—males and C—females. Figure S2: Scatterplots of chronological vs. epigenetic age by Horvath's, Hannum's, PhenoAge and Skin and Blood clocks. Black line corresponds to the predicted age equal to the chronological age. Figure S3: Correlation chart for the chronological age and four DNAm age predictions. The panels on the main diagonal show distributions of the CA and DNAm clock results, the panels below the diagonal are scatter plots with a fitted line, the panels above the diagonal show the corresponding Pearson correlation coefficients with significance level below 0.001. Figure S4: Density plots and boxplots of the age acceleration distribution for (A) Horvath's, (B) Hannum's, (C) PhenoAge, (D) Skin and Blood epigenetic clocks for sex- and case-control-specific groups. The numbers on the right side of the figure corresponds to t-test p-values. Table S1: Relationship between MI/ACS and epigenetic age acceleration, per 1–year increment of the difference between baseline EA minus CA in men and women (men, $n = 171$, women, $n = 135$). Table S2: Distribution of baseline covariates among cases of incident MI/ACS and expanded control sample (cases, $n = 129$ and controls, $n = 265$). Table S3: Relationship between MI/ACS and epigenetic age acceleration, per 1–year increment of the difference between baseline EA and CA in the expanded sample (cases, $n = 129$ and controls, $n = 265$). Table S4: Relationship between MI/ACS and epigenetic age acceleration in the expanded sample, by tertiles of the difference between baseline EA and CA (cases, $n = 129$ and controls, $n = 265$).

Author Contributions: Conceptualization, S.M., M.B., O.C., S.B.; methodology, S.M., O.C., T.T., H.P.; software, O.C., H.P.; validation, O.C., H.P., V.G.; formal analysis, S.M., O.C.; investigation, S.M., V.M., A.R., V.G.; resources, M.B., S.M., V.M.; data curation, S.M., O.C., H.P.; writing—original draft preparation, S.M.; writing—review and editing, O.C., V.M., T.T., A.R., V.G., J.A.H., H.P., S.B., M.B.; visualization, S.M., O.C., A.R.; supervision, S.M., M.B.; project administration, S.M.; funding acquisition, M.B., S.M., T.T. All authors have read and agreed to the published version of the manuscript.

Funding: This study was supported by the Russian Scientific Foundation (20–15–00371); the baseline HAPIEE study was funded by the Wellcome Trust (WT064947, WT081081, 106554/Z/14/Z) and the US National Institute of Aging (1RO1AG23522).

Institutional Review Board Statement: The study was conducted according to the guidelines of the Declaration of Helsinki, and approved by the ethics committee of IIPM—Branch of IC&G SB RAS (Institute of Internal and Preventive Medicine—Branch of Federal State Budgeted Research Institution, 'Federal Research Center, Institute of Cytology and Genetics, Siberian Branch of the Russian Academy of Sciences'), Protocol no. 1 from 14 March 2002 and Protocol no. 12 from 8 December 2020. The study did not involve humans or animals.

Informed Consent Statement: Informed consent was obtained from all subjects involved in the study.

Data Availability Statement: The data presented in this study are available in tabulated form on request. The data are not publicly available due to ethical restrictions and project regulations.

Acknowledgments: O. Chervova and S. Beck were supported by grants from the Frances and Augustus Newman Foundation (172074). O. Chervova, S. Beck, M. Bobak and H. Pikhart were supported by EU-H2020 Project 'CETOCOEN Excellence' (857560). S. Malyutina, V. Maximov, A. Ryabikov and V. Gafarov were supported by the Russian Academy of Science, State Assignment (AAAA–A17–117112850280–2). J.A. Hubacek is supported by project No. 00023001 (ICEM MH CR).

Conflicts of Interest: The authors declare no conflict of interest.

References

1. United Nations, Department of Economic and Social Affairs, Population Division (2017). World Population Prospects: The 2017 Revision, Key Findings and Advance Tables. Working Paper No. ESA/P/WP/248. Available online: https://population.un.org/wpp/Publications/Files/WPP2017_KeyFindings.pdf (accessed on 29 October 2021).
2. WHO/Global Status Report on Noncommunicable Diseases. 2014. Available online: https://www.who.int/publications/i/item/9789241564854 (accessed on 29 October 2021).
3. Jylhävä, J.; Pedersen, N.L.; Hägg, S. Biological Age Predictors. *EBioMedicine* **2017**, *21*, 29–36. [CrossRef]
4. Horvath, S.; Raj, K. DNA methylation-based biomarkers and the epigenetic clock theory of ageing. *Nat. Rev. Genet.* **2018**, *19*, 371–384. [CrossRef] [PubMed]
5. Riggs, A.D.; Martienssen, R.F.; Russo, V.E.A. *Introduction. Epigenetic Mechanisms of Gene Regulation*; Cold Spring Harbor Laboratory Press: Cold Spring Harbor, NY, USA, 1996.
6. Jones, M.J.; Goodman, S.J.; Kobor, M. DNA methylation and healthy human aging. *Aging Cell* **2015**, *14*, 924–932. [CrossRef]
7. Bock, C. Analysing and interpreting DNA methylation data. *Nat. Rev. Genet.* **2012**, *13*, 705–719. [CrossRef] [PubMed]
8. Horvath, S.; Zhang, Y.; Langfelder, P.; Kahn, R.S.; Boks, M.P.; Van Eijk, K.; Van den Berg, L.H.; Ophoff, R.A. Aging effects on DNA methylation modules in human brain and blood tissue. *Genome Biol.* **2012**, *13*, R97. [CrossRef]
9. Hannum, G.; Guinney, J.; Zhao, L.; Zhang, L.; Hughes, G.; Sadda, S.; Klotzle, B.; Bibikova, M.; Fan, J.-B.; Gao, Y.; et al. Genome-wide Methylation Profiles Reveal Quantitative Views of Human Aging Rates. *Mol. Cell* **2012**, *49*, 359–367. [CrossRef] [PubMed]
10. Weidner, C.I.; Lin, Q.; Koch, C.M.; Eisele, L.; Beier, F.; Ziegler, P.; Bauerschlag, D.O.; Jöckel, K.-H.; Erbel, R.; Mühleisen, T.W.; et al. Aging of blood can be tracked by DNA methylation changes at just three CpG sites. *Genome Biol.* **2014**, *15*, R24. [CrossRef]
11. Bell, C.G.; Lowe, R.; Adams, P.D.; Baccarelli, A.A.; Beck, S.; Bell, J.T.; Christensen, B.C.; Gladyshev, V.N.; Heijmans, B.T.; Horvath, S.; et al. DNA methylation aging clocks: Challenges and recommendations. *Genome Biol.* **2019**, *20*, 249. [CrossRef]
12. Horvath, S. DNA methylation age of human tissues and cell types. *Genome Biol.* **2013**, *14*, R115. [CrossRef]
13. Levine, M.E.; Lu, A.T.; Quach, A.; Chen, B.H.; Assimes, T.L.; Bandinelli, S.; Hou, L.; Baccarelli, A.A.; Stewart, J.D.; Li, Y.; et al. An epigenetic biomarker of aging for lifespan and healthspan. *Aging* **2018**, *10*, 573–591. [CrossRef]
14. Horvath, S.; Oshima, J.; Martin, G.M.; Lu, A.T.; Quach, A.; Cohen, H.; Felton, S.; Matsuyama, M.; Lowe, D.; Kabacik, S.; et al. Epigenetic clock for skin and blood cells applied to Hutchinson Gilford Progeria Syndrome and ex vivo studies. *Aging* **2018**, *10*, 1758–1775. [CrossRef]
15. Oblak, L.; van der Zaag, J.; Higgins-Chen, A.T.; Levine, M.E.; Boks, M.P. A systematic review of biological, social and environmental factors associated with epigenetic clock acceleration. *Ageing Res. Rev.* **2021**, *69*, 101348. [CrossRef]

16. Lee, Y.; Haftorn, K.L.; Denault, W.R.P.; Nustad, H.E.; Page, C.M.; Lyle, R.; Lee-Odegard, S.; Moen, G.-H.; Prasad, R.B.; Groop, L.C.; et al. Blood-based epigenetic estimators of chronological age in human adults using DNA methylation data from the Illumina MethylationEPIC array. *BMC Genom.* **2020**, *21*, 747. [CrossRef]
17. Lu, A.T.; Quach, A.; Wilson, J.G.; Reiner, A.P.; Aviv, A.; Raj, K.; Hou, L.; Baccarelli, A.A.; Li, Y.; Stewart, J.D.; et al. DNA methylation GrimAge strongly predicts lifespan and healthspan. *Aging* **2019**, *11*, 303–327. [CrossRef]
18. Shireby, G.L.; Davies, J.P.; Francis, P.T.; Burrage, J.; Walker, E.M.; Neilson, G.W.A.; Dahir, A.; Thomas, A.J.; Love, S.; Smith, R.G.; et al. Recalibrating the epigenetic clock: Implications for assessing biological age in the human cortex. *Brain* **2020**, *143*, 3763–3775. [CrossRef]
19. Christiansen, L.; Lenart, A.; Tan, Q.; Vaupel, J.; Aviv, A.; McGue, M.; Christensen, K. DNA methylation age is associated with mortality in a longitudinal Danish twin study. *Aging Cell* **2015**, *15*, 149–154. [CrossRef] [PubMed]
20. Perna, L.; Zhang, Y.; Mons, U.; Holleczek, B.; Saum, K.-U.; Brenner, H. Epigenetic age acceleration predicts cancer, cardiovascular, and all-cause mortality in a German case cohort. *Clin. Epigenet.* **2016**, *8*, 64. [CrossRef] [PubMed]
21. Dugué, P.-A.; Bassett, J.K.; Joo, J.H.E.; Baglietto, L.; Jung, C.-H.; Wong, E.M.; Fiorito, G.; Schmidt, D.; Makalic, E.; Li, S.; et al. Association of DNA Methylation-Based Biological Age With Health Risk Factors and Overall and Cause-Specific Mortality. *Am. J. Epidemiol.* **2018**, *187*, 529–538. [CrossRef] [PubMed]
22. Marioni, R.E.; Shah, S.; McRae, A.F.; Chen, B.H.; Colicino, E.; Harris, S.E.; Gibson, J.; Henders, A.K.; Redmond, P.; Cox, S.R.; et al. DNA methylation age of blood predicts all-cause mortality in later life. *Genome Biol.* **2015**, *16*, 25. [CrossRef]
23. Chen, B.H.; Marioni, R.E.; Colicino, E.; Peters, M.J.; Ward-Caviness, C.K.; Tsai, P.C.; Roetker, N.S.; Just, A.C.; Demerath, E.W.; Guan, W.; et al. DNA methylation-based measures of biological age: Meta-analysis predicting time to death. *Aging* **2016**, *8*, 1844–1865. [CrossRef]
24. Fransquet, P.D.; Wrigglesworth, J.; Woods, R.L.; Ernst, M.E.; Ryan, J. The epigenetic clock as a predictor of disease and mortality risk: A systematic review and meta-analysis. *Clin. Epigenet.* **2019**, *11*, 62. [CrossRef]
25. Horvath, S.; Gurven, M.; Levine, M.E.; Trumble, B.C.; Kaplan, H.; Allayee, H.; Ritz, B.R.; Chen, B.; Lu, A.T.; Rickabaugh, T.M.; et al. An epigenetic clock analysis of race/ethnicity, sex, and coronary heart disease. *Genome Biol.* **2016**, *17*, 171. [CrossRef] [PubMed]
26. EUROSTAT. Mortality and Life Expectancy Statistics. 2021. Available online: https://ec.europa.eu/eurostat/statistics-explained/index.php?title=Mortality_and_life_expectancy_statistics (accessed on 30 October 2021).
27. Global Age Watch Index 2015: Insight report. Available online: https://www.helpage.org/global-agewatch/reports/global-agewatch-index-2015-insight-report-summary-and-methodology/ (accessed on 29 October 2021).
28. Bobak, M.; Malyutina, S.; Horvat, P.; Pajak, A.; Tamosiunas, A.; Kubinova, R.; Simonova, G.; Topor-Madry, R.; Peasey, A.; Pikhart, H.; et al. Alcohol, drinking pattern and all-cause, cardiovascular and alcohol-related mortality in Eastern Europe. *Eur. J. Epidemiol.* **2016**, *31*, 21–30. [CrossRef]
29. Tillmann, T.; Pikhart, H.; Peasey, A.; Kubínová, R.; Pajak, A.; Tamošiūnas, A.; Malyutina, S.; Steptoe, A.; Kivimäki, M.; Marmot, M.; et al. Psychosocial and socioeconomic determinants of cardiovascular mortality in Eastern Europe: A multicentre prospective cohort study. *PLoS Med.* **2017**, *14*, e1002459. [CrossRef] [PubMed]
30. Stefler, D.; Brett, D.; Sarkadi-Nagy, E.; Kopczynska, E.; Detchev, S.; Bati, A.; Scrob, M.; Koenker, D.; Aleksov, B.; Douarin, E.; et al. Traditional Eastern European diet and mortality: Prospective evidence from the HAPIEE study. *Eur. J. Nutr.* **2021**, *60*, 1091–1100. [CrossRef]
31. Ryabikov, A.; Maksimov, V.; Holmes, M.; Bobak, M.; Malyutina, S. The association between epigenetic age and progression of subclinical atherosclerosis in ageing cohort. *Atheroscler* **2020**, *315*, e132. [CrossRef]
32. Peasey, A.; Bobak, M.; Kubinova, R.; Malyutina, S.; Pajak, A.; Tamosiunas, A.; Pikhart, H.; Nicholson, A.; Marmot, M. Determinants of cardiovascular disease and other non-communicable diseases in Central and Eastern Europe: Rationale and design of the HAPIEE study. *BMC Public Health* **2006**, *6*, 255–264. [CrossRef]
33. Fortin, J.-P.; Triche, T.J., Jr.; Hansen, K.D. Preprocessing, normalization and integration of the Illumina HumanMethylationEPIC array with minfi. *Bioinformatics* **2016**, *33*, 558–560. [CrossRef]
34. Tian, Y.; Morris, T.J.; Webster, A.; Yang, Z.; Beck, S.; Feber, A.; Teschendorff, A. ChAMP: Updated methylation analysis pipeline for Illumina BeadChips. *Bioinformatics* **2017**, *33*, 3982–3984. [CrossRef]
35. Xu, Z.; Langie, S.A.S.; De Boever, P.; Taylor, J.A.; Niu, L.; De Boever, P. RELIC: A novel dye-bias correction method for Illumina Methylation BeadChip. *BMC Genom.* **2017**, *18*, 4. [CrossRef]
36. Chervova, O.; Conde, L.; Guerra-Assunção, J.A.; Moghul, I.; Webster, A.P.; Berner, A.; Cadieux, E.L.; Tian, Y.; Voloshin, V.; Jesus, T.F.; et al. The Personal Genome Project-UK, an open access resource of human multi-omics data. *Sci. Data* **2019**, *6*, 257. [CrossRef] [PubMed]
37. Fix, E.; Hodges, J.L., Jr. Discriminatory Analysis. Nonparametric Discrimination: Consistency Properties. *Int. Stat. Rev.* **1989**, *57*, 238–247. [CrossRef]
38. Altman, N.S. An Introduction to Kernel and Nearest-Neighbor Nonparametric Regression. *Am. Stat.* **1992**, *46*, 175. [CrossRef]
39. Ryan, J.; Wrigglesworth, J.; Loong, J.; Fransquet, P.; Woods, R.L. A Systematic Review and Meta-analysis of Environmental, Lifestyle, and Health Factors Associated With DNA Methylation Age. *J. Gerontol. Ser. A Boil. Sci. Med. Sci.* **2020**, *75*, 481–494. [CrossRef] [PubMed]

40. Marioni, R.; Shah, S.; McRae, A.; Ritchie, S.J.; Terrera, G.M.; Harris, S.E.; Gibson, J.; Redmond, P.; Cox, S.R.; Pattie, A.; et al. The epigenetic clock is correlated with physical and cognitive fitness in the Lothian Birth Cohort 1936. *Int. J. Epidemiol.* **2015**, *44*, 1388–1396. [CrossRef] [PubMed]
41. Levine, M.E.; Lu, A.T.; Bennett, D.A.; Horvath, S. Epigenetic age of the pre-frontal cortex is associated with neuritic plaques, amyloid load, and Alzheimer's disease related cognitive functioning. *Aging* **2015**, *7*, 1198–1211. [CrossRef]
42. Levine, M.E.; Lu, A.T.; Chen, B.H.; Hernandez, D.G.; Singleton, A.B.; Ferrucci, L.; Bandinelli, S.; Salfati, E.; Manson, J.E.; Quach, A.; et al. Menopause accelerates biological aging. *Proc. Natl. Acad. Sci. USA* **2016**, *113*, 9327–9332. [CrossRef]
43. Wang, C.; Ni, W.; Yao, Y.; Just, A.; Heiss, J.; Wei, Y.; Gao, X.; Coull, B.A.; Kosheleva, A.; Baccarelli, A.A.; et al. DNA methylation-based biomarkers of age acceleration and all-cause death, myocardial infarction, stroke, and cancer in two cohorts: The NAS, and KORA F4. *EBioMedicine* **2021**, *63*, 103151. [CrossRef] [PubMed]
44. Roetker, N.S.; Pankow, J.; Bressler, J.; Morrison, A.C.; Boerwinkle, E. Prospective Study of Epigenetic Age Acceleration and Incidence of Cardiovascular Disease Outcomes in the ARIC Study (Atherosclerosis Risk in Communities). *Circ. Genom. Precis. Med.* **2018**, *11*, e001937. [CrossRef] [PubMed]
45. Horvath, S.; Erhart, W.; Brosch, M.; Ammerpohl, O.; von Schönfels, W.; Ahrens, M.; Heits, N.; Bell, J.; Tsai, P.-C.; Spector, T.D.; et al. Obesity accelerates epigenetic aging of human liver. *Proc. Natl. Acad. Sci. USA* **2014**, *111*, 15538–15543. [CrossRef]
46. Pagiatakis, C.; Musolino, E.; Gornati, R.; Bernardini, G.; Papait, R. Epigenetics of aging and disease: A brief overview. *Aging Clin. Exp. Res.* **2021**, *33*, 737–745. [CrossRef] [PubMed]
47. Fernández-Sanlés, A.; Baixeras, S.S.; Subirana, I.; Degano, I.R.; Elosua, R. Association between DNA methylation and coronary heart disease or other atherosclerotic events: A systematic review. *Atherosclerosis* **2017**, *263*, 325–333. [CrossRef] [PubMed]
48. Fernández-Sanlés, A.; Sayols-Baixeras, S.; Curcio, S.; Subirana, I.; Marrugat, J.; Elosua, R. DNA Methylation and Age-Independent Cardiovascular Risk, an Epigenome-Wide Approach. *Arter. Thromb. Vasc. Biol.* **2018**, *38*, 645–652. [CrossRef]
49. Gonzalez-Jaramillo, V.; Portilla-Fernandez, E.; Glisic, M.; Voortman, T.; Bramer, W.; Chowdhury, R.; Roks, A.J.; Danser, A.H.J.; Muka, T.; Nano, J.; et al. The role of DNA methylation and histone modifications in blood pressure: A systematic review. *J. Hum. Hypertens.* **2019**, *33*, 703–715. [CrossRef]
50. Hartman, R.J.G.; Huisman, S.; Ruijter, H.M.D. Sex differences in cardiovascular epigenetics-a systematic review. *Biol. Sex Differ.* **2018**, *9*, 19. [CrossRef]
51. Xia, Y.; Brewer, A.; Bell, J.T. DNA methylation signatures of incident coronary heart disease: Findings from epigenome-wide association studies. *Clin. Epigenet.* **2021**, *13*, 186. [CrossRef]

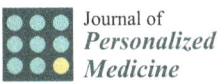

Article

The Role of Cumulative LDL Cholesterol in Cardiovascular Disease Development in Patients with Familial Hypercholesterolemia

Victoria Korneva [1,*], Tatyana Kuznetsova [1] and Ulrich Julius [2]

[1] Faculty Therapy Department, Petrozavodsk State University, Lenin Avenue, 33, 185000 Petrozavodsk, Russia; eme@karelia.ru
[2] Lipidology and Lipoprotein Apheresis Center, Department of Internal Medicine III, University Hospital Carl Gustav Carus, Technische Universität Dresden, Fetscherstr. 74, 01307 Dresden, Germany; ulrich.julius@ukdd.de
* Correspondence: vikkorneva@mail.ru

Abstract: In patients with familial hypercholesterolemia (FH) the exposure of very high LDL-C concentration and cumulative LDL-C level (cum LDL-C) can play a significant role in the prognosis. Objective: to analyze the contribution of "cum LDL-C for all life" and the index "cum LDL-C/age" to the development of coronary heart disease (CHD), myocardial infarction (MI), and a combined end point: MI, stroke, unstable angina in FH patients. Methods: 188 patients (mean age 49.2 years, males 45.7%) with FH were examined (Dutch Lipid Clinic Criteria). We had evaluated cumulative LDL-C and index "cum DL-C/age" along with other classical risk factors. Cum LDL-C was calculated as LDL-Cmax × (age at initiating of hypolipidemic therapy) + LDL-C at inclusion age at initiation/correction therapy). Cumulative LDL-C and "cum LDL-C/age" were calculated as the ratio cum LDL-C to age. The follow-up period was 5.4 (from 3 to 10) years. Results: The index "cum LDL-C/age" was higher in patients with CHD 58.7 ± 10.4 mmol/L/years vs. 40.1 ± 11.7 mmol/L/years in patients without CHD ($p < 0.001$). According to our data based on the results of the logistic regression analysis in patients with FH, cumulative LDL-C and the cumulative index "cum LDL–C/age" played a strong predictive role in the development of CHD in FH patients; it was greater than the role of TC and LDL-C concentrations. We present ROC curves for CHD, MI and combined end point in FH patients, and a prognostic scale for CHD development, which is based on classical cardiovascular risk factors. Conclusion: cumulative LDL-C level plays an important role in the development of CHD in FH patients.

Keywords: familial hypercholesterolemia; cumulative LDL-C level; prognosis

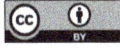

1. Introduction

Familial hypercholesterolemia (FH) is an autosomal codominant genetic disease, which is characterized by an elevation of low-density lipoprotein cholesterol (LDL-C) and a deposition of LDL-derived cholesterol in tendons (xanthomatosis) and arteries, and which leads to premature cardiovascular disease [1–4]. However, cardiovascular risk among these patients can vary widely, even in those who belong to the same family or share the same mutation [5–7]. FH patients refer to the high and very high cardiovascular risk categories, but scales, such as SCORE and the Framingham Risk Score, cannot be applied in these subjects [8,9]. Classic cardiovascular risk factors can contribute with high variability to the presence of cardiovascular disease. Although the use of statins reduces the cardiovascular risk, FH patients have still a high residual risk [5]. In patients with FH the exposure of very high LDL-C concentration since birth [10] and cumulative LDL-C level (cum LDL-C) can play a significant role in the prognosis of the disease.

2. Aim

To analyze the contribution of "cum LDL-C for all life" and the index "cum LDL-C/age" to the development of coronary heart disease (CHD), myocardial infarction (MI), and a combined end point (MI, stroke, unstable angina) in addition to classic cardiovascular risk factors in FH patients.

3. Methods

One hundred and eighty-eight patients (mean age 49.2 (range 18–64) years, males 86 (45.7%) with FH were examined (Dutch Lipid Clinic Criteria). In 118 patients, a definite FH was diagnosed (62.7%), a genetic test was performed in 102 patients (54.2%). We had evaluated cumulative LDL-C and index "cum LDL-C/age" along with classical risk factors (total cholesterol (TC), LDL-C, HDL-C, triglycerides (TG), body mass index (BMI), burdened heredity for cardiovascular diseases, age, gender, smoking). For calculation of cumulative LDL-C we used formula: Cum LDL-C = LDL − Cmax × age at initiation of hypolipidemic therapy + LDL-C at inclusion-age at initiation/correction therapy) [11]. Index cumulative LDL-C and index "cum LDL-C/age" were calculated as ratio cum LDL-C to age of patients.

Additional laboratory criteria were lipoprotein(a) (Lp(a)), creatinine and glomerular filtration rate calculated according to CKD-EPI formula. In the follow-up period of 5.4 (from 3 to 10) years, we analyzed the development of CHD, MI and calculated the combined end point (CEP). CHD was diagnosed according to typical clinical symptoms (angina pectoris), ischemic criteria on ECG monitoring and stress test. If there were indications for a coronary angiography this was performed. MI was diagnosed in the presence of medical history data, ECG chance and positive troponin test.

Patients who stopped smoking were considered non-smokers.

Positive family history was considered if acute coronary syndromes were also observed in relatives of men under the age of 55 and woman under the age of 65.

Arterial hypertension was diagnosed when blood pressure was detected above 140 and 90 mmHg before the start of therapy. Further, the patient was considered to have arterial hypertension, despite the blood pressure figures on the background of treatment.

The study was conducted according to the guidelines of the Declaration of Helsinki, and approved by Ethics Committee of the Ministry of Health and Petrozavodsk State University (date of approval 14 November 2013), protocol code No. 29.

All patients included in the study signed informed consent. The principles of the study comply with the Helsinki Declaration.

For 15 years we have maintained a register of FH patients in Karelia Republic. (It now includes 380 patients). All patients have been observed by us on the basis of the lipid center created at the medical institute of Petrozavodsk state university. We had two sources for our register: the first one was patients who were treated in emergency care hospital in Petrozavodsk (28,225 patients) and the second was patients with severe dyslipidemia, who were forwarded to our clinic by outpatient cardiologists for special consultation.

4. Results

Non-lipid risk factors in FH patients with CHD are presented in Table 1. Lipid risk factors in FH patients with CHD are given in Table 2. FH patients with CHD were older than patients without CHD: mean age was 58.7(range 34–84) years and 40.1 (range 18–64) years, respectively ($p < 0.0001$).

TC concentrations in FH patients with CHD were 9.9 ± 1.8 mmol/L, in patients without CHD 9.3 ± 1.8 mmol/L; $p = 0.003$. LDL-C in CHD patients was 7.2 ± 1.6 mmol/L, without CHD 6.6 ± 1.2 mmol/L; $p = 0.004$. TG in CHD patients was 1.79 ± 0.6 mmol/L vs. 1.48 ± 0.6 mmol/L; $p = 0.004$. HDL-C in CHD was 1.4 ± 0.4 mmol/L vs. 1.7 ± 0.5 mmol/L, $p = 0.0007$. The mean age at the start of a hypolipidemic therapy in FH patients with CHD was 54.2 ± 10.0 years vs. 42.2 ± 10.3 years without CHD, $p < 0.001$. Cum LDL-C in FH patients with CHD was 409.4 ± 126.3 mmol/L × age vs. 261.1 ± 85.8 mmol/L × age, $p < 0.001$.

The index "cum LDL-C/age" was higher in patients with CHD 58.7 ± 10.4 mmol/L/years vs. 40.1 ± 11.7 mmol/L/years in patients without CHD ($p < 0.001$).

Table 1. Non-lipid risk factors and CHD development in FH patients.

	With CHD (n = 102)	Without CHD (n = 86)	p
Age, years	58.7 ± 10.4	40.1 ± 11.7	<0.0001
Males, n (%)	44 (43.1%)	42 (48.8%)	0.436
Creatinine, umol/L	92.1 ± 20	76.3 ± 14.2	<0.001
Glomerular Filtration Rate (GFR, CKD-EPI), ml/min/1.73 m^2	70.2 ± 17.1	100.1 ± 17.4	<0.001
Glucose level, mmol/L	5.4 ± 1.9	4.9 ± 0.6	0.03
BMI, kg/m^2	28.2 ± 3.9	26.5 ± 3.7	0.005
Waist size, cm	87.7 ± 12	75.2 ± 12	<0.001
Hypertension, n (%)	87 (85.2%)	36 (41.9%)	<0.0001
Smoking, n (%)	33 (32.4%)	19 (22%)	0.153
Positive family history, n (%)	80 (78.4%)	50 (58.1%)	0.005

The data are presented in the form of mean and standard deviation.

Table 2. Lipid risk factors and CHD development in FH patients.

	With CHD (n = 102)	Without CHD (n = 86)	p
Lp(a), g/l	0.55 ± 0.5	0.27 ± 0.4	0.005
Total Cholesterol (TC) initial, mmol/L	9.9 ± 1.8	9.3 ± 1.2	0.003
Low density cholesterol (LDL-C) initial, mmol/L	7.2 ± 1.6	6.6 ± 1.2	0.004
High density cholesterol (HDL-C) initial, mmol/L	1.4 ± 0.4	1.7 ± 0.5	0.0007
Triglycerides (TG) initial, mmol/L	1.8 ± 0.7	1.5 ± 0.7	0.004
TC on treatment, mmol/L	7.2 ± 2.3	8.1 ± 1.9	0.004
LDL-C on treatment, mmol/L	4.8 ± 2.1	5.6 ± 1.7	0.008
HDL-C on treatment, mmol/L/	1.4 ± 0.4	1.6 ± 0.5	<0.001
TG on treatment, mmol/L	2.1 ± 1.3	1.5 ± 0.6	<0.001
Percentage of TC reduction, %	26.6 ± 22.9	11.9 ± 20.1	<0.001
Percentage of LDL-C reduction, %	32.9 ± 28.9	14.7 ± 24.3	<0.001
Cum LDL-C, mmol/L × years	409.4 ± 126.3	261.1 ± 85.8	<0.001
Index "cum LDL-C/age", mmol/L × years	58.7 ± 10.4	40.1 ± 11.7	<0.001
Age at hypolipidemic therapy start, years	54.2 ± 10.0	42.2 ± 10.3	<0.001

The data are presented in the form of means and standard deviation.

Glucose concentrations in patients with CHD were higher: 5.4 ± 1.9 mmol/L vs. 4.9 ± 0.6 mmol/L, $p = 0.03$. BMI in CHD patients was higher: 28.2 ± 3.9 kg/m^2 vs. 26.5 ± 3.7, $p = 0.005$; the waist size (WS) in CHD was 87.7 ± 12 cm vs. 75.2 ± 12 cm ($p < 0.001$). Additionally, 85.2% of CHD patients had a hypertension vs. 41.9% of patients without CHD, $p < 0.0001$. A positive family history of cardiovascular diseases was found in 80 (78.4%) of patients with CHD compared to 50 (58.1%) in patients without CHD, $p = 0.005$.

The creatinine concentration in patients with CHD was 92.1 ± 20 umol/L, in patients without CHD it was 76.3 ± 14.2 ($p < 0.001$) and the glomerular filtration rate (GFR) according to the CKD-EPI formula was lower in FH patients with CHD: 70.2 ± 17.1 mL/min/1.73 m^2 vs. 100.1 ± 17.4 mL/min/1.73 m^2, $p < 0.001$).

It was found by logistic regression that the cum LDL-C level and the index "cum LDL-C/age" had a greater prognostic value for the development of CHD in FH patients compared to TC and LDL–C concentrations. Other significant prognostic factors included gender, TG initial, hypertension and positive family history of CHD (Table 3).

Table 3. Statistical significance of coefficients in calculating the odds ratio of IHD in FH patients (logistic regression analysis).

Predictors	Coefficient	Statistical Error	OR	p
Deviation	−4.66	1.47	0.009	0.0015
Positive family history of CHD	1.46	0.45	4.35	0.001
Male gender	0.97	0.44	2.64	0.027
Cum LDL-C	0.018	0.003	1.02	<0.0001
Cum LDL/age	−0.71	0.24	0.49	0.003
TG initial	0.75	0.30	2.12	0.011
Hypertension	0.77	0.44	2.16	0.084

Formula for calculating OR and probability of CHD: OR(CHD) = exp(−4.66 + 1.46 × Family history + 0.97 × male sex + 0.018 × cum LDL-C − 0.71 × cum LDL-C/age + 0.75 × TG initial + 0.77 × Hypertension. p (CHD) = 1/(1 + (1/OR)). The threshold classification = 0.45. If p (CHD) < 0.45, the absence of CHD is predicted. If p (CHD) ≥ 0.45, CHD is predicted. At the accepted threshold, the sensitivity is 84.8%; specificity is 75.0%.

Thus, the cumulative level of LDL-C plays an important prognostic role in the CHD development along with classic risk factors. Figure 1 shows the ROC curve in the prognostic model of the CHD outcome in patients with complex risk factors, including cum LDL-C.

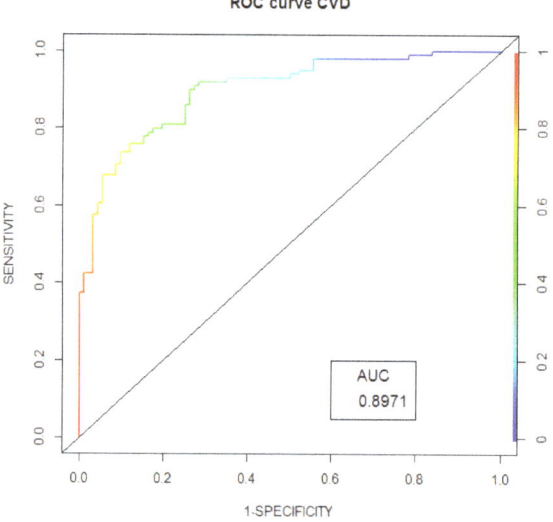

Figure 1. ROC curve in the prognostic model of the coronary heart disease (CHD) outcome when taking into account the index "cum LDL-C" in FH patients.

The characteristics of non-lipid risk factors in FH patients with MI are presented in Table 4, and lipid factors are presented in Table 5.

Table 4. Non-lipid risk factors and MI in FH patients.

Predictors	With MI (n = 52)	Without MI (n = 126)	p
Age, years	56.9 ± 11.9	47 ± 15	0.987
Males, n (%)	31 (59.6%)	47 (37.3%)	0.007
Creatinine, umol/L	96.2 ± 22.3	79 ± 15	0.0002
GFR, ml/min/1.73 m^2	70.4 ± 17.7	90 ± 23	0.0003
Glucose, mmol/L	5.0 ± 2.0	5.5 ± 1.2	0.172
BMI, kg/m^2	28.2 ± 37	27.0 ± 4.0	0.225
Waist size, cm	88.0 ± 11.9	80.0 ± 14.0	0.038
Age of onset of CHD, years	51.7 ± 0.18	58.0 ± 8.0	0.013
Hypertension, n (%)	41 (78.8%)	89 (70.6%)	0.063
Smoking, n (%)	22 (43.1%)	22 (18.2%)	0.001
Positive family history of CHD, n (%)	52 (100%)	71 (59.1%)	0.001

The data are presented in the form of average and standard deviation.

Table 5. Lipid risk factors and MI in FH patients.

Predictors	With MI (n = 52)	Without MI (n = 126)	p
Lp(a), g/L	0.67 ± 0.7	0.3 ± 0.42	0.008
TC initial, mmol/L	9.6 ± 1.7	10.0 ± 1.0	0.987
LDL-C initial, mmol/L	6.9 ± 1.4	7.0 ± 1.0	0.151
HDL-C initial, mmol/L	1.5 ± 0.5	2.0 ± 0.1	0.318
TG initial, mmol/L	1.8 ± 0.6	2.0 ± 1.0	0.574
TC on treatment, mmol/L	7 ± 2.2	8.0 ± 2.0	0.055
LDL-C on treatment, mmol/L	4.7 ± 2.0	5.0 ± 2.0	0.146
HDL-C on treatment, mmol/L/	17.0 ± 22	25.3 ± 23.6	0.047
TG on treatment, mmol/L	1.9 ± 0.7	2.0 ± 1.0	0.464
Percentage of TC reduction, %	17 ± 22	25.5 ± 14.6	0.048
Percentage of LDL-C reduction, %	46.8 ± 14.6	56.9 ± 11.9	<0.001
Cum LDL-C, mmol/L × years	50.0 ± 12.0	52.6 ± 10.3	0.500

The data are presented in the form of means and standard deviation.

In patients with MI the Lp(a) level was 0.67 ± 0.7 g/L, compared with 0.3 ± 0.42 mmol/L in patients without MI, p = 0.008. The TC and LDL-C concentrations were not significantly different in patients with and without MI. It should be noted that although the age of lipid-lowering therapy initiation in both groups did not differ, in patients with MI the lipid-lowering therapy was less intense. The percentage of TC and LDL-C reduction was 17.0 ± 22% and 21.0 ± 27.0% in patients with MI after 1 year, and 25.3 ± 23.6% (p = 0.047) and 31.5 ± 29.9% in patients without MI (p = 0.048). Gender differences were found between these subgroups: the number of men was more 31 (59.6%) in patients with MI than 47 (37.3%) in patients without MI, p = 0.007.

A positive family history of CHD was found in 52 (100%) patients with MI and 71 (59.1%) in patients without MI, p = 0.001.

Creatinine concentrations in patients with MI were significantly higher: 96.2 ± 22.3 umol/L vs. 79 ± 15 (p = 0.0002). The GFR according to the CKD-EPI formula was lower 70.4 ± 17.7 mL/min/1.73 m^2 in patients with MI compared with 90 ± 23 mL/min/1.73 m^2 in FH patients without MI, p = 0.0003. Additionally, among patients with MI the number of smokers was significantly higher: 22 (43.1%) compared with 22 (18.2%) in patients without MI, $p = 0.001$.

The logistic regression shows the most significant factors which determine the probability of MI in patients with FH: positive family history of CHD, gender, initial TC level, cum LDL-C/age, the presence of hypertension and smoking (Table 6).

Table 6. Statistical significance of coefficients in calculating the odds ratio of MI in FH patients (logistic regression).

Predictor	Coefficient	Statistical Error	OR	p
Deviation	−4.59	1.34	0.01	0.0006
Positive family history of CHD	1.69	0.46	5.42	0.0002
Male gender	1.11	0.43	3.03	0.010
TC initial	0.35	0.19	1.41	0.061
Cum LDL-C/age	−0.43	0.22	0.65	0.051
Hypertension	1.75	0.44	5.75	<0.0001
Smoking	1.07	0.44	2.92	0.015

Formula for calculating OR and MI probability: OR(MI) = exp − 4.59 + 1.69 × Family history + 0.35 × TC − 0.43 × cum LDL-C/age + 1.75 × Hypertension + 1.07 × smoking. P(MI) = 1/(1 + (1/OR)). The threshold classification = 0.19. If p (MI) < 0.19, MI is not predicted. If p (MI) ≥ 0.19, the MI is predicted. At the accepted threshold, the sensitivity is 81.8%; the specificity is 70.7%.

Figure 2 shows the ROC curve in the prognostic model of MI outcome in FH patients.

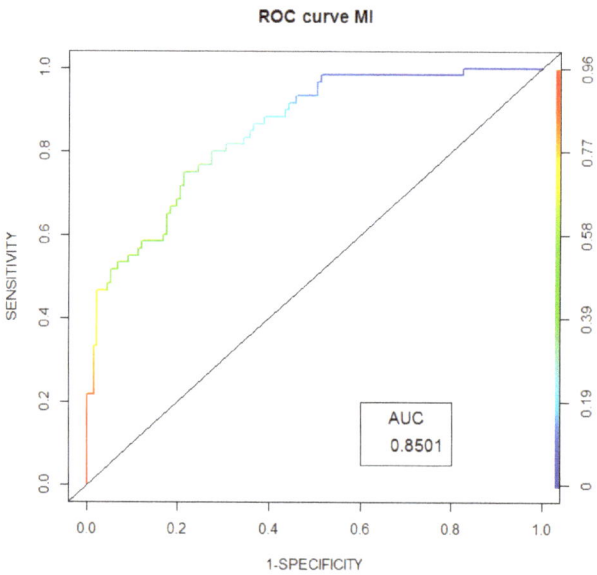

Figure 2. ROC curve of prognostic model of MI outcome in FH patients.

The combined end point (CEP) included MI, unstable angina, and ischemic stroke.

Non-lipid risk factors in patients with CP and FH are presented in Table 7; the lipid factors are presented in Table 8.

Table 7. Assessment of the global non-lipid risk factors impact for the development of the combined end point (CEP).

	With CEP (n = 68)	Without CEP (n = 120)	p
Age, years	57.4 ± 11.0	46.1 ± 14.5	<0.001
Males, n (%)	38 (55.9%)	47 (39.2%)	0.028
Creatinine, umol/L	93.4 ± 20.6	78.9 ± 15.6	<0.001
GFR, mL/min/1.73 m^2	71.6 ± 17.0	91.6 ± 22.6	<0.001
Glucose, mmol/L	5.4 ± 1.1	5.0 ± 1.7	0.128
BMI, kg/m^2	28.1 ± 4.1	27.0 ± 3.7	0.084
Waist size, cm	87.5 ± 11.9	79.9 ± 13.6	0.007
Age of CHD onset, years	51.1 ± 10.3	58.1 ± 7.5	<0.001
Hypertension, n (%)	58 (85.2%)	64 (53.3%)	<0.0001
Smoking, n (%)	30 (44.1%)	22 (18.3%)	0.0003
Positive family history of CHD, n (%)	60 (88.2%)	69 (57.5%)	<0.0001
CHD, n (%)	67 (98.5%)	34 (28.3%)	<0.0001

The data are presented in the form of means and standard deviation.

Table 8. Lipid risk factors in FH patients with combined end point (CEP).

	With CEP (n = 68)	Without CEP (n = 120)	p
Lp(a), g/L	0.63 ± 0.59	0.29 ± 0.42	0.001
TC initial, mmol/L	10.0 ± 1.9	9.4 ± 1.3	0.022
LDL initial, mmol/L	7.2 ± 1.6	6.8 ± 1.3	0.030
HDL initial, mmol/L	1.5 ± 0.5	1.6 ± 0.5	0.040
TG initial, mmol/L	1.8 ± 0.6	1.6 ± 0.7	0.293
TC on treatment, mmol/L	7.0 ± 2.2	8.0 ± 2.0	0.002
LDL-C on treatment, mmol/L	4.7 ± 2.1	5.4 ± 1.8	0.012
Percentage of TC reduction, %	28.3 ± 23.9	14.7 ± 20.6	0.00006
Percentage of LDL-C reduction, %	34.7 ± 30.0	18.3 ± 25.6	0.0001
Cum LDL-C, mmol/L × years	397.8 ± 125.4	309.2 ± 124.8	<0.001
Index "Cum LDL-C/age", mmol/L × years	57.4 ± 11.0	46.1 ± 14.5	<0.001
Age of hypolipidemic therapy start, years	52.5 ± 10.5	49.8 ± 12.0	0.173

The data are presented in the form of average and standard deviation.

In patients with CEP, the Lp(a) level was higher: 0.63 ± 0.59 g/L compared with 0.29 ± 0.42 g/L without CP, $p = 0.001$. A similar trend was noted for the TC and LDL-C concentrations. HDL-C concentrations were higher in patients without CEP: 1.6 ± 0.5 mmol/L compared with 1.5 ± 0.5 mmol/L in patients with CEP ($p = 0.040$). The cum LDL-C was significantly higher in FH patients with CEP: 397.8 ± 125.4 mmol/L × years compared to 309.2 ± 124.8 without CEP ($p < 0.001$). The ratio "cum LDL-C/age" was also higher in patients with CP: 57.4 ± 11.0 vs. 46.1 ± 14.5 ($p < 0.001$).

It should be noted that the age of lipid-lowering therapy initiation in both groups did not differ; however, the lipid-lowering therapy in patients with CEP was started later, and it was more intensive (the percentage of TC reduction was 28.3 ± 23.9% compared to 14.7 ± 20.6%, $p = 0.00006$). A similar trend was observed for the LDL-C level: 34.7 ± 30.0% in patients with CEP and 18.3 ± 25.6% in patients without CEP ($p = 0.0001$).

The age of CHD onset in patients without CEP was higher, at 58.1 ± 7.5 years compared to 51.1 ± 10.3 in patients with CEP ($p < 0.001$). There were gender differences between the subgroups with and without CEP; the number of men was equal to 55.9% in patients with CEP and to 39.2% in patients without CEP, $p = 0.028$.

Positive family history of CHD was found in more patients with CEP: 60 (88.2%) vs. 69 (57.5%), $p < 0.0001$. The BMI did not differ between the groups; the waist size was significantly higher in patients with CEP: 87.5 ± 11.9 cm vs. 79.9 ± 13.6 ($p = 0.007$).

The creatinine concentration in patients with CEP was significantly higher: 93.4 ± 20.6 umol/L vs. 78.9 ± 15.6 umol/L ($p < 0.001$), and GFR (CKD-EPI formula) was 71.6 ± 17.0 mL/min/1.73 m² in patients with CEP, and 91.6 ± 22.6 mL/min/1.73 m² in patients without CEP, $p < 0.001$. There was a significantly higher number of smokers among patients with CEP: 30 (44.1%) vs. (18.3%), $p = 0.0003$. The number of patients with hypertension was higher in patients with CEP: 58 (85.2%) vs. 64 (53.3%) in patients without CEP, $p < 0.0001$.

The logistic regression shows the most significant factors which determine the probability of CEP in patients with FH: positive family history of IHD, gender (male), age, hypertension and smoking (Table 9).

Table 9. Statistical significance of coefficients in calculating the odds ratio of the combined end point (CEP) in patients with FH.

Indicator	Coefficient	Statistical Error	OR (Exp)	p
Deviation	−8.03	1.32	0.0003	<0.0001
Positive family history of CHD	2.16	0.48	8.67	<0.0001
Male gender	1.18	0.48	3.25	0.014
Age	0.08	0.02	1.08	<0.0001
Hypertension	1.07	0.46	2.92	0.021
Smoking	1.09	0.48	2.97	0.024

Note: It can be stated that increasing the age by 10 years leads to an increase in the OR (CEP) by 2.16 times. Formula for calculating OR and CEP probability: OR (CEP) = exp(−8.03 + 2.16 × Family history of CHD + 1.18 × male Sex + 0.08 × Age + 1.07 × Hypertension + 1.09 × Smoking. R (CEP) = 1/(1 + (1/OR)). The classification threshold = 0.45. If p (CEP) is <0.45, the CEP is not predicted. If p (CEP) is ≥0.45, the development of a CEP is predicted. The sensitivity is 67.6%; the specificity is 81.3%.

Figure 3 shows ROC curve in the prognostic model of CEP outcome in FH patients.

The scale for assessing the risk of a combined end point developing in patients with certain and probable FH was developed using a prognostic formula, obtained by step-by-step logistic regression. All factors are available for evaluation in general clinical practice: age, gender, smoking, burdened heredity for cardiovascular diseases and the presence of arterial hypertension. The scale is presented separately for men and women. Of course, genetic analysis is an important prognostic factor in FH patients, but in real clinical practice a doctor usually only has information about the phenotypic manifestation of the disease.

Tables 10 and 11 are showing the scale for assessing the risk of CEP in patients with defined and probable FH for men and women.

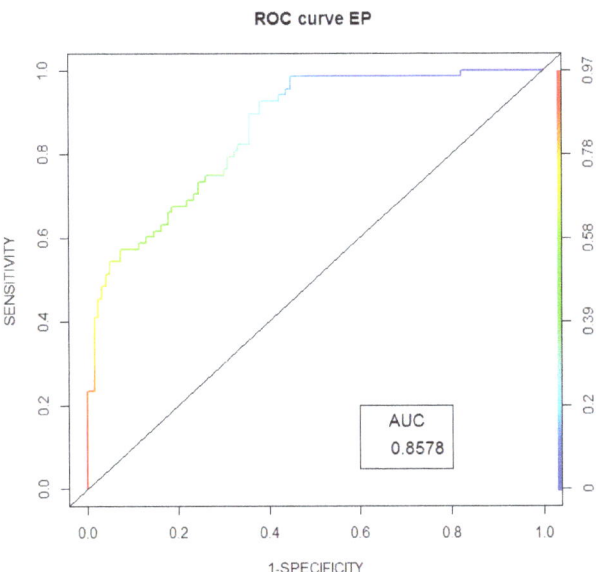

Figure 3. ROC curve in the prognostic model of CEP outcome in FH patients.

Table 10. Scale for assessing the risk of CEP developing in men with defined and probable familial hypercholesterolemia (FH).

	Men (Risk CEP Minimum)					
	Age < 30 years					
Positive family history	Yes	Yes	Yes	No	Yes	No
Hypertension	Yes	No	Yes	Yes	No	No
Smoking	Yes	Yes	No	Yes	No	No
	Age 30–42 years					
Positive family history	Yes	Yes	Yes	No	Yes	No
Hypertension	Yes	No	Yes	Yes	No	No
Smoking	Yes	Yes	No	Yes	No	No
	Age 43–56 years					
Positive family history	Yes	Yes	Yes	No	Yes	No
Hypertension	Yes	No	Yes	Yes	No	No
Smoking	Yes	Yes	No	Yes	No	No
	Age 56–83 years					
Positive family history	Yes	Yes	Yes	No	Yes	No
Hypertension	Yes	No	Yes	Yes	No	No
Smoking	Yes	Yes	No	Yes	No	No
	Age > 84 years					
Positive family history	Yes	Yes	Yes	No	Yes	No
Hypertension	Yes	No	Yes	Yes	No	No
Smoking	Yes	Yes	No	Yes	No	No

Note. Yes—the presence of a cardiovascular risk factors in the patient; no—the absence of a cardiovascular risk factors in the patient. Yellow background—high probability of CEP development (CEP development is predicted). Green background—low probability of CEP development (CEP development is not predicted).

Table 11. Scale for assessing the risk of combined end point developing in women with defined and probable FH.

	Women (Risk CP Minimum)					
	Age < 44 years					
Positive family history	Yes	Yes	No	Yes	No	No
Hypertension	Yes	No	Yes	No	No	No
Smoking	Yes	Yes	Yes	No	Yes	No
	Age 44–57 years					
Positive family history	Yes	Yes	No	Yes	No	No
Hypertension	Yes	No	Yes	No	No	No
Smoking	Yes	Yes	Yes	No	Yes	No
	Age 58–70 years					
Positive family history	Yes	Yes	No	Yes	No	No
Hypertension	Yes	No	Yes	No	No	No
Smoking	Yes	Yes	Yes	No	Yes	No
	Age 71–84 years					
Positive family history	Yes	Yes	No	Yes	No	No
Hypertension	Yes	No	Yes	No	No	No
Smoking	Yes	Yes	Yes	No	Yes	No
	Age ≥ 85 years					
Heredity	Yes	Yes	No	Yes	No	No
Hypertension	Yes	No	Yes	No	No	No
Smoking	Yes	Yes	Yes	No	Yes	No

Note. Yes—the presence of a cardiovascular risk factors in the patient; no—the absence of cardiovascular risk factors in the patient. Yellow background—high probability of CEP development (CEP development is predicted). Green background—low probability of CEP development (CEP development is not predicted).

Based on gender and age, one must look at the appropriate verse in Table 10 or Table 11 and ask whether the patient had the following three risk factors: positive family history, hypertension and smoking. Then evaluate the risk of combined end point developing in FH patients.

Limitations

The number of patients including in this study was not too big. The analysis performed validates a CV risk equation in a population of FH patients with either genetic or clinical diagnosis of FH. The study included only individuals living in northwestern part of Russia. The lack of a control group of patients with CV events and not affected by familial hypercholesterolemia can limit the strength of the findings.

5. Discussion

Classical cardiovascular risk factors and the Lp(a) concentration in FH patients play an important role in prognosis, but their contribution in FH may differ from the general population. Besides the genetic nature of the disease, other risk factors contribute, such as cumulative LDL levels. It was shown that LDL-C levels are more important than the type of mutation, reinforcing the concept that the phenotype is more important than the genotype in the risk of patients with familial hypercholesterolemia [12].

According to our data based on the results of the logistic regression analysis in patients with FH, cumulative LDL-C and the cumulative index "cum LDL-C/age" played a strong predictive role in the development of CHD in FH patients; it was greater than the role of TC and LDL-C concentrations.

Several predictive scales for FH patients were suggested, such as the Montreal—FH-Score and SAFEHEART registry; however, they were based only on classical risk factors (age, HDL-C, gender, hypertension and smoking). It is also important to take into account the indicator "cumulative level of LDL-C" for patients with FH [13,14].

The role of cum LDL-C was discussed in the literature [11,15]. The cholesterol-year-score is a simple tool which evaluates the duration and intensity of vascular exposure to elevated cholesterol levels [16], and it is a similar to that in which pack-year is used to measure lifelong exposure to tobacco [11]. An increased prevalence of early atherosclerotic burden has been observed in young FH subjects who present a high vascular cholesterol burden [17]. The cholesterol-year-score was first used in homozygous FH subjects [16] but its validation in FH patients has not been reported to date [11].

Early initiating of lipid-lowering therapy is very important. The cumulative burden of 6250 mg-years of LDL by age 50 years means that person has very likely already developed a large atherosclerotic plaque burden. As a result, lowering LDL-C after this cumulative exposure can reduce the risk of cardiovascular events, but this person will remain at relatively high "residual" risk of experiencing an acute cardiovascular event because one of the existing plaques can still disrupt and cause an acute coronary syndrome [15]. After the cumLDL-C exposure threshold has been exceeded, the incidence of MI appears to double with each increasing decade of exposure to the same plasma level of LDL-C. For example, the risk of MI increases from 1% after 5000 mg-years (129.2 mmol-years) of cumulative exposure to LDL-C by age 40 years, to 2% after 6250 mg-years (156.3 mmol-years) of exposure by the age 50 years, to 4% after 7500 mg-years (187.5 mmol-years) of exposure by the age 60 years [14].

In the study of Gallo A. the LDL-year score was a strong predictor of CV events in FH patients, especially in primary prevention. The CV risk is multiplied by 5.7-fold for patients with a cholesterol-year-score between 6000 and 16,000 mg/dL and by 17.4 for those with a cholesterol-year-score above 16,000 mg/dL. More interestingly, we observed that a LDL-C-year-score above 6000 mg/dL provided a similar CV risk to that in patients who had already suffered from a CV event, suggesting that earlier initiation of lipid lowering therapy might contribute to reduction in the incidence of CV events [16].

6. Conclusions

The "cum LDL-C" level plays a more important role in the development of CHD in FH patients than LDL-C. The index "cum LDL-C/age" has a still higher significance in the development of MI in FH patients, than LDL-C.

We present ROC-curves for CHD, MI and CEP in FH patients. We also present a prognostic scale for CHD development, which is based on classical cardiovascular risk factors.

Author Contributions: V.K.: substantial contributions to the conception of the work; analysis and interpretation of data for the work, analysis and interpretation of data for the work; agreement to be accountable for all aspects of the work. T.K.: analysis and interpretation of data for the work; final approval of the version to be published; agreement to be accountable for all aspects of the work. U.J.: substantial contributions to the conception of the work; analysis and interpretation of data for the work; final approval of the version to be published; agreement to be accountable for all aspects of the work. All authors have read and agreed to the published version of the manuscript.

Funding: This research received no external funding.

Institutional Review Board Statement: The study was conducted according to the guidelines of the Declaration of Helsinki, and approved by Ethics Committee of the Ministry of Health and Petrozavodsk State University (date of approval 14 November 2013), protocol code № 29. All patients included in the study signed informed consent. The principles of the study comply with the Helsinki Declaration.

Informed Consent Statement: Informed consent was obtained from all subjects involved in the study. Written informed consent has been obtained from the patient(s) to publish this paper.

Conflicts of Interest: The authors declare no conflict of interest.

References

1. Celermajer, D.; Sorensen, K.; Gooch, V.; Spiegelhalter, D.; Miller, O.; Sullivan, I.; Lloyd, J.; Deanfield, J. Non-invasive detection of endothelial dysfunction in children and adults at risk of atherosclerosis. *Lancet* **1992**, *340*, 1111–1115. [CrossRef]
2. Marais, A.D. Familial hypercholesterolemia. *Clin. Biochem. Rev.* **2004**, *5*, 49–68.
3. Nordestgaard, B.G.; Chapman, M.J.; Humphries, S.E.; Ginsberg, H.N.; Masana, L.; Descamps, O.S.; Wiklund, O.; Hegele, R.A.; Raal, F.J.; Defesche, J.C.; et al. European Atherosclerosis Society Consensus Panel. Familial hypercholesterolaemia is underdiagnosed and undertreated in the general population: Guidance for clinicians to prevent coronary heart disease: Consensus statement of the European Atherosclerosis Society. *Eur. Heart J.* **2013**, *34*, 3478–3490a. [PubMed]
4. Umans-Eckenhausen, M.A.; Sijbrands, E.; Kastelein, J.J.; Defesche, J.C. Low-Density Lipoprotein Receptor Gene Mutations and Cardiovascular Risk in a Large Genetic Cascade Screening Population. *Circulation* **2002**, *106*, 3031–3036. [CrossRef] [PubMed]
5. Sharifi, M.; Higginson, E.; Bos, S.; Gallivan, A.; Gallivan, D.; Li, K.W.; Abeysekera, A.; Haddon, A.; Ashby, H.; Shipman, K.E.; et al. Greater preclinical atherosclerosis in treated monogenic familial hypercholesterolemia vs. polygenic hypercholesterolemia. *Atherosclerosis* **2017**, *263*, 405–411. [CrossRef] [PubMed]
6. Mata, P.; Alonso, R.; Pérez de Isla, L. Atherosclerotic cardiovascular disease risk assessment in familial hypercholesterolemia: Does one size fit all? *Curr. Opin. Lipidol.* **2018**, *29*, 445–452. [CrossRef] [PubMed]
7. Genest, J.; Hegele, R.A.; Bergeron, J.; Brophy, J.; Carpentier, A.; Couture, P.; Davignon, J.; Dufour, R.; Frohlich, J.; Gaudet, D.; et al. Canadian Cardiovascular Society position statement on familial hypercholesterolemia. *Can. J. Cardiol.* **2014**, *30*, 1471–1481. [CrossRef] [PubMed]
8. Watts, G.F.; Gidding, S.; Wierzbicki, A.S.; Toth, P.P.; Alonso, R.; Brown, W.V.; Bruckert, E.; Defesche, J.; Lin, K.K.; Livingston, M.; et al. International Familial Hypercholesterol Foundation Integrated guidance on the care of familial hypercholesterolemia from the International FH Foundation. *Eur. J. Prev. Cardiol.* **2015**, *22*, 849–854. [CrossRef] [PubMed]
9. Gidding, S.S.; Champagne, M.A.; de Ferranti, S.D.; Ito, M.K.; Knowles, J.W.; McCrindle, B.; Raal, F.; Rader, D.; Santos, R.D.; Lopes-Virella, M.; et al. The agenda for familial hypercholesterolemia: A scientific statement from the American Heart Association. *Circulation* **2015**, *132*, 2167–2192. [CrossRef] [PubMed]
10. Gallo, A.; Charriere, S.; Vimont, A.; Chapman, M.J.; Angoulvant, D.; Boccara, F.; Cariou, B.; Carreau, V.; Carrié, A.; Bruckert, E.; et al. SAFEHEART risk-equation and cholesterol-year-score are powerful predictors of cardiovascular events in French patients with familial hypercholesterolemia. *Atherosclerosis* **2020**, *306*, 41–49. [CrossRef] [PubMed]
11. Santos, R.D.; Gidding, S.S.; Hegele, R.A.; Cuchel, M.A.; Barter, P.J.; Watts, G.F.; Baum, S.J.; Catapano, A.L.; Chapman, M.J.; Defesche, J.C.; et al. Defining severe familial hypercholesterolemia and the implications for clinical management: a consensus statement from the International Atherosclerosis Society Severe Familial Hypercholesterolemia Panel. *Lancet Diabetes Endocrinol.* **2016**, *4*, 850–861. [CrossRef]
12. Paquette, M.; Brisson, D.; Dufour, R.; Khoury, E.; Gaudet, D.; Baass, A. Cardiovascular disease in familial hypercholesterolemia: Validation and refinement of the Montreal-FH-SCORE. *J. Clin. Lipidol.* **2017**, *11*, 1161–1167. [CrossRef] [PubMed]
13. De Isla, L.P.; Alonso, R.; Mata, N.; Fernández-Pérez, C.; Muñiz, O.; Díaz-Díaz, J.L.; Saltijeral, A.; Fuentes-Jiménez, F.; de Andrés, R.; Zambón, D.; et al. Predicting Cardiovascular Events in Familial Hypercholesterolemia The SAFEHEART Registry (Spanish Familial Hypercholesterolemia Cohort Study). *Circulation* **2017**, *135*, 2133–2144. [CrossRef] [PubMed]
14. Ference, B.A.; Phill, M.; Graham, I.; Tokgozoglu, L.; Catapano, A.L. Impact of lipids on cardiovascular health. *J. Am. Coll. Cardiol.* **2018**, *10*, 1141–1156. [CrossRef] [PubMed]
15. Schmidt, H.H.; Hill, S.; Makariou, E.V.; Feuerstein, I.M.; Dugi, K.A.; Hoeg, J.M. Relation of cholesterol-year score to severity of calcific atherosclerosis and tissue deposition in homozygous familial hypercholesterolemia. *Am. J. Cardiol.* **1996**, *15*, 575–580. [CrossRef]
16. Gallo, A.; Giral, P.; Carrie, A.; Carreau, V.; Béliard, S.; Pharm, R.B.; Maranghi, M.; Arca, M.; Cluzel, P.; Redheuil, A.; et al. Early coronary calcifications are related to cholesterol burden in heterozygous familial hypercholesterolemia. *J. Clin. Lipidol.* **2017**, *11*, 704–711.e2. [CrossRef] [PubMed]
17. Mozaffarian, D.; Benjamin, E.J.; Go, A.S.; Arnett, D.K.; Blaha, M.J.; Cushman, M.; Das, S.R.; de Ferranti, S.; Després, J.P.; Fullerton, H.J.; et al. Executive Summary: Heart Disease and Stroke Statistics—2016 Update: A Report From the American Heart Association. *Circulation* **2016**, *133*, 447–454. [CrossRef] [PubMed]

Article

Associations of Antioxidant Enzymes with the Concentration of Fatty Acids in the Blood of Men with Coronary Artery Atherosclerosis

Viktoriya S. Shramko [1,*], Eugeniia V. Striukova [1], Yana V. Polonskaya [1], Ekaterina M. Stakhneva [1], Marina V. Volkova [1], Alexey V. Kurguzov [2], Elena V. Kashtanova [1] and Yuliya I. Ragino [1]

[1] Research Institute of Internal and Preventive Medicine, Branch of the Institute of Cytology and Genetics, Siberian Branch of Russian Academy of Sciences (IIPM–Branch of IC&G SB RAS), 175/1 B. Bogatkova Str., 630089 Novosibirsk, Russia; stryukova.j@mail.ru (E.V.S.); yana-polonskaya@yandex.ru (Y.V.P.); stahneva@yandex.ru (E.M.S.); marina_volkova91@mail.ru (M.V.V.); elekastanova@yandex.ru (E.V.K.); ragino@mail.ru (Y.I.R.)

[2] Federal State Budgetary Institution "National Medical Research Center Named Academician E.N. Meshalkin", Ministry of Health of the Russian Federation, Rechkunovskaya Str., 15, 630055 Novosibirsk, Russia; aleksey_kurguzov@mail.ru

* Correspondence: nosova@211.ru or shramko-90@inbox.ru

Abstract: Objective: To identify associations of fatty acids (FAs) with the antioxidant enzymes in the blood of men with coronary atherosclerosis and ischemic heart disease (IHD). Methods: The study included 80 patients: control group—20 men without IHD, the core group—60 men with IHD. The core group was divided into subgroups: subgroup A—with the presence of vulnerable atherosclerotic plaques, subgroup B—with the absence of vulnerable atherosclerotic plaques. We analyzed the levels of FAs, free radicals, superoxide dismutase (SOD), catalase (CAT), and glutathione peroxidase (GPx) in the blood. Results. Patients with IHD, compared with the control group: (1) had higher levels of SOD, CAT, myristic, palmitic, palmitoleic, and octadecenoic FAs; (2) had lower levels of GPx, α-linolenic, docosapentaenoic, docosahexaenoic, and arachidonic FAs. In subgroup A there were found: (1) negative associations of SOD—with linoleic, eicosatrienoic, arachidonic, eicosapentaenoic, docosapentaenoic and docosahexaenoic FAs, positive associations—with palmitic acid; (2) positive correlations of CAT level with palmitoleic and stearic acids; (3) negative associations between of GPx and palmitic, palmitoleic, stearic and octadecenoic FAs. Conclusions: Changes in the levels of antioxidant enzymes, and a disbalance of the FAs profile, probably indicate active oxidative processes in the body and may indicate the presence of atherosclerotic changes in the vessels.

Keywords: coronary atherosclerosis; ischemic heart disease; saturated fatty acids; monounsaturated fatty acids; polyunsaturated fatty acids; oxidative stress; superoxide dismutase; catalase; glutathione peroxidase

1. Introduction

It is widely acknowledged that atherosclerosis is a pathophysiological process that leads to the development of ischemic heart disease (IHD) [1,2]. According to data for 2013, the total incidence of IHD increased by 13.25% over 10 years, and the number of deaths amounted to 7.4 million people, which is a third of all deaths [3–5].

Currently, there is a unanimous opinion that oxidative stress plays a significant role in the pathogenesis of atherosclerosis [6]. A disbalance between pro-oxidants and the antioxidant defense of the body leads to the activation of the inflammatory signal and mitochondrial-mediated apoptosis, which, in turn, contributes to the occurrence and development of IHD [7]. Superoxide dismutase (SOD), catalase (CAT), and glutathione peroxidase (GPx) are some of the key enzymes of the antioxidant system.

The SOD is the most active enzyme against reactive oxygen species (ROS) in the myocardium [8]. Due to its antioxidant and anti-apoptotic properties, as well as the ability to inhibit cell hypertrophy, SOD plays a potential protective role against the occurrence of atherosclerosis [9]. However, it should be noted that the role of SOD in preventing free radical oxidation is not entirely obvious. Despite the high specificity of the enzyme, under certain conditions, SOD can interact with H_2O_2 and play the role of a pro-oxidant [10]. The CAT is a hydroperoxidase. CAT can interfere with apoptosis by attenuating the H_2O_2 signal, and thereby increase the life span of the cell [11,12]. Lei et al. [13] reported that overexpression of CAT protects against cardiovascular dysfunction. The GPx is a selenoprotein enzyme that protects the body from oxidative damage and supports vascular homeostasis [14,15]. GPx deficiency is associated with an increase in the number of oxidants associated with peroxide and subsequent chronic diseases, such as atherogenesis [16] and cardiovascular events [17].

There is evidence that changes in the level of fatty acids (FAs) can disrupt the redox state of cells, not only by increasing the production of ROS, but also by reducing the activity of antioxidant enzymes [18]. Accordingly, FAs are probably one of the physiological factors controlling oxidative stress [19]. Therefore, in our study, we decided to evaluate the relationship of the antioxidant system indicators with the FA concentration in the blood in coronary atherosclerosis.

2. Materials and Methods

The study was conducted in the framework of the research work program "IIPM–branch of IC&G SB RAS" jointly with the Federal State Budgetary Institution "National Medical Research Center named after Academician E.N. Meshalkin" of the Ministry of Health of the Russian Federation, as well as with the Novosibirsk Institute of Organic Chemistry SB RAS. The present study has a "descriptive" design.

The local Ethics Committee of the Research Institute of Internal and Preventive Medicine—Branch of the Institute of Cytology and Genetics, Siberian Branch of Russian Academy of Sciences approved the study (protocol №2, approval on 3 July 2017). Each patient gave written informed consent to participate in the study and for the processing of their data.

2.1. Subjects

The study included 80 people. The core group consisted of 60 men with coronary angiographically verified atherosclerosis of the coronary arteries, with IHD, with stable angina pectoris and without acute coronary syndrome (ACS), who was admitted to the clinic of the E. N. Meshalkin National Medical Research Center of the Ministry of Health of the Russian Federation for coronary bypass surgery (CBS). The age of the patients was 59.43 ± 7.38 years.

Inclusion criteria were male gender, diagnosis of IHD, verified by coronary angiography data, history of a previous myocardial infarction (MI) or episodes of stable angina pectoris (more than six months before admission), documented by the description of the clinical picture, the results of ECG and biochemical blood tests.

Exclusion criteria were being of female gender, clinically significant severe concomitant pathology in the acute stage (chronic infectious and inflammatory diseases, kidney failure, respiratory failure, liver failure), known active oncological diseases, hyperparathyroidism, toxic damage by heavy metals, and taking steroid and non-steroidal anti-inflammatory drugs.

As a control group, 20 men were taken from a population sample of Novosibirsk without IHD, comparable to the core group in terms of age and body mass index (BMI). Inclusion criteria were being of male gender, the absence of IHD, being verified by the results of a complete clinical and instrumental examination, and the absence of therapy with cardiovascular drugs. The screening of the control group was carried out based on IIPM—a branch of ICIG SB RAS. Table 1 presents the characteristics of patients in the core and control groups.

Table 1. Characteristics of patients in the core and control groups.

Parameter	Control Group (n = 20)	Core Group (n = 60)	p
Mean age, years (M ± SD)	56.7 ± 2.65	59.4 ± 7.38	0.116
BMI, kg/m² (M ± SD)	27.18 ± 2.49	29.05 ± 4.55	0.266
Systolic BP, mmHg (M ± SD)	130.64 ± 11.47	135.8 ± 11.45	0.204
Diastolic BP, mmHg (M ± SD)	83.33 ± 8.35	82.07 ± 9.64	0.741
Heart rate, beats per minute (M ± SD)	66.13 ± 7.21	68.16 ± 8.38	0.372
Tobacco use (absolute in %)	15%	15%	0.956
Alcohol use (absolute in %)	45%	50%	0.770
Lipid profile (M ± SD):			
Cholesterol, mg/dL	171.6 ± 10.75	202.83 ± 6.76	0.175
Triglycerides, mg/dL	87.45 ± 14.71	153.9 ± 11.38	0.005
HDL, mg/dL	47.6 ± 2.27	32.7 ± 1.17	0.010
LDL, mg/dL	110.5 ± 9.92	131.8 ± 7.14	0.092
Content of LPO in LDL after 30-min oxidation, nM MDA/mg LDL protein	16.43 ± 2.41	22.71 ± 10.25	0.053

Footnote: BMI—body mass index; BP—blood pressure; HDL—high-density lipoprotein; LDL—low-density lipoprotein; LPO—lipid peroxidation products; M—mean; MDA—malonic dialdehyde; SD—standard deviation.

According to the results of the histological analysis of intima-media pieces, 45% of the patients in the core group had vulnerable atherosclerotic plaques in coronary arteries (subgroup A), whereas in 55% of patients, no vulnerable atherosclerotic plaques were detected (subgroup B). Table 2 presents the clinical-biochemical characteristics of patients of the studied subgroups.

2.2. Methods

2.2.1. Histological Analysis

During CBS, patients underwent endarterectomy of the coronary arteries strictly according to intraoperative indications. All endarterectomy samples were sent for histological analysis to the pathomorphological laboratory of the "National Medical Research Center named after Academician E.N. Meshalkin". Each endarterectomy material containing the intima-media of the coronary arteries was divided longitudinally and transversely into 3–5 fragments for histological studies. The pathologist performed a macroscopic description of the samples (the prevalence of atherosclerotic plaque, the degree of the artery lumen narrowing, hemorrhages in the structures of atherosclerotic plaque, calcification sites, blood clots) and standard hematoxylin-eosin and Van Gieson staining, following which histological analysis of intima-media fragments was made using an Axiostar Plus binocular microscope.

A vulnerable atherosclerotic plaque was differentiated according to the following criteria: the thickness of the fibrous covering being less than 65 microns, infiltration by macrophages, and T-lymphocytes (more than 25 cells in the field of view of 0.3 mm), as well as a large lipid nucleus (more than 40%) [20].

2.2.2. Fatty Acids Analysis

The Laboratory of Environmental Research and Chromatographic Analysis of the Novosibirsk Institute of Organic Chemistry named after N. N. Vorozhtsov, SB RAS, carried out the determination of the qualitative and quantitative composition of FAs. After extraction and methanolysis, the composition of FAs was studied in all samples using high-efficiency capillary gas-liquid chromatography on an Agilent Technologies (AT) 6890N chromatograph with a flame ionization detector and chromatography-mass spectrometry on an AT 6890N chromatograph with an AT 5975N mass-selective detector. Studied the content of saturated FAs: myristic (C14:0), palmitic (C16:0), stearic (C18:0) and unsaturated FAs (essential unsaturated fatty acids): palmitoleic (C16:1, ω-7), octadecenoic (C18:1, ω-9), eicosenoic (C20:1, ω-9), linoleic (C18:2, ω-6), α-linolenic (C18:3, ω-3), γ-linolenic (C18:3, ω-6), eicosatrienoic (C20:3, ω-6), eicosapentaenoic (C20:5, ω-3), docosapentaenoic (C22:5, ω-3), docosahexaenoic (C22:6, ω-3) and arachidonic (C20:4, ω-6).

Table 2. Clinical-biochemical characteristics of patients of the subgroups.

Parameter	Subgroup A (n = 27)	Subgroup B (n = 33)	p
Mean age, years (M ± SD)	60.5 ± 6.48	58.6 ± 8.03	0.307
BMI, kg/m^2 (M ± SD)	29.91 ± 3.78	28.35 ± 5.05	0.191
Systolic BP, mmHg (M ± SD)	137.57 ± 12.75	134 ± 10.18	0.222
Diastolic BP, mmHg (M ± SD)	82.82 ± 9.86	81.45 ± 9.58	0.589
Heart rate, beats per minute (M ± SD)	69.63 ± 9.37	66.96 ± 7.4	0.222
Hypertensive disease (absolute in %):	96%	82%	0.362
History of heart attack (absolute in %)	81%	61%	0.082
Angina pectoris (absolute in %): II FC III FC IV FC	7% 70% 11%	21% 42% 12%	0.141 0.031 0.906
Multivessel coronary artery disease (absolute in %)	89%	82%	0.518
Tobacco use (absolute in %)	7%	21%	0.141
Alcohol use (absolute in %)	44%	56%	0.585
Dyslipidemia (absolute in %)	70%	73%	0.844
Lipid profile (M ± SD): Cholesterol, mg/dL Triglycerides, mg/dL HDL, mg/dL LDL, mg/dL Content of LPO in LDL after 30-min oxidation, nM MDA/mg LDL protein	202.5 ± 7.39 170.3 ± 12.44 32.5 ± 1.71 131.4 ± 6.47 21.71 ± 10.12	203.1 ± 11.01 171.4 ± 20.14 33 ± 1.6 132.1 ± 7.33 23.59 ± 10.57	0.963 0.993 0.855 0.945 0.601
History of type II diabetes (absolute in %)	37%	22%	0.241

Footnote: BMI—body mass index; BP—blood pressure; FC—functional class; HDL—high-density lipoprotein; LDL—low-density lipoprotein; LPO—lipid peroxidation products; M—mean; MDA—malonic dialdehyde; NYHA—New York Heart Association functional classification; SD—standard deviation.

2.2.3. Biochemical Studies

Peripheral (venous) blood sampling was performed in all patients included in the study (for patients of the core group before the CBS), at least 12 h after the last meal with a night's rest, as well as abstinence from physical exertion, stressful situations, physiotherapy, medication, alcohol use, smoking, and fatty foods. The blood was kept at room temperature for 30 min, then centrifuged at a speed of 1900 g for 15 min. Then, the blood specimens were separated into plasma or serum, and stored at −70 °C until analysis.

The Laboratory of Clinical Biochemical and Hormonal Studies of Therapeutic Diseases of IIPM–branch of IC&G SB RAS carried out the biochemical studies. The concentration of total cholesterol, triglycerides, and high-density lipoprotein (HDL) was determined by the enzymatic method using the Thermo Fisher Scientific kits on the Konelab Prime 30i biochemical analyzer (Thermo Fisher Scientific, Finland). The levels of LDL were calculated using the Friedwald formula. The level of lipid peroxidation products (LPO) in LDL isolated from blood serum was evaluated by the content of TBA-reactive products in LDL by the fluorimetric method on the Versafluor spectrofluorimeter, Bio-Rad. The free radical detection test (FORT) was evaluated using the FORM Plus CR3000 analyzer

(Callegary, Italy). The FORT colorimetric test is based on the ability of transition metals to catalyze the cleavage of hydroxyperoxides (ROOH) with the formation of free radicals. The reading of the FORT test results was based on a linear kinetic reaction. The absorption value was automatically converted into conventional units, called units H2O2. The CAT and GPx1 concentrations were evaluated by enzyme immunoassay (ELISA) using standard ELISA test systems (Cloud-Clone Corp., USA), Hu Cu/ZnSOD (SOD1) concentrations were evaluated using ELISA test systems (Bender MedSystems, Austria), on the MultiscanEX ELISA analyzer (Thermo Labsystem, Finland). These ELISA methods were designed for the quantitative determination of enzymes in serum, plasma, cell lysates, and so forth.

2.2.4. Statistical Methods

Statistical processing of the results was carried out using the IBM SPSS Statistics software package (version 20.0). The Kolmogorov–Smirnov test was used to assess the distribution of quantitative features. A comparative study of clinical and anamnestic characteristics in the groups was carried out using Student's t-test. In the text, these characteristics are presented in the form of an arithmetic mean (M) and a standard deviation (SD). In the presence of an abnormal distribution of signs (study of fatty acids and antioxidant enzymes), the nonparametric Mann–Whitney U-test was used (for two independent groups). The obtained data are presented in the form of a median (Me) with the interquartile range—the 25th and 75th percentiles. The Spearman rank correlation coefficient (r_s) was used to analyze the dependence of quantitative features of sample data from aggregates. Multiple logistic regression was used to assess the probability of the unstable atherosclerotic plaques presence in the coronary arteries. In the Table, the results are presented as a ratio of chances (OR) with a 95% confidence interval for OR. The difference in proportions and the nature of associations was evaluated by the Pearson criterion χ^2. The criterion of the statistical reliability of the obtained data was set at the level of $p < 0.05$.

3. Results

When assessing the levels of the lipid spectrum, men with IHD, compared with the control group, had increased levels of triglycerides by 1.7 times ($p = 0.005$) and decreased levels of HDL by 1.45 times ($p = 0.010$). The level of LPO increased by 1.4 times ($p = 0.053$) (Table 1).

When analyzing the clinical characteristics of the subgroups, it was revealed that a history of MI occurred in 81% of cases in subgroup A and 61% in subgroup B, but there was no statistically significant difference (Table 2). The angina pectoris of functional class (FC) III was established in 70% of men from subgroup A, which differed from subgroup B by 1.7 times ($p = 0.031$). To describe the severity of the chronic heart failure (CHF) symptoms was used FC classification following the criteria proposed by the New York Association of Cardiologists (NYHA) [21]. In subgroup A, the number of people with CHF of FC III was 92%, which significantly differed from subgroup B, where the number of people with CHF of FC III was 69% ($p = 0.027$). According to the results of coronary angiography, hemodynamically significant severe stenosis was found in all patients (>70% for all coronary arteries, except for the left main coronary artery, where stenosis > 50% is considered significant) [22].

When evaluating free radicals in the subgroups, we revealed significant differences from the Control group values ($p < 0.05$), but there were no significant differences between patients with the presence/absence of vulnerable atherosclerotic plaques (Figure 1).

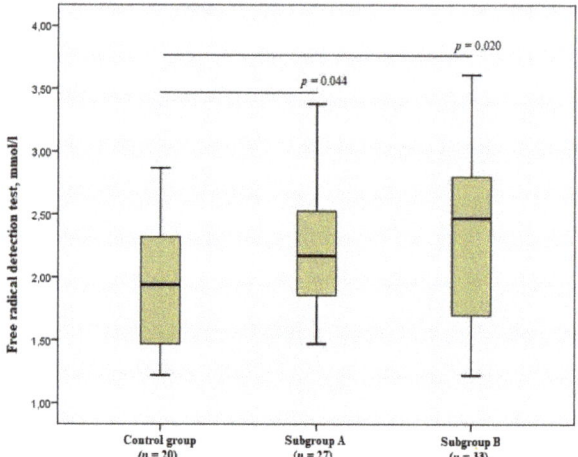

Figure 1. Free radical detection test in the group of men without ischemic artery disease (Control group), in the subgroup of men with ischemic artery disease and the presence of vulnerable atherosclerotic plaques in the coronary arteries (Subgroup A), and the subgroup of men with ischemic artery disease and the absence of vulnerable atherosclerotic plaques (Subgroup B), Me (25%; 75%). p—the significance of difference in comparison with the Control group.

When studying antioxidant enzymes, there was an increase in the level of SOD1 in subgroup A by 2.8 times and subgroup B by 2.5 times compared to the control group ($p < 0.001$) (Figure 2), however, there was no statistical difference between the subgroups.

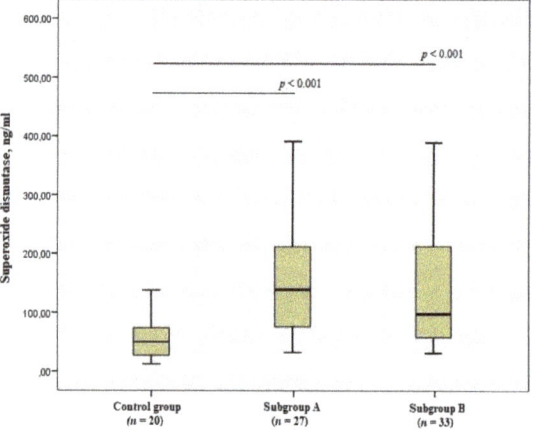

Figure 2. The content of superoxide dismutase in the blood of men without ischemic artery disease (Control group), men with ischemic artery disease and the presence of vulnerable atherosclerotic plaques in the coronary arteries (Subgroup A) and men with ischemic artery disease and the absence of vulnerable atherosclerotic plaques (Subgroup B), Me (25%; 75%). p—the significance of difference in comparison with the Control group.

There was a significant increase in the level of CAT in subgroup A by 1.3 times ($p = 0.019$) and subgroup B by 1.5 times ($p = 0.010$) compared to the control group (Figure 3), but there was no difference in the content of CAT between the subgroups ($p > 0.05$).

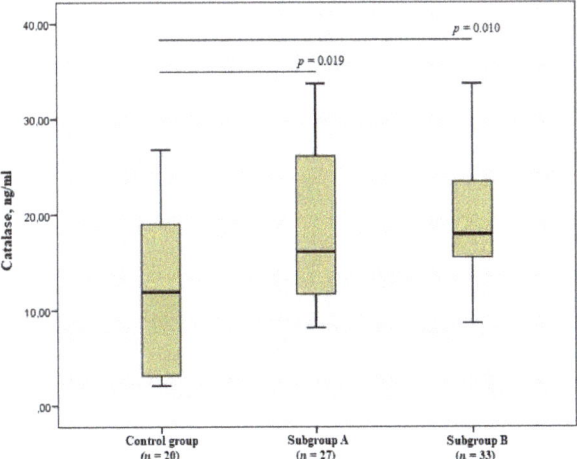

Figure 3. The blood catalase levels in the group of men without ischemic artery disease (Control group), in the subgroup of men with ischemic artery disease and the presence of vulnerable atherosclerotic plaques in the coronary arteries (Subgroup A) and the subgroup of men with ischemic artery disease and the absence of vulnerable atherosclerotic plaques (Subgroup B), Me (25%; 75%). p—the significance of difference in comparison with the Control group.

When studying GPx1, we obtained the opposite results—a significant decrease in the level of the enzyme in patients of the subgroups by 1.7 times compared with the control group ($p < 0.01$) (Figure 4).

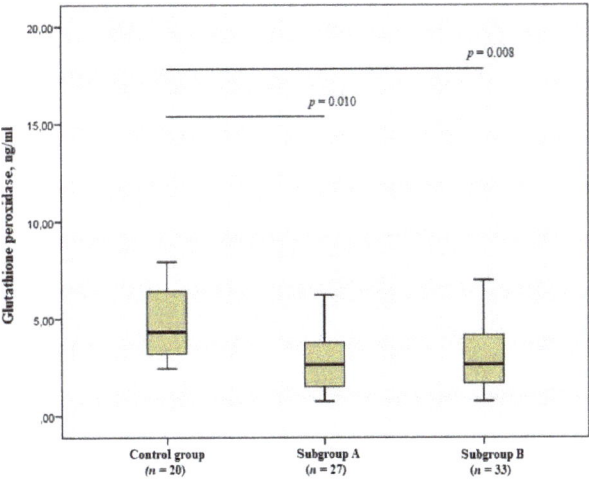

Figure 4. The concentrations of glutathione peroxidase in the blood of men without ischemic artery disease (Control group), men with ischemic artery disease and the presence of vulnerable atherosclerotic plaques in the coronary arteries (Subgroup A) and men with ischemic artery disease and the absence of vulnerable atherosclerotic plaques in the coronary arteries (Subgroup B), Me (25%; 75%). p—the significance of difference in comparison with the Control group.

When studying the distribution of FAs in blood serum, the comparative analysis showed a statistically significant increase in the total content of the saturated FAs (SFAs) fraction by 12% in subgroup A ($p < 0.01$) and by 8% in the subgroup B ($p < 0.05$) compared with the control group (Figure 5).

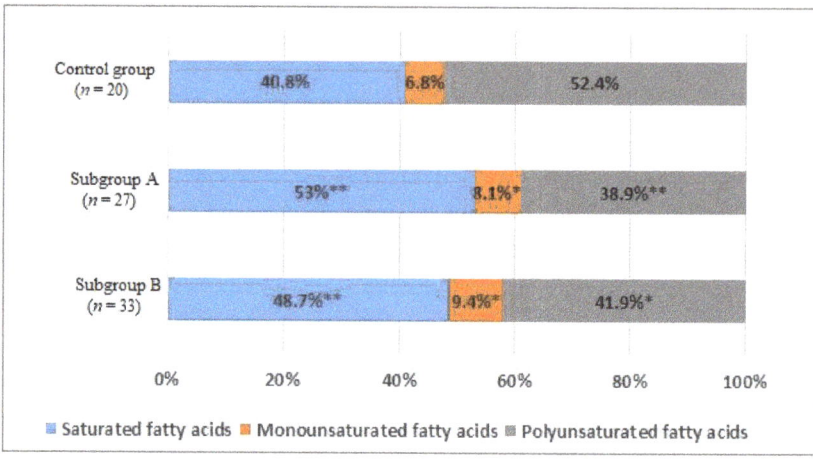

Figure 5. The percentage of saturated (SFAs), monounsaturated (MUFAs), and polyunsaturated fatty acids (PUFAs) of the total content of fatty acids in the blood of men without ischemic artery disease (Control group), men with ischemic artery disease and the presence of vulnerable atherosclerotic plaques in the coronary arteries (Subgroup A) and men with ischemic artery disease and the absence of vulnerable atherosclerotic plaques in the coronary arteries (Subgroup B), %. *—$p < 0.05$, **—$p < 0.01$, p—the significance of difference in comparison with the Control group.

Mainly due to an increase in the level of myristic acid by 1.3 and 1.8 times, respectively ($p < 0.05$), and the level of palmitic acid by 1.6 and 1.3 times, respectively ($p < 0.05$) (Table 3).

There was an increase in the total content of monounsaturated FAs (MUFAs) ($p < 0.05$) in subgroups compared with the group of men without IHD (Figure 5). An increase in the level of palmitoleic acid (1.6 times, $p < 0.01$) and octadecenoic acid (1.3 times, $p < 0.05$) was found (Table 3).

In addition, there was a decrease in the total content of polyunsaturated FAs (PUFAs) by 13.5% in subgroup A ($p < 0.01$) and by 10.5% in subgroup B ($p < 0.05$) (Figure 5). The level of ω-6 arachidonic acid in subgroup A decreased by 1.35 times, in subgroup B by 1.5 times ($p < 0.05$). The content of ω-3 docosapentaenoic acid in subgroup A was lower in 1.55 times, in subgroup B—1.9 times ($p < 0.05$); docosahexaenoic acid—1.4 and 1.7 times, respectively ($p < 0.05$). The level of α-linolenic acid only in subgroup A differed significantly from the values of the control group 1.6 times ($p < 0.05$) (Table 3).

The analysis of the FAs content did not reveal statistically significant differences between the subgroups.

Table 4 shows the results of the correlation analysis between the content of FAs and the antioxidant system enzymes in men of subgroup A.

Table 3. The content of FAs in the blood of men in Subgroups and in the Control group, Me (25%; 75%), mg/dL.

Fatty Acids	Control Group (n = 20)	Subgroup A (n = 27)	Subgroup B (n = 33)
Saturated fatty acids			
Myristic (C 14:0)	2.57 (1.01; 4.58)	3.37 (2.69; 6.21) *	4.72 (2.24; 5.49) *
Palmitic (C 16:0)	84.68 (37.42; 134.25)	132.66 (81.62; 145.8) *	105.65 (88.93; 142.72) *
Stearic (C 18:0)	29.34 (14.84; 49.39)	38.46 (23.9; 42.59)	33.79 (23.87; 38.79)
Monounsaturated fatty acids			
Palmitoleic (C 16:1, ω-7)	6.4 (2.23; 10.45)	10.13 (5.69; 15.45) **	10.3 (7.35; 12.76) **
Octadecenoic (C 18:1, ω-9)	11.97 (7.1; 15.18)	15.43 (12.78; 19.32) *	16.26 (11.9; 18.44) *
Eicosenoic (C 20:1, ω-9)	1.07 (0.42; 1.77)	1.1 (0.82; 1.32)	1.14 (0.85; 1.56)
Omega-3 polyunsaturated fatty acids			
α-linolenic (C 18:3, ω-3)	5.52 (1.22; 9.31)	3.32 (2.43; 3.51) *	3.86 (2.83; 4.96) *
Eicosapentaenoic (C 20:5, ω-3)	1.97 (1.32; 3.42)	2.3 (1.06; 3.09)	1.56 (0.91; 2.72)
Docosapentaenoic (C 22:5, ω-3)	1.77 (0.9; 2.73)	1.14 (0.62; 2.12) *	0.93 (0.57; 1.83) *
Docosahexaenoic (C 22:6, ω-3)	6.58 (3.38; 10.3)	4.62 (2.5; 8.57) *	3.96 (2.6; 7.12) *
Omega-6 polyunsaturated fatty acids			
Linoleic (C 18:2, ω-6)	110.94 (63.45; 179.86)	97.13 (72.34; 124.78)	96.94 (69.33; 120.92)
Arachidonic (C 20:4, ω-6)	16.65 (11.77; 35.94)	12.3 (8.24; 22.57) *	11.33 (7.67; 19.76) *
γ-linolenic (C 18:3, ω-6)	1.14 (0.75; 4.03)	1.47 (0.75; 2.29)	1.27 (0.56; 1.79)
Eicosatrienoic (C 20:3, ω-6)	5.27 (2.59; 8.12)	5.74 (3.59; 7.29)	4.24 (3.19; 6.74)

Footnote: * ($p < 0.05$); ** ($p < 0.01$) —the significance of difference in comparison with the Control group.

Table 5 shows the results of the correlation analysis between the content of FAs and the antioxidant system enzymes in men of subgroup B.

Significant inverse associations were established between the indicators of FORT and PUFAs—arachidonic and docosahexaenoic acids ($p < 0.05$) from the studied spectrum of FAs in the blood of patients with vulnerable plaques. When studying the indicators of the antioxidant system, negative correlations of the SOD level with PUFAs—linoleic, arachidonic, eicosapentaenoic, eicosatrienoic, docosapentaenoic, and docosahexaenoic ($p < 0.05$), and positive associations with palmitic acid ($p < 0.01$) were revealed. The positive correlations of the CAT level with the content of palmitoleic and stearic acids ($p < 0.05$) were revealed. The negative correlations were established between the concentrations of GPx and palmitic, palmitoleic, octadecenoic, and stearic acids ($p < 0.05$).

In men with atherosclerosis of the coronary arteries and the absence of vulnerable atherosclerotic plaques, the results of the correlation analysis were markedly different. The negative associations were established between FORT and all the PUFAs. For eicosenoic acid, a direct relationship was found; for eicosatrienoic, an inverse relationship with the SOD level was found ($p < 0.05$). The CAT levels are inversely dependent on the level of eicosatrienoic acid and directly on the level of octadecenoic acid ($p < 0.05$). In the subgroup of patients without vulnerable plaques, no significant associations with GPx were found.

Table 4. The associations between the content of FAs and the antioxidant system enzymes in men with ischemic artery disease and the presence of vulnerable atherosclerotic plaques in the coronary arteries (Subgroup A).

Fatty Acids	Rank Coefficients of Spearman Correlation (r_s)			
	FORT	SOD	CAT	GPx
Palmitic (C 16:0)	—	r = 0.515 p = 0.005	—	r = −0.339 p = 0.059
Palmitoleic (C 16:1, ω-7)	—	—	r = 0.373 p = 0.040	r = −0.331 p = 0.060
Stearic (C 18:0)	—	—	r = 0.412 p = 0.033	r = −0.375 p = 0.039
Octadecenoic (C 18:1, ω-9)	—	—	—	r = −0.372 p = 0.041
Linoleic (C 18:2, ω-6)	—	r = −0.430 p = 0.025	—	—
Eicosatrienoic (C 20:3, ω-6)	—	r = −0.453 p = 0.018	—	—
Arachidonic (C 20:4, ω-6)	r = −0.362 p = 0.043	r = −0.407 p = 0.035	—	—
Eicosapentaenoic (C 20:5, ω-3)	—	r = −0.464 p = 0.015	—	—
Docosapentaenoic (C 22:5, ω-3)	—	r = −0.464 p = 0.015	—	—
Docosahexaenoic (C 22:6, ω-3)	r = −0.388 p = 0.036	r = −0.549 p = 0.003	—	—

Footnote: CAT—catalase; FORT—free radical detection test; GPx—glutathione peroxidase; SOD—superoxide dismutase

To assess the probability of atherosclerotic changes in the coronary arteries depending on the content of antioxidant enzymes (Table 6), we used multivariate logistic regression analysis. The presence of vulnerable atherosclerotic plaques in the coronary arteries toward their absence was used as a dependent variable. The content of free radicals and all the antioxidant enzymes studied by us was used as independent variables.

Table 5. The associations between the content of FAs and the antioxidant system enzymes in men with ischemic artery disease and the absence of vulnerable atherosclerotic plaques in the coronary arteries (Subgroup B).

Fatty Acids	Rank Coefficients of Spearman Correlation (r_s)		
	FORT	SOD	CAT
Octadecenoic (C 18:1, ω-9)	—	—	r = 0.405 p = 0.019
Linoleic (C 18:2, ω-6)	r = −0.448 p = 0.009	—	—
α-linolenic (C 18:3, ω-3)	r = −0.390 p = 0.033	—	—
γ-linolenic (C 18:3, ω-6)	r = −0.388 p = 0.031	—	—

Table 5. Cont.

Fatty Acids	Rank Coefficients of Spearman Correlation (r_s)		
	FORT	SOD	CAT
Eicosenoic (C 20:1, ω-9)	—	r = 0.413 p = 0.017	—
Eicosatrienoic (C 20:3, ω-6)	r = −0.397 p = 0.022	r = −0.414 p = 0.017	r = −0.307 p = 0.053
Arachidonic (C 20:4, ω-6)	r = −0.512 p = 0.002	—	—
Eicosapentaenoic (C 20:5, ω-3)	r = −0.471 p = 0.006	—	—
Docosapentaenoic (C 22:5, ω-3)	r = −0.518 p = 0.002	—	—
Docosahexaenoic (C 22:6, ω-3)	r = −0.588 p = 0.0001	—	—

Footnote: CAT—catalase; FORT—free radical detection test; SOD—superoxide dismutase.

Table 6. Results of a multivariate logical regression analysis for predicting coronary artery atherosclerosis by the activity of antioxidant enzymes.

Antioxidant Enzymes	B	Exp(B)	95.0% C.I. for Exp(B)		p
			Lower	Upper	
FORT	0.396	1.485	0.428	5.157	0.533
SOD	0.020	1.020	1.003	1.037	0.019
CAT	0.107	1.113	1.001	1.239	0.050
GPx	−0.096	0.908	0.753	1.095	0.314

Footnote: CAT—catalase; C.I.—confidence interval, Exp(B)—odds ratio; FORT—free radical detection test; GPx—glutathione peroxidase; SOD—superoxide dismutase.

The results showed that an increase in the content of SOD and CAT in the blood is associated with a relative risk of having vulnerable atherosclerotic plaques in the coronary arteries.

4. Discussion

The study of the lipid profile, including the FAs profile, is a promising direction in clinical diagnostics for the early detection of persons with a high risk of CVD.

We have obtained data on the increase in the level of myristic and palmitic SFAs in the blood of patients with IHD, which is consistent with the data in the literature. Lausada et al. [23] identified that in the blood plasma of patients with IHD, there is a significant increase in SFAs, mainly due to palmitic acid, and, to a lesser extent, oleic and stearic acids, compared with the control groups. In a large-scale study, CIRCS [24], the authors found that high levels of saturated myristic and palmitic FAs had the most adverse effect on the development of CVD. Björck et al. [25], in their study, concluded that an increase in the consumption of SFAs affects the growth of total cholesterol in the blood and, therefore, positively influenced mortality from IHD. Conversely, even a moderate decrease in the SFA content and replacing them with PUFAs in the diet significantly reduced the risk of developing CVD [26].

Therefore, the determination of the content of SFAs in the blood, especially palmitic and myristic, can be used in the clinical diagnosis of atherosclerosis-associated diseases.

When studying the content of MUFAs, we obtained a significant increase in the content of palmitoleic and octadecenoic FAs in the group of patients with atherosclerosis, which probably indicates that these FAs are associated with CVD risk. Several researchers have found an association between palmitoleic acid and cardiovascular risk factors [27].

Chei et al. [24] found that high levels of palmitoleic acid increased the risk of IHD. On the contrary, data from some controlled randomized trials have shown that MUFAs have a beneficial effect on the profile of lipoproteins in the blood, and as a consequence, on reducing the risk of CVD [28]. The results obtained may cast doubt on the supposed positive effects of MUFAs in the body, particularly in IHD.

Increasingly more studies are being published showing the influence not only of SFAs, and some MUFAs on CVD, but also the effect of PUFAs [26]. According to our data, in the core group of men with IHD, the content of very long-chain omega-3 PUFAs (such as docosapentaenoic and docosahexaenoic FAs) and arachidonic omega-6 PUFA was significantly lower when compared with the control group. That suggests that even in the subgroups of PUFAs, specific individual FAs may have a different impact on the risk of developing IHD [24]. In addition, in recent years, the complex biochemistry of eicosanoids has become clearer, so the very class of omega-6 PUFAs can no longer be so simply considered as pro-inflammatory [29].

On the one hand, obtained high levels of SFAs and MUFAs can probably block the bioavailability of PUFAs for cells and form a deficiency of PUFAs in cells, which contributes to the development of the atherosclerotic process [30]. On the other hand, the high degree of unsaturation of PUFAs makes these FAs very susceptible to oxidation, which makes them "harmful" and leads to an increase in the number of oxidative molecules that trigger inflammatory reactions [19,31].

Oxidative stress occurs due to an imbalance between the production of ROS and a decrease in the overall antioxidant capacity. We studied the levels of free radicals and antioxidant indicators as markers of oxidative stress. Excessive formation of H_2O_2 was found in patients with atherosclerosis and, accordingly, a high degree of oxidative damage by free radicals. The reduced content of individual PUFAs in the blood of patients with atherosclerosis, as well as increased lipid peroxidation, confirms the influence of oxidative stress on the pathogenesis of IHD.

Currently, increasingly more attention is being paid to the quantitative assessment of antioxidant enzymes. Under normal conditions, SOD is the first line of defence against oxidative stress [7]. A meta-analysis conducted by Flores-Mateo et al. [32], which included 26 case-control studies, evaluated the relationship between the level of activity of SOD and IHD. In most studies, inverse associations between SOD and the outcome of IHD were found, although they were not always statistically significant [32]. In our study, there was a significant increase in the level of the SOD enzyme in the blood serum of patients with IHD, compared with the control group. Vichova et al. [33], in their work, reported that oxidative stress directly triggers the cascade of inflammation and accelerates the oxidation of lipids containing PUFAs, causing vulnerability of atherosclerotic plaques. This explains the direct relationship between we obtained the SOD level and a lower PUFAs content in patients with vulnerable plaques since the high production of the SOD enzyme is aimed at neutralizing oxidative damage by free radicals.

Whenever ROS are involved, CAT, together with other enzymes, forms a reliable defence of the body [34,35]. Overexpression of CAT has been reported to prevent the stimulation of ROS and protect against cardiovascular dysfunction or injury [14,36]. A study by Gupta et al. [37] showed that in the early stages of IHD, the levels of SOD and CAT increased to protect and prevent lipid peroxidation. Our study also shows an increase in SOD and CAT levels in patients with IHD, despite the prolonged course of the disease. Animal studies have shown that oleic acid (C 18: 1) induces an increase in the level of H_2O_2 [38]. In our study, the increased level of CAT was directly related to the content of octadecenoic acid (C 18:1) in the group of patients with atherosclerosis. We suggest that this may be due to excessive production of H_2O_2 in the vessels of these patients.

SOD oxidation (mainly by H_2O_2) can affect His residues (oxidized to 2-oxo derivatives), and catalase can be oxidatively modified after reaction with H_2O_2 or malondialdehyde (which results from the OH radical generated by either the Haber-Weiss or Fenton reactions). It is likely that the measured circulating concentrations of these enzymes may not be strictly related to endogenous antioxidant defences, as the mentioned modifications lead to decreased activity of these enzymes.

The GPx is another intracellular antioxidant, the deficiency of which is associated with atherogenesis [17] and the occurrence of IHD [39]. A meta-analysis, which included 32 case-control studies and two prospective cohort studies, showed there was significant heterogeneity in the direction and magnitude of the relationship between GPx and the outcomes of IHD, although, in most studies, an inverse relationship with IHD was found [32]. In our study, the GPx level in men with atherosclerosis was significantly lower than in the control group. Codoñer-Franch et al. [40] showed that following a diet with a reduced content of SFAs for six months significantly improved the antioxidant ability in the form of increased activity of SOD, CAT, and GPx. In our study, we obtained an inverse association between the GPx level and the SFAs content in patients with vulnerable plaques, which probably indicates a violation of the antioxidant defence system and contributes to the development of cardiovascular complications.

In addition, we wanted to assess the probability of the presence of vulnerable atherosclerotic plaques in the coronary arteries, depending on the content of antioxidant enzymes. According to multivariate regression analysis, it can be assumed that in patients with IHD, high levels of SOD and CAT in the blood are associated with a relative risk of destabilization of atherosclerotic plaques. Therefore, it is necessary to carry out a complex of preventive and therapeutic measures to prevent the development of acute coronary syndrome.

Limitations

One of the limitations of our study is the small sample size, since our study is a pilot. Our findings need further confirmation in a larger study, with a sufficient sample size to allow meta-analyses to determine specific risk profiles. In addition, frozen biomaterial was used in this work. Therefore, it was decided to determine the concentrations of antioxidant enzymes without studying their activity. Since the measured circulating concentrations do not determine the true antioxidant capacity, and an increased activity may normalize or aggregate the differences that are currently observed, it is necessary to measure activity in follow-up studies. Finally, this type of study cannot demonstrate a causal relationship because it is a descriptive, not an experimental study.

5. Conclusions

Changes in the levels of antioxidant enzymes, and a disbalance in the FA profile, may probably indicate active oxidative processes in the body and indicate the presence of atherosclerotic changes in the vessels. In addition, changes in the levels of SOD and CAT in the blood of patients with an already established diagnosis of IHD may indicate the presence of destabilizing (i.e., vulnerable) atherosclerotic plaques in the coronary arteries, which requires further study.

Author Contributions: Conceptualization, V.S.S. and Y.V.P.; methodology, Y.I.R.; software, E.V.K.; validation, E.V.S. and E.V.K.; formal analysis, E.M.S. and M.V.V.; investigation, V.S.S. and Y.V.P.; resources, A.V.K.; data curation, A.V.K. and E.V.K.; writing—original draft preparation, V.S.S. and E.V.S.; writing—review and editing, Y.V.P., E.M.S. and E.V.K.; visualization, V.S.S.; supervision, Y.V.P. and Y.I.R.; project administration, Y.I.R.; funding acquisition, Y.I.R. All authors have read and agreed to the published version of the manuscript.

Funding: The study was conducted within the framework of: budget topic under State Task No. AAAA-A17-117112850280-2, with the support of bioresource collections; financial support from the Government of the Novosibirsk Region and RFBR grant No. 19-315-90013 (2019–2021).

Institutional Review Board Statement: This study was approved by the local Ethics Committee of the Research Institute of Internal and Preventive Medicine—Branch of the Institute of Cytology and Genetics, Siberian Branch of Russian Academy of Sciences (protocol №2, approval on 3 July 2017).

Informed Consent Statement: Informed consent was obtained from all subjects involved in the study.

Data Availability Statement: The datasets before and after analysis in this study are available from the corresponding author on reasonable request.

Conflicts of Interest: The authors declare no conflict of interest. The funders had no role in the design of the study; in the collection, analyses, or interpretation of data; in the writing of the manuscript, or in the decision to publish the results.

References

1. Ling, P.; Shan, W.; Zhai, G.; Qiu, C.; Liu, Y.; Xu, Y.; Yang, X. Association between glutathione peroxidase-3 activity and carotid atherosclerosis in patients with type 2 diabetes mellitus. *Brain Behav.* **2020**, *10*, e01773. [CrossRef]
2. Souiden, Y.; Mallouli, H.; Meskhi, S.; Chaabouni, Y.; Rebai, A.; Chéour, F.; Mahdouani, K. MnSOD and GPx1 polymorphism relationship with coronary heart disease risk and severity. *Biol. Res.* **2016**, *49*, 22. [CrossRef] [PubMed]
3. Bogachevskaia, S.A.; Bondar, V.Y.; Kapitonenko, N.A.; Kapitonenko, K.A.; Bogatchevskiy, A.N. Epidemiology of the circulatory system diseases requiring high-technology medical care in the Russian Federation over the past 10 years. statistical "gaps". *Far East. Med. J.* **2015**, *2*, 112–116. (In Russian)
4. Yang, X.; Li, Y.; Ren, X.; Xiong, X.; Wu, L.; Li, J.; Wang, J.; Gao, Y.; Shang, H.; Xing, Y. Effects of exercise-based cardiac rehabilitation in patients after percutaneous coronary intervention: A meta-analysis of randomized controlled trials. *Sci. Rep.* **2017**, *7*, srep44789. [CrossRef] [PubMed]
5. Kelly, B.B.; Narula, J.; Fuster, V. Recognizing Global Burden of Cardiovascular Disease and Related Chronic Diseases. *Mt. Sinai J. Med. A J. Transl. Pers. Med.* **2012**, *79*, 632–640. [CrossRef] [PubMed]
6. Goncharov, N.V.; Avdonin, P.V.; Nadeev, A.D.; Zharkikh, I.L.; Jenkins, R.O. Reactive Oxygen Species in Pathogenesis of Atherosclerosis. *Curr. Pharm. Des.* **2015**, *21*, 1134–1146. [CrossRef]
7. Soto, M.E.; Soria-Castro, E.; Guarner-Lans, V.; Ontiveros, E.M.; Mejía, B.I.H.; Hernandez, H.J.M.; García, R.B.; Herrera, V.; Pérez-Torres, I. Analysis of Oxidative Stress Enzymes and Structural and Functional Proteins on Human Aortic Tissue from Different Aortopathies. *Oxidative Med. Cell. Longev.* **2014**, *2014*, 760694. [CrossRef] [PubMed]
8. Dubois-Deruy, E.; Peugnet, V.; Turkieh, A.; Pinet, F. Oxidative Stress in Cardiovascular Diseases. *Antioxidants* **2020**, *9*, 864. [CrossRef]
9. Peng, J.-R.; Lu, T.-T.; Chang, H.-T.; Ge, X.; Huang, B.; Li, W.-M. Elevated Levels of Plasma Superoxide Dismutases 1 and 2 in Patients with Coronary Artery Disease. *BioMed Res. Int.* **2016**, *2016*, 3708905. [CrossRef]
10. Svistunov, A.A.; Chesnokova, N.P.; Barsukov, V.Y.; Selezneva, T.D.; Zyablov, E.V. Activation of Lipoperoxidation Pro-cesses as a Typical Process of Cell Biomembrane Destabilization at Neoplasias of Different Localization. *Saratov J. Med. Sci. Res.* **2010**, *6*, 267–270. (In Russian)
11. Dias, A.E.M.S.; Melnikov, P.; Cônsolo, L.Z.Z. Oxidative stress during coronary bypass artery grafting. *Rev. Bras. Cir. Cardiovasc.* **2015**, *30*, 417–424. [CrossRef]
12. Tehrani, H.S.; Moosavi-Movahedi, A.A. Catalase and its mysteries. *Prog. Biophys. Mol. Biol.* **2018**, *140*, 5–12. [CrossRef]
13. Lei, X.G.; Zhu, J.-H.; Cheng, W.-H.; Bao, Y.; Ho, Y.-S.; Reddi, A.R.; Holmgren, A.; Arnér, E. Paradoxical Roles of Antioxidant Enzymes: Basic Mechanisms and Health Implications. *Physiol. Rev.* **2016**, *96*, 307–364. [CrossRef]
14. Lee, Y.S.; Kim, A.Y.; Choi, J.W.; Kim, M.; Yasue, S.; Son, H.J.; Masuzaki, H.; Park, K.S.; Kim, J.B. Dysregulation of Adipose Glutathione Peroxidase 3 in Obesity Contributes to Local and Systemic Oxidative Stress. *Mol. Endocrinol.* **2008**, *22*, 2176–2189. [CrossRef] [PubMed]
15. Voetsch, B.; Loscalzo, J.; Westerbacka, J.; Bergholm, R.; Tiikkainen, M.; Yki-Järvinen, H. Genetic Determinants of Arterial Thrombosis. *Arter. Thromb. Vasc. Biol.* **2004**, *24*, 216–229. [CrossRef]
16. Wickremasinghe, D.; Peiris, H.; Chandrasena, L.G.; Senaratne, V.; Perera, R. Case control feasibility study assessing the association between severity of coronary artery disease with Glutathione Peroxidase-1 (GPX-1) and GPX-1 polymorphism (Pro198Leu). *BMC Cardiovasc. Disord.* **2016**, *16*, 111. [CrossRef]
17. Pastori, D.; Pignatelli, P.; Farcomeni, A.; Menichelli, D.; Nocella, C.; Carnevale, R.; Violi, F. Aging-Related Decline of Glutathione Peroxidase 3 and Risk of Cardiovascular Events in Patients with Atrial Fibrillation. *J. Am. Heart Assoc.* **2016**, *5*, e003682. [CrossRef] [PubMed]
18. Azevedo-Martins, A.K.; Curi, R. Fatty acids decrease catalase activity in human leukaemia cell lines. *Cell Biochem. Funct.* **2007**, *26*, 87–94. [CrossRef] [PubMed]
19. Catalá, A. A synopsis of the process of lipid peroxidation since the discovery of the essential fatty acids. *Biochem. Biophys. Res. Commun.* **2010**, *399*, 318–323. [CrossRef] [PubMed]
20. Waksman, R.; Seruys, P.W. *Handbook of the Vulnerable Plaque*; CRC Press: London, UK, 2004.
21. Aronov, D.M.; Lupanov, V.P. Atherosclerosis and coronary heart disease: Some aspects of pathogenesis. *Atheroscler. Dyslipidemia* **2011**, *1*, 48–56. (In Russian)
22. Cury, R.C.; Abbara, S.; Achenbach, S.; Agatston, A.; Berman, D.S.; Budoff, M.J.; Dill, K.E.; Jacobs, J.E.; Maroules, C.D.; Rubin, G.; et al. Coronary Artery Disease—Reporting and Data System (CAD-RADS). *JACC Cardiovasc. Imaging* **2016**, *9*, 1099–1113. [CrossRef] [PubMed]
23. Lausada, N.R.; Boullón, S.; Boullón, F.; de Gomez Dumm, I.T. Erythrocyte membrane, plasma and atherosclerotic plaque lipid pattern in coro-nary heart disease. *Med. B. Aires* **2007**, *67*, 451–457.
24. Chei, C.-L.; Yamagishi, K.; Kitamura, A.; Kiyama, M.; Sankai, T.; Okada, T.; Imano, H.; Ohira, T.; Cui, R.; Umesawa, M.; et al. Serum Fatty Acid and Risk of Coronary Artery Disease—Circulatory Risk in Communities Study (CIRCS). *Circ. J.* **2018**, *82*, 3013–3020. [CrossRef]

25. Björck, L.; Rosengren, A.; Winkvist, A.; Capewell, S.; Adiels, M.; Bandosz, P.; Critchley, J.; Boman, K.; Guzman-Castillo, M.; O'Flaherty, M.; et al. Changes in Dietary Fat Intake and Projections for Coronary Heart Disease Mortality in Sweden: A Simulation Study. *PLoS ONE* **2016**, *11*, e0160474. [CrossRef]
26. Shramko, V.S.; Polonskaya, Y.V.; Kashtanova, E.V.; Stakhneva, E.M.; Ragino, Y.I. The Short Overview on the Relevance of Fatty Acids for Human Cardiovascular Disorders. *Biomolecules* **2020**, *10*, 1127. [CrossRef] [PubMed]
27. Frigolet, M.E.; Gutiérrez-Aguilar, R. The Role of the Novel Lipokine Palmitoleic Acid in Health and Disease. *Adv. Nutr.* **2017**, *8*, 173S–181S. [CrossRef]
28. Joris, P.J.; Mensink, R.P. Role of cis-Monounsaturated Fatty Acids in the Prevention of Coronary Heart Disease. *Curr. Atheroscler. Rep.* **2016**, *18*, 38. [CrossRef] [PubMed]
29. Wang, Y.; Wang, H.; Howard, A.G.; Tsilimigras, M.C.; Avery, C.L.; Meyer, K.A.; Sha, W.; Sun, S.; Zhang, J.; Su, C.; et al. Gut Microbiota and Host Plasma Metabolites in Association with Blood Pressure in Chinese Adults. *Hypertension* **2020**, *77*, 706–717. [CrossRef]
30. Titov, V.N. Cholesterol, biological role at phylogenetic stages, mechanisms of sterol synthesis inhibition by statins, phar-macogenomics factors and diagnostic value of low-density lipoprotein cholesterol. *Eurasian J. Cardiol.* **2016**, *1*, 56–66. (In Russian)
31. Mesa, M.; Olza, J.; Gonzalez-Anton, C.; Aguilera, C.; Moreno-Torres, R.; Jimenez, A.; de la Cruz, A.P.; Ruperez, A.I.; Gil, A. Changes in Oxidative Stress and Inflammatory Biomarkers in Fragile Adults over Fifty Years of Age and in Elderly People Exclusively Fed Enteral Nutrition. *Oxidative Med. Cell. Longev.* **2015**, *2015*, 5709312. [CrossRef] [PubMed]
32. Flores-Mateo, G.; Carrillo-Santisteve, P.; Elosua, R.; Guallar, E.; Marrugat, J.; Bleys, J.; Covas, M.-I. Antioxidant Enzyme Activity and Coronary Heart Disease: Meta-analyses of Observational Studies. *Am. J. Epidemiol.* **2009**, *170*, 135–147. [CrossRef] [PubMed]
33. Vichova, T.; Motovska, Z. Oxidative stress: Predictive marker for coronary artery disease. *Exp. Clin. Cardiol.* **2013**, *18*, e88–e91. [PubMed]
34. Orsi, N.M.; Leese, H.J. Protection against reactive oxygen species during mouse preimplantation embryo development: Role of EDTA, oxygen tension, catalase, superoxide dismutase and pyruvate. *Mol. Reprod. Dev.* **2001**, *59*, 44–53. [CrossRef]
35. Birben, E.; Sahiner, U.M.; Sackesen, C.; Erzurum, S.; Kalayci, O. Oxidative Stress and Antioxidant Defense. *World Allergy Organ. J.* **2012**, *5*, 9–19. [CrossRef]
36. Maiellaro-Rafferty, K.; Weiss, D.; Joseph, G.; Wan, W.; Gleason, R.L.; Taylor, W.R. Catalase overexpression in aortic smooth muscle prevents pathological mechanical changes underlying abdominal aortic aneurysm formation. *Am. J. Physiol. Circ. Physiol.* **2011**, *301*, H355–H362. [CrossRef]
37. Gupta, S.; Sodhi, S.; Mahajan, V. Correlation of antioxidants with lipid peroxidation and lipid profile in patients suffering from coronary artery disease. *Expert Opin. Ther. Targets* **2009**, *13*, 889–894. [CrossRef] [PubMed]
38. Schönfeld, P.; Wojtczak, L. Fatty acids as modulators of the cellular production of reactive oxygen species. *Free Radic. Biol. Med.* **2008**, *45*, 231–241. [CrossRef]
39. Schnabel, R.; Lackner, K.J.; Rupprecht, H.J.; Espinola-Klein, C.; Torzewski, M.; Lubos, E.; Bickel, C.; Cambien, F.; Tiret, L.; Münzel, T.; et al. Glutathione Peroxidase-1 and Homocysteine for Cardiovascular Risk Prediction: Results from the AtheroGeneStudy. *J. Am. Coll. Cardiol.* **2005**, *45*, 1631–1637. [CrossRef]
40. Codoñer-Franch, P.; Alberola, A.B.; Camarasa, J.V.D.; Moya, M.C.E.; Bellés, V.V. Influence of dietary lipids on the erythrocyte anti-oxidant status of hypercholesterolaemic children. *Eur. J. Pediatr.* **2009**, *168*, 321–327. [CrossRef]

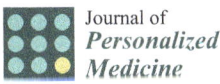

Article

Analysis of Rare Variants in Genes Related to Lipid Metabolism in Patients with Familial Hypercholesterolemia in Western Siberia (Russia)

Elena Shakhtshneider [1,2,*], Dinara Ivanoshchuk [1,2], Olga Timoshchenko [1,2], Pavel Orlov [1,2], Sergey Semaev [1,2], Emil Valeev [1], Andrew Goonko [3], Nataliya Ladygina [3] and Mikhail Voevoda [1]

[1] Institute of Cytology and Genetics (ICG), Siberian Branch of Russian Academy of Sciences (SB RAS), 10 Prospekt Ak. Lavrentyeva, 630090 Novosibirsk, Russia; dinara@bionet.nsc.ru (D.I.); lentis@yandex.ru (O.T.); orlovpavel86@gmail.com (P.O.); sse85@ngs.ru (S.S.); emil@bionet.nsc.ru (E.V.); mvoevoda@ya.ru (M.V.)

[2] Institute of Internal and Preventive Medicine (IIPM)—Branch of ICG SB RAS, 175/1 Borisa Bogatkova Str., 630089 Novosibirsk, Russia

[3] Department of Automation, Novosibirsk State Technical University, 20 Prospekt K. Marksa, 630073 Novosibirsk, Russia; gun@ait.cs.nstu.ru (A.G.); natskanzler@gmail.com (N.L.)

* Correspondence: shakhtshneyderev@bionet.nsc.ru

Abstract: The aim of this work was to identify genetic variants potentially involved in familial hypercholesterolemia in 43 genes associated with lipid metabolism disorders. Targeted high-throughput sequencing of lipid metabolism genes was performed (80 subjects with a familial-hypercholesterolemia phenotype). For patients without functionally significant substitutions in the above genes, multiplex ligation-dependent probe amplification was conducted to determine bigger mutations (deletions and/or duplications) in the *LDLR* promoter and exons. A clinically significant variant in some gene associated with familial hypercholesterolemia was identified in 47.5% of the subjects. Clinically significant variants in the *LDLR* gene were identified in 19 probands (73.1% of all variants identified in probands); in three probands (11.5%), pathogenic variants were found in the *APOB* gene; and in four probands (15.4%), rare, clinically significant variants were identified in genes *LPL*, *SREBF1*, *APOC3*, and *ABCG5*. In 12 (85.7%) of 14 children of the probands, clinically significant variants were detectable in genes associated with familial hypercholesterolemia. The use of clinical criteria, targeted sequencing, and multiplex ligation-dependent probe amplification makes it possible to identify carriers of rare clinically significant variants in a wide range of lipid metabolism genes and to investigate their influence on phenotypic manifestations of familial hypercholesterolemia.

Keywords: familial hypercholesterolemia; targeted sequencing technologies; multiplex ligation-dependent probe amplification; *LDLR*; *APOB*; *ABCG5*; *APOC3*; *LPL*; *SREBF1*; rare variants

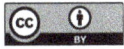

1. Introduction

Familial hypercholesterolemia is a condition caused by a type of genetic defect leading to a decreased rate of removal of low-density lipoproteins from the bloodstream and a pronounced increase in the blood level of total cholesterol [1]. Familial hypercholesterolemia is one of the most common congenital metabolic disorders [2]. With very rare exceptions, familial hypercholesterolemia is an autosomal dominant disorder [3]. In patients with familial hypercholesterolemia, there is a significantly higher total serum cholesterol level (from birth) and a significantly higher low-density lipoprotein cholesterol (LDL-C) concentration, while triglyceride levels are normal or moderately elevated [4]. Familial hypercholesterolemia poses a substantial risk of the early onset of complications such as coronary heart disease and atherosclerotic lesions in the vessels of the brain and arteries of the lower extremities [5]. In people with a high blood level of LDL-C and a confirmed mutation associated with familial hypercholesterolemia, the incidence of cardiovascular diseases is 22-fold higher than that in people with a normal level of LDL-C and no mutation [6]. Despite the considerable prevalence of this disease and the availability of effective treatments, familial hypercholesterolemia often remains undiagnosed and untreated, especially in children [7].

LDLR, *APOB*, and *PCSK9* are the genes whose mutations underlie the pathogenesis of the autosomal dominant type of familial hypercholesterolemia. Mutations in the *LDLR* gene are present in 80–85% of cases in which a molecular genetic cause of familial hypercholesterolemia has been identified; *APOB* mutations are present in 5–7% of the patients; and *PCSK9* mutations have been identified in fewer than 5% of the patients. Mutations in genes associated with the autosomal recessive type of familial hypercholesterolemia—for example, in the *LDLRAP1* gene—are seen in <1% of the cases [8,9]. A negative result of genetic screening for mutations of *LDLR*, *APOB*, *PCSK9*, *LDLRAP1*, and some other genes does not rule out familial hypercholesterolemia. In 5–30% of its cases, molecular genetic testing does not show changes in the above-mentioned genes: some cases of phenotypic familial hypercholesterolemia may be caused by mutations in other genes (currently not known to be associated with this disease) or may have a polygenic cause, in contrast to the autosomal dominant type of this disease [10–14].

More than 250 loci associated with dyslipidemia are known thanks to exome sequencing [15–17]. Targeted sequencing of a set of genes of interest is a fast and cost-effective alternative to exome sequencing and is widely used in clinical laboratories. The aim of the present work was to identify genetic variants potentially involved in familial hypercholesterolemia in 43 genes associated with lipid metabolism disorders; for this purpose, we analyzed patients having a phenotype of familial hypercholesterolemia.

2. Materials and Methods

2.1. Patients

Patients with familial hypercholesterolemia were recruited in the Clinical Diagnostic Department of the Institute of Internal and Preventive Medicine (IIPM)—a branch of the Institute of Cytology and Genetics, Siberian Branch of Russian Academy of Sciences (ICG SB RAS). The study protocol was approved by the Ethics Committee of the IIPM—a branch of the ICG SB RAS (session No. 68 of 4 June 2019). Written informed consent to be examined and to participate in the study was obtained from each patient or his/her parent or legal guardian.

The study included 80 patients referred by a clinical lipidologist for molecular genetic testing after a diagnosis of familial hypercholesterolemia. This diagnosis was made using the Dutch Lipid Clinic Network (DLCN) Criteria [Geneva: World Health Organization; 1999]. To calculate the total score in accordance with the DLCN criteria, the Familial Hypercholesterolemia Calculator software was used, which has been developed in the Department of Automation of the Faculty of Automation and Computer Engineering at Novosibirsk State Technical University (https://lipidcenter.iimed.ru/o-lipidnom-tsentre/calc.html [accessed on 1 November 2021]). In this software, the likelihood of familial hypercholesterolemia in a patient is computed from the sum of subscores obtained in each group of criteria. For these calculations, LDL-C levels of first-degree relatives that are known to exceed the age- and sex-specific 95th percentile are analyzed by the software according to populational age- and sex-specific LDL-C data from Russia [1]. Familial hypercholesterolemia is designated as "definite," "probable," or "possible" according to the total score (hereafter: DLCN score). All three subtypes are referred to as a "phenotype of familial hypercholesterolemia" below. A JavaScript v.1.5 function is employed to compute the total score. Taking into account the DLCN criteria and the results of molecular genetic testing, an electronic database was compiled for this study.

In this way, in the total of 80 participants, 34 subjects were assigned to the "definite" familial hypercholesterolemia group (DLCN score > 8), five subjects to the "probable" familial hypercholesterolemia group (DLCN score: 6–8), and 41 subjects to the "possible" familial hypercholesterolemia group (DLCN score: 3–5). The study included 60 probands and 20 first-degree relatives of the probands. Among these relatives, 70% ($n = 14$) were children of the probands.

The patients underwent a medical examination and ultrasonographic testing, and blood samples were collected for biochemical tests (the lipid profile and general biochemical indicators) and molecular genetic testing. The testing of the probands and their first-degree relatives was carried out according to the principles of cascade genetic screening [18].

Blood samples for biochemical tests were taken once from the cubital vein in the morning on an empty stomach (12 h after a meal). The lipid parameters (levels of total cholesterol, triglycerides, LDL-C, and high-density lipoprotein cholesterol [HDL-C]) and blood glucose concentration were determined by enzymatic methods on an automatic biochemical analyzer KoneLab300i (Vantaa, Finland) with Termo Fisher reagents (Vantaa, Finland). The LDL-C level was calculated using the Friedewald formula; when LDL-C concentration was >4.5 mmol/L, direct LDL-C measurement was employed. Means ± standard deviation were computed in the SPSS software for Windows for the data on biochemical testing of the subjects over 18 years of age.

2.2. Isolation of Genomic DNA

To isolate DNA from blood, phenol–chloroform extraction was used [19]. The quality of the extracted DNA was assessed by means of an Agilent 2100 Bioanalyzer capillary electrophoresis system (Agilent Technologies Inc., Santa Clara, CA, USA).

2.3. Genome Library Preparation, Sequencing, and Bioinformatic Analysis

Targeted high-throughput sequencing of lipid metabolism genes was performed on the whole participants ($n = 80$, all had a diagnosis of familial hypercholesterolemia to various degrees of certainty). The custom panel of genes for the testing consisted of 43 genes (*LDLR, APOB, PCSK9, LDLRAP1, CETP, LPL, HMGCR, NPC1L1, PPARA, MTTP, LMF1, SAR1B, ABCA1, ABCG5, ABCG8, CYP7A1, STAP1, LIPA, PNPLA5, APOA1, APOA5, APOC2, APOE, LCAT, ANGPTL3, LIPC, APOA4, APOC3, SREBF1, LMNA, PPARG, PLIN1, POLD1, LPA, SMAD1, SMAD2, SMAD3, SMAD4, SMAD5, SMAD6, SMAD7, SMAD9*, and *LIPG*). Genes *LDLR*, *APOB*, and *PCSK9* are associated with the autosomal dominant type of familial hypercholesterolemia; genes *LDLRAP1*, *ABCG5*, *ABCG8*, and *CYP7A1* with the autosomal recessive type of familial hypercholesterolemia; and genes *STAP1*, *LIPA*, and *PNPLA5* are associated with phenotypic variations of familial hypercholesterolemia, including the development of hypertriglyceridemia. Rare variants in the genes of apolipoproteins and other genes related to lipid metabolism can cause a familial-hypercholesterolemia-like phenotype in patients [20–24].

Targeted high-throughput sequencing (next-generation sequencing) was performed with NimbleGen SeqCap Target Enrichment (Roche, Basel, Switzerland) on a MySeq sequencer (Illumina, San Diego, CA, USA). The coverage was 97%.

The bioinformatic processing pipeline included the following steps. After we removed adapters from sequencing data via cutadapt (available online: https://cutadapt.readthedocs.io/en/stable/ [accessed on 4 October 2021]), sequencing reads were mapped with a Burrow–Wheeler Alignment tool (BWA) v.0.7.17 (available online: http://bio-bwa.sourceforge.net/ [accessed on 4 October 2021]); we used human genome assembly GRCh38 as a reference. At the second stage, sequencing data were improved: we removed PCR-generated duplicates with MarkDuplicates by Picard (available online: https://broadinstitute.github.io/picard/ [accessed on 4 October 2021]), and recalibrated base quality with BQSR tools of Genome Analysis Toolkit (GATK) v.3.3 (available online: https://gatk.broadinstitute.org/hc/en-us [accessed on 4 October 2021]). At the third stage, we performed single-nucleotide variant (SNV) calling via HaplotypeCaller tool of GATK.

Finally, SNVs were annotated and filtered. Annotation was performed by means of the ANNO-VAR tool (available online: https://annovar.openbioinformatics.org/en/latest/ [accessed on 4 October 2021]); we utilized the following databases:

- Big population frequency databases, such as gnomAD (available online: https://gnomad.broadinstitute.org/ [accessed on 4 October 2021]), with some help of databases on specific populations, like Greater Middle East (GME) Variome Project (available online: http://igm.ucsd.edu/gme/ [accessed on 4 October 2021]), AbraOM (Brazilian genomic variants) (available online: https://abraom.ib.usp.br/ [accessed on 4 October 2021]), and Korean Personal Genome Project (available online: http://opengenome.net/Main_Page [accessed on 4 October 2021]).
- Databases representing in silico prediction tools, such as dbNSFP (available online: https://sites.google.com/site/jpopgen/dbNSFP [accessed on 4 October 2021]), which contains data from more than 30 pathogenicity prediction tools (e.g., MutationTaster2, SIFT, PROVEAN, and Polyphen2), and from 10 conservation prediction tools (e.g., phastCons, GERP++, and SiPhy). For pathogenicity prediction tools, we set thresholds according to respective authors' recommendations; additionally, for conservation prediction tools, we used one common threshold, 0.7; therefore, we assumed a variant to be conserved if its conservation score was greater than the scores of $\geq 70\%$ other variants. Additionally, we used databases dbscSNV and regSNP-intron for variants that may have an effect on splicing. Nevertheless, all these databases were only a supplementary tool, and they contributed little to the summary measure of pathogenicity.
- Gene-based phenotype databases (e.g., OMIM).
- Clinical significance databases: ClinVar (available online: https://www.ncbi.nlm.nih.gov/clinvar/ [accessed on 4 October 2021]), Human Gene Mutation Database (HGMD) (available online: http://www.hgmd.cf.ac.uk/ [accessed on 4 October 2021]), and Leiden Open Variation Database (available online: https://www.lovd.nl/ [accessed on 4 October 2021]); variants described as benign (B) or likely benign (LB) were also excluded from further analysis.
- PubMed (available online: https://pubmed.ncbi.nlm.nih.gov/ [accessed on 4 October 2021]) and some other article databases as a source of information on specific clinical cases.

We estimated pathogenicity of each novel candidate mutation according to the recommendations of the American College of Medical Genetics and Genomics (ACMG) and the Association for Molecular Pathology [25].

2.4. Verification of Findings

All selected rare SNVs were verified by Sanger direct automatic sequencing on an ABI 3500 DNA sequencer (Thermo Fisher Scientific, Waltham, MA, USA) by means of the BigDye Terminator v3.1 Cycle Sequencing Kit (Thermo Fisher Scientific, Waltham, MA, USA). Primer design for the selected SNVs was performed in the Primer-Blast software (available online: https://www.ncbi.nlm.nih.gov/tools/primer-blast/ [accessed on 4 October 2021]). Targeted Sanger sequencing was carried out to detect mutations in the relatives of the probands.

2.5. Multiplex Ligation-Dependent Probe Amplification (MLPA)

For patients without functionally significant point substitutions in the above genes, MLPA was conducted to find possible bigger mutations (deletions and/or duplications) in the *LDLR* promoter and exons. The MLPA analysis was performed using SALSA MLPA Kit P062 (MRCHolland, Amsterdam, The Netherlands) followed by the separation of fluorescently labeled fragments by capillary electrophoresis (on an ABI3500 sequencer). The Coffalyser.Net software (MRCHolland, Amsterdam) was utilized to interpret the MLPA results.

3. Results

In the subjects over 18 years of age ($n = 69$; all participants [$n = 80$] had a phenotype of familial hypercholesterolemia), the total cholesterol level was 8.6 ± 3.4 mmol/L (mean $\pm$ standard deviation), with a maximum of 25 mmol/L (Table 1). This relatively low total cholesterol concentration is due to the fact that at the time of the initial medical examination by the clinical lipidologist in the Clinical Diagnostic Department of the IIPM (a branch of the ICG SB RAS), lipid-lowering drugs were taken by 41% of the probands. All lipid-lowering drugs were statins. One proband did not tolerate lipid-lowering medication of the statin class. According to the medical examination, in 42% of the subjects, tendon xanthomas were present. Three probands (4.9%) had comorbid type 2 diabetes mellitus.

Table 1. Data on biochemical testing of the subjects over 18 years of age, $n = 69$.

	M ± SD *	Minimum	Maximum
Glucose, mmol/L	5.7 ± 1.2	4.0	10.4
Total cholesterol, mmol/L (mg/dL)	8.6 ± 3.4 (332.5 ± 131.4)	3.4 (131.4)	25.0 (966.5)
Triglycerides, mmol/L (mg/dL)	1.8 ± 1.4 (157.5 ± 122.5)	0.4 (35.0)	17.4 (1522.5)
HDL-C, mmol/L (mg/dL)	1.4 ± 0.4 (54.1 ± 15.5)	0.54 (20.9)	2.2 (85.1)
LDL-C, mmol/L (mg/dL)	5.6 ± 2.3 (216.5 ± 88.9)	1.11 (42.9)	11.94 (461.6)
Body–mass index, m^2/kg	27.2 ± 4.6	19.0	39.0
Age, years	46.0 ± 13.9	20	73

* M ± SD: mean ± standard deviation.

A clinically significant variant in some genes associated with familial hypercholesterolemia was identified in 47.5% of the subjects. Clinically significant variants in the *LDLR* gene were identified in 19 probands (73.1% of all variants identified in probands); in three probands (11.5%), pathogenic variants were found in the *APOB* gene, and in four probands (15.4%), rare, clinically significant variants were identified in genes *LPL*, *SREBF1*, *APOC3*, and *ABCG5*. In 12 (85.7%) of 14 children of the probands, clinically significant variants were detectable in genes associated with familial hypercholesterolemia: in 10 cases, in the *LDLR* gene; in one case, in the APOB gene; and in one case, in the *SREBPF1* gene. Among the other six first-degree relatives of the probands (mother, father, or sibling), a pathogenic variant in the *LDLR* gene was identified in one case.

3.1. LDLR

Structural changes in the *LDLR* gene in patients with a phenotype of familial hypercholesterolemia are presented in Table 2. All missense variants were heterozygous. Some of the identified variants (Cys352Tyr, Cys340Phe, and Leu401His) have been described in patients with familial hypercholesterolemia in Russia [26–30]. The variant most common in our participations—rs121908038—was found in three unrelated families (six subjects total).

Table 2. The genetic variants identified in Western Siberia patients with a phenotype of Familial Hypercholesterolemia. MAF: minor allele frequency.

Patient ID	dbSNP ID	Position on Chromosome (GRCh38)	Nucleotide Substitution	Amino Acid Substitution	MAF According to Database GnomAD	Clinical Effect According to Database ClinVar	References for Russia
				LDLR Gene			
P28, P40, P41, P42, P55, P56	rs121908038	19:11113293	c.1202T > A	p.Leu401His	ND	Likely Pathogenic	Zakharova et al., 2005 [26]; Shakhtshneider et al., 2017 [27]; Shakhtshneider et al., 2019 [28]; Vasilyev et al., 2020 [29]; Miroshnikova et al., 2021 [30]
P45	rs137853964	19:11129602	c.2479G > A	p.Val827Ile	A = 0.001006	Likely Pathogenic	Shakhtshneider et al., 2017 [27]; Shakhtshneider et al., 2019 [28]; Vasilyev et al., 2020 [29]
22, P36, P58	rs28942078	19:11113376	c.1285G > A	p.Val429Met	A = 0.000012	Pathogenic/Likely Pathogenic	-

Table 2. Cont.

Patient ID	dbSNP ID	Position on Chromosome (GRCh38)	Nucleotide Substitution	Amino Acid Substitution	MAF According to Database GnomAD	Clinical Effect According to Database ClinVar	References for Russia
			LDLR Gene				
P65	rs539080792	19:11221396	c.1009G > A	p.Glu337Lys	A = 0.000104	Uncertain Significance	Shakhtshneider et al., 2017 [27]; Shakhtshneider et al., 2019 [28]; Vasilyev et al., 2020 [29]
P47	rs570942190	19:11113337	c.1246C > T	p.Arg416Trp	T = 0.000024	Not reported in ClinVar	Shakhtshneider et al., 2017 [27]; Shakhtshneider et al., 2019 [28]; Vasilyev et al., 2020 [29]
P67, P68	rs755757866	19:11110730	c.1019G > T	p.Cys340Tyr	T = 0.000008	Likely Pathogenic	Shakhtshneider et al., 2017 [27]; Shakhtshneider et al., 2019 [28]; Vasilyev et al., 2020 [29]
7	rs761954844	19:11110697	c.986G > A	p.Cys329Tyr	A = 0.000016	Likely Pathogenic	Zakharova et al., 2005 [26]; Shakhtshneider et al., 2019 [28]; Semenova et al., 2020 [31]; Vasilyev et al., 2020 [29]; Miroshnikova et al., 2021 [30]
P35	rs879254566	19:11105440	c.534TT > G	p.Asp178Glu	ND	Pathogenic/ Likely Pathogenic	Shakhtshneider et al., 2019 [28]; Vasilyev et al., 2020 [29]
P38, P39	rs879254721	19:11107496	c.922G > A	p.Glu308Lys	ND	Pathogenic	Semenova et al., 2020 [31]; Vasilyev et al., 2020 [30];
P2	rs879254980	19:11116179	c.1672G > T	p.Glu558Ter	ND	Pathogenic	-
P24, P25, P26, P81, P82	rs879255191	19:11128090	c.2389 + 5G > A	-	ND	Conflicting Interpretations of Pathogenicity	Meshkov et. Al. [32]; Shakhtshneider et al., 2019 [28]; Vasilyev et al., 2020 [29]
P52	rs875989907	19:11106666	c.796G > A	p.Asp266Asn	A = 0.000012	Pathogenic	Shakhtshneider et al., 2017 [27]
	rs879254769	19:11110765	c.1054T > C	p.Cys352Ser	ND	Likely Pathogenic	Shakhtshneider et al., 2017 [27]
P10	rs875989894	19:11213415	c.266G > C	p.Cys89Ser	ND	Pathogenic/Likely Pathogenic	-
	ND	19:11222252	c.1123T > G	p.Tyr375Asp	ND	Novel variant	-
			APOB Gene				
P11, P15, P71	rs5742904	2:21006288	c.10580G > A	p.Arg3527Gln	T = 0.000275	Pathogenic	Voevoda et al. 2014 [33]; Shakhtshneider et al., 2019 [28]; Miroshnikova et al., 2021 [30]
			ABCG5 Gene				
P74	rs145164937	2:43832056	c.293C > G	p.Ala98Gly	C = 0.002223	Conflicting interpretations of pathogenicity	-
			APOC3 Gene				
P59	rs138326449	11:116830638	c.55 + 1G > A	-	C = 0.002244	Conflicting interpretations of pathogenicity	-
			LPL Gene				
P9	rs118204077	8:19955873	c.808C > T	p.Arg270Cys	C = 0.0001	Pathogenic	-
			SREBF1 Gene				
P83, P84	rs115855236	17:17820281	c.422C > T	p.Pro141Leu	A = 0.001210	Not reported in ClinVar	-

Two unrelated probands were compound heterozygotes in terms of the *LDLR* gene and showed a clinical course corresponding to the homozygous type of the disease. In the first case, a 28-year-old (patient P52) got a diagnosis of "definite" familial hypercholesterolemia (DLCN score of 18, a history of myocardial infarction at the age of 24; percutaneous transluminal coronary angioplasty at ages 25 and 26 years); rare variants chr19:11217342 and chr19:11221441 were identified in exons 5 and 7 of the *LDLR* gene (Table 2). The patient had been taking lipid-lowering medication, and the total cholesterol level was 18.6 mmol/L, and LDL-C 15.2 mmol/L.

In the second case, a 35-year-old (patient P10) got a diagnosis of "definite" familial hypercholesterolemia (DLCN score of 18, a history of myocardial infarction at the age of 24; mammary coronary artery bypass grafting at the age of 24; a second myocardial infarction at 34 years of age); rare variants were identified in exons 3 and 8 of the *LDLR* gene. One of these variants is located at position chr19:11213415 (NM_000527:exon3:c.G266C:p.C89S), earlier, a rare "pathogenic" variant (rs875989894) has been described at this position: a G > A substitution (available online: https://databases.lovd.nl/shared/variants/00000921 11#00011039 [accessed on 1 October 2021]). The other variant is located at chr19:11222252; it is described for the first time: NM_000527:exon8:c.T1123G:p.Y375D (Table 2). Before treatment with lipid-lowering medication was started, the total cholesterol level was 25.0 mmol/L, and LDL-C 11.94 mmol/L.

The clinical signs of the homozygous type of familial hypercholesterolemia, including early onset of severe complications in the cardiovascular system, are typical for patients who are compound heterozygotes in the *LDLR* gene, as shown in various populations [34].

The rs879255191 variant in the regulatory region of *LDLR* has previously been described by us in proband P24 with familial hypercholesterolemia and in his two children (patients P25 and P26) with hyperlipidemia (7 and 8 years old) [35,36]. Variant c.2389 + 5G > A is located in highly conserved dinucleotide AG at the splice donor site of intron 16 of *LDLR*. Functional significance of the detected substitution was evaluated in the SPANR software (available online: http://tools.genes.toronto.edu/ [accessed on 4 October 2021]). According to the SPANR analysis, the change in the probability of exon inclusion in mRNA in various tissues when this variant is present is -13.47 points, meaning that the probability of inclusion of exons 14–16 in gene transcripts is lower than 100%. Previously, rs879255191 has already been detected in patients with familial hypercholesterolemia, including in Russia [32]. In the present study, the rs879255191 variant was also detected in a sibling (patient P81) and a nephew (P82) of the proband (P24) who has clinical signs of familial hypercholesterolemia (Figure 1). Patient P81 had a myocardial infarction at age 44 years.

3.2. Identification of Deletions and Duplications in the LDLR Gene by MLPA

Forty-two patients, without functionally significant point substitutions in lipid metabolism genes, were subjected to MLPA analysis to find possible structural changes (deletions or duplications) in the *LDLR* promoter and exons. This analysis revealed deletions in DNA samples from two unrelated patients. In the first case, deletion NM_000527.4:c.(67+1_68-1)_(1586+1_1587-1)del in a heterozygous state eliminated a region spanning exons 2 to 10 (Figure 2a). In the second case, the patient was a carrier of a deletion of exon 15 in the *LDLR* gene NM_000527.4:c.(2140+1_2141-1)_(2311+1_2312-1)del in a heterozygous state (Figure 2b).

Patient P33 (31 years old) with an exon 2–10 deletion had a total cholesterol level of 10.96 mmol/L, and LDL-C 7.76 mmol/L (DLCN score: 6), with a family history of deaths from myocardial infarction before the age of 50 on the paternal side. At the time of the medical examination, she was not taking lipid-lowering medication. This deletion was first described in 2010 in the French Autosomal Dominant Hypercholesterolemia Research Network study [37].

In patient P5 (69 years old) with an exon 15 deletion, the total cholesterol level was 6.6 mmol/L and LDL-C 3.8 mmol/L while the patient was on 10 mg of rosuvastatin. A similar deletion of *LDLR* exon 15 has been described by Koivisto P.V. et al. [38].

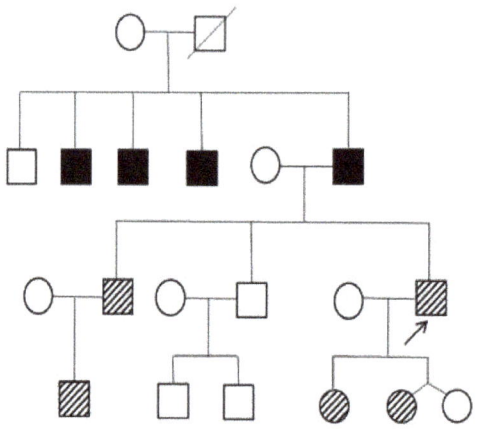

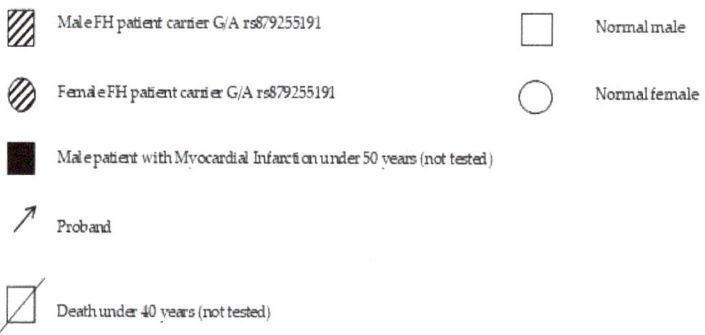

Figure 1. The screened family with variant rs879255191 identified in the *LDLR* gene.

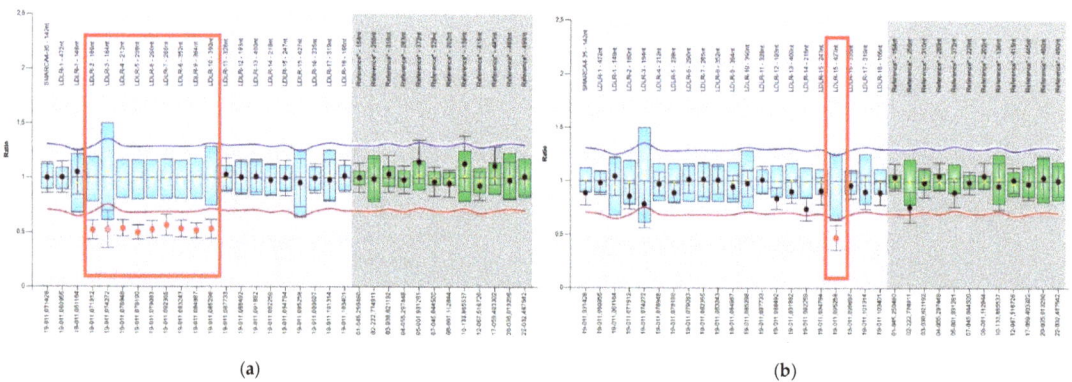

Figure 2. MLPA analysis shows a heterozygous deletion (ratio of ~1.5) of *LDLR* exons 2–10 in patient P33 (**a**) and of *LDLR* exon 15 in patient P5 (**b**). The ratio charts of the patients with a familial hypercholesterolemia phenotype were generated by means of SALSA MLPA Kit P062. Each red dot below the red curve represents a deletion. The probes whose data do not go outside the blue and red curves represent two wild-type copies of the *LDLR* gene.

3.3. APOB

In the molecular genetic test, we detected some structural changes in the *APOB* gene in patients with a phenotype of familial hypercholesterolemia (Table 2). In three patients from two unrelated families (a proband and a son of the proband from one family and a proband from another family), variant rs5742904 was found: NM_000384.3(APOB):c.10580G > A (p.Arg3527Gln). Minor allele frequency was T = 0.000275 according to database GnomAD.

In the first family, patient P71 (36 years old) carried the rs5742904 variant, and the total cholesterol level was 7.75 mmol/L and LDL-C 5.76 mmol/L while on 10 mg of rosuvastatin (DLCN score: 12; examination revealed xanthomas). The patient's father had a myocardial infarction at age 50 and died of a second myocardial infarction at age 62; the father's mother died of ischemic stroke at age 60. The son (13 years old, patient P11) of patient P71—had a total cholesterol level of 6.9 mmol/L and carried the rs5742904 variant.

In the second family, patient P15 (25 years old) carried the rs5742904 variant, and the total cholesterol level was 7.5 mmol/L, LDL-C 5.7 mmol/L, and the DLCN score was 11.

The clinical effect of rs5742904 has conflicting interpretations of pathogenicity in the literature: likely pathogenic (three studies), pathogenic (27 studies), and uncertain significance (one study) according to database ClinVar [39].

3.4. ABCG5

A rare variant, rs145164937, in the *ABCG5* gene in a heterozygous state was detected in one of the probands (patient P74, woman, 38 years old) with a total cholesterol level of 8.3 mmol/L, LDL-C of 5.4 mmol/L, and a DLCN score of 3 (Table 2). Minor allele frequency (MAF) of allele C is 0.002223 for Europeans (non-Finnish) according to the GnomAD database [40]. A known disease-associated mutation at this position is HGMD ID CM169023. When the rs145164937 (NM_022436; p.Ala98Gly; c.293C > G) variant was analyzed in PolyPhen-2, it showed a high probability of a damaging effect on the protein product (a score of 0.977). Earlier, an association of rs145164937 with non-high-density lipoprotein cholesterol levels has been demonstrated [41].

3.5. APOC3

Analysis of the targeted-high-throughput-sequencing data from the *APOC3* gene revealed variant rs138326449 (IVS2 + 1G > A) in a heterozygous state (Table 2). MAF of allele C is 0.002244 for Europeans (non-Finnish) according to the GnomAD database. This substitution is located in a highly conserved dinucleotide at a splice donor site, thereby leading to alternative splicing and a dysfunctional protein [42]. A.B. Jorgensen et al. have reported an association of the IVS2 + 1G > A variant with low triglyceride levels and a low risk of coronary heart disease [42]. In our study, variant IVS2 + 1G > A of *APOC3* was detected in a 65-year-old subject (patient P59) with hypercholesterolemia (total cholesterol 8.2 mmol/L, LDL-C 5.45 mmol/L) and normal levels of triglycerides (0.7 mmol/L) and HDL-C (2.4 mmol/L), with a DLCN score of 5. In the ClinVar database, rs138326449 is listed as pathogenic for apolipoprotein C-III deficiency.

3.6. LPL

Analysis of the targeted-high-throughput-sequencing results from the *LPL* gene revealed a rare variant: rs118204077 (NM_000237; p.Arg270Cys, c.808C > T) in a heterozygous state (Table 2). MAF of allele C is 0.0001 for Europeans (non-Finnish) according to the GnomAD database. Its clinical significance is indicated as pathogenic in the ClinVar database. A known disease-associated mutation at this position is HGMD ID CM941054. When the rs118204077 variant was analyzed in PolyPhen-2, the probability of a damaging effect on the protein product turned out to be 1.000 (very high score).

The rs118204077 variant in *LPL* was identified in a 45-year-old (patient P9) with hypercholesterolemia (12.4 mmol/L), hypertriglyceridemia (17.4 mmol/L), and a DLCN score of 5. Previously, at this locus, variants associated with hypertriglyceridemia have been described in the literature [43,44].

3.7. SREBF1

A rare variant of the *SREBF1* gene (rs115855236, chr17:17820281) was identified in proband P83 and a son of this proband (patient P84) with clinical signs of familial hypercholesterolemia (Table 2). MAF of allele A is 0.001210 for Europeans (non-Finnish) according to the GnomAD database. In other genes associated with familial hypercholesterolemia, pathogenic and probably pathogenic variants were not identified in these patients. *SREBF1* encodes a transcription factor of the basic helix-loop-helix-leucine zipper family (bHLH-Zip); this protein binds to a sterol regulatory element (SRE1) and regulates the biosynthesis of fatty acids and cholesterol. One of the target genes for transcription factor SREBF1 is *LDLR*.

4. Discussion

In this study, the prevalence of detected "pathogenic" and "probably pathogenic" mutations was 47.5% among the analyzed probands with a phenotype of familial hypercholesterolemia from the Western Siberia region (Russia) and 85.7% among their tested children who also had a phenotype of familial hypercholesterolemia. As in other studies, this finding confirms the effectiveness of cascade genetic screening [45–50].

Among 34 subjects with a diagnosis of "definite" familial hypercholesterolemia (DLCN score > 8), pathogenic variants in *LDLR* (76.5%) or *APOB* (8.8%) were identified in 29 subjects. In five subjects (14.7%), no pathogenic variants were found in the genes included in the tested panel.

Among the five subjects with a diagnosis of "probable" familial hypercholesterolemia (DLCN scores 6–8), two subjects were found to have pathogenic variants in the *LDLR* gene, including deletion NM_000527.4:c.(67+1_68-1)_(1586+1_1587-1)del in a heterozygous state.

Among 41 subjects with a diagnosis of "possible" familial hypercholesterolemia (DLCN score: 3–5), rare "pathogenic" and "probably pathogenic" variants in the analyzed genes of lipid metabolism were identified in only 15% of cases. In two subjects, pathogenic variants in the *LDLR* gene were identified, including a deletion of the 15th exon NM_000527.4:c.(2140+1_2141-1)_(2311+1_2312-1)del; in one subject, a pathogenic variant was found in the *APOB* gene, and in four probands, in other lipid metabolism genes (*ABCG5*, *LPL*, *APOC3*, or *SREBF1*). A negative result of genetic screening for *LDLR*, *APOB*, and *PCSK9* mutations does not rule out the presence of familial hypercholesterolemia in a patient. In ~40% of cases, molecular genetic testing fails to determine the cause of familial hypercholesterolemia [51] or an elevated LDL-C level that may have a polygenic type of inheritance [52,53]. Despite the lower prevalence of detected mutations among our subjects with "possible" familial hypercholesterolemia, they should also be monitored by a doctor and receive appropriate lipid-lowering therapy because of the high risk of cardiovascular events at elevated LDL-C levels and/or with a family history of an early cardiovascular disease [54–56].

Molecular genetic research on familial hypercholesterolemia in Russia has been conducted for more than 30 years in different regions of the country [29]. It is worth mentioning some variants of the *LDLR* gene that not only occur in most regions of Russia but are also the most common variants of this gene: rs121908038 and rs761954844 [28–32,57]. Additionally, these variants have been found in populations of Northern and Central Europe (rs121908038) and in populations of Central and Eastern Europe, Southeast Asia, and North America (rs761954844) [40].

The most common limitation of such studies is a small sample size [29]. We should also mention low accessibility of molecular genetic testing in some regions of Russia and the high cost of these tests. The small sample sizes do not allow us to assess clinical-course features of the disease that are associated with various pathogenic variants in lipid metabolism genes and to evaluate the spectrum of pathogenic variants in lipid metabolism genes in the population of Russia. Targeted sequencing can be useful not only for rapid and cost-effective diagnosis of familial hypercholesterolemia, but also for investigation of rare variants of lipid metabolism genes and their influence on the patients' phenotype [30,57,58].

This method may help to combine the efforts of physicians and investigators from different regions for the research on familial hypercholesterolemia.

MLPA is necessary for the diagnosis of familial hypercholesterolemia in patients without functionally significant point substitutions in relevant genes to which one of the sequencing methods has been applied [59]. Wider use of the MLPA method should help to identify 2–3% more probands with familial hypercholesterolemia. As revealed by research on the practice of molecular genetic diagnostics, patients who carry a confirmed pathogenic variant in a relevant gene are more likely to lead a healthy lifestyle and to regularly take lipid-lowering medication [18].

The use of clinical criteria, targeted sequencing, and MLPA makes it possible to identify carriers of rare clinically significant variants in a wide range of lipid metabolism genes and to investigate their influence on phenotypic manifestations of familial hypercholesterolemia.

Author Contributions: Conceptualization, E.S. and M.V.; data curation, E.S. and O.T.; investigation, D.I., P.O. and S.S.; methodology, E.S., D.I., E.V. and A.G.; project administration, E.S.; validation, N.L., E.V. and P.O.; writing—original draft, E.S., D.I. and A.G.; writing—review and editing, E.S. and M.V. All authors have read and agreed to the published version of the manuscript.

Funding: This study was conducted within the framework of the publicly funded topic in state assignment No. AAAA-A19-119100990053-4 (0259-2019-0009), and the bioinformatic analyses are financially supported as Russian Foundation for Basic Research project No. 19-015-00458.

Institutional Review Board Statement: The study protocol was approved by the Ethics Committee of the IIPM—a branch of the ICG SB RAS, session No. 68 of 4 June 2019.

Informed Consent Statement: Informed consent was obtained from each subject or his/her parent or legal guardian.

Data Availability Statement: The data presented in this study are available on request from the corresponding author. The data are not publicly available due to privacy concerns.

Conflicts of Interest: The authors declare that they have no conflict of interest related to the publication of this article.

References

1. Ezhov, M.V.; Bazhan, S.S.; Ershova, A.I.; Meshkov, A.N.; Sokolov, A.A.; Kukharchuk, V.V.; Gurevich, V.S.; Voevoda, M.I.; Sergienko, I.V.; Shakhtshneider, E.V.; et al. Clinical guidelines for familial hypercholesterolemia. *Ateroskleroz* **2019**, *15*, 58–98. [CrossRef]
2. Nordestgaard, B.G.; Chapman, M.J.; Humphries, S.E.; Ginsberg, H.N.; Masana, L.; Descamps, O.S.; Wiklund, O.; Hegele, R.A.; Raal, F.J.; Defesche, J.C.; et al. European Atherosclerosis Society Consensus Panel. Familial hypercholesterolaemia is underdiagnosed and undertreated in the general population: Guidance for clinicians to prevent coronary heart disease: Consensus statement of the European Atherosclerosis Society. *Eur. Heart J.* **2013**, *34*, 3478–3490. [CrossRef] [PubMed]
3. Sjouke, B.; Kusters, D.M.; Kindt, I.; Besseling, J.; Defesche, J.C.; Sijbrands, E.J.; Roeters van Lennep, J.E.; Stalenhoef, A.F.; Wiegman, A.; de Graaf, J.; et al. Homozygous autosomal dominant hypercholesterolemia in the Netherlands: Prevalence, genotype–phenotype relationship, and clinical outcome. *Eur. Heart J.* **2015**, *36*, 560–565. [CrossRef] [PubMed]
4. Borén, J.; Chapman, M.J.; Krauss, R.M.; Packard, C.J.; Bentzon, J.F.; Binder, C.J.; Daemen, M.J.; Demer, L.L.; Hegele, R.A.; Nicholls, S.J.; et al. Low-density lipoproteins cause atherosclerotic cardiovascular disease: Pathophysiological, genetic, and therapeutic insights: A consensus statement from the European Atherosclerosis Society Consensus Panel. *Eur. Heart J.* **2020**, *41*, 2313–2330. [CrossRef]
5. Santos, R.D.; Gidding, S.S.; Hegele, R.A.; Cuchel, M.A.; Barter, P.J.; Watts, G.F.; Baum, S.J.; Catapano, A.L.; Chapman, M.J.; Defesche, J.C.; et al. International Atherosclerosis Society Severe Familial Hypercholesterolemia Panel. Defining severe familial hypercholesterolaemia and the implications for clinical management: A consensus statement from the International Atherosclerosis Society Severe Familial Hypercholesterolemia Panel. *Lancet Diabetes Endocrinol.* **2016**, *4*, 850–861. [CrossRef]
6. Wiegman, A. Lipid Screening, Action, and Follow-up in Children and Adolescents. *Curr Cardiol. Rep.* **2018**, *20*, 80. [CrossRef]
7. Wiegman, A.; Gidding, S.S.; Watts, G.F.; Chapman, M.J.; Ginsberg, H.N.; Cuchel, M.; Ose, L.; Averna, M.; Boileau, C.; Borén, J.; et al. European Atherosclerosis Society Consensus Panel. Familial hypercholesterolaemia in children and adolescents: Gaining decades of life by optimizing detection and treatment. *Eur. Heart J.* **2015**, *36*, 2425–2437. [CrossRef]
8. Brautbar, A.; Leary, E.; Rasmussen, K.; Wilson, D.P.; Steiner, R.D.; Virani, S. Genetics of familial hypercholesterolemia. *Curr. Atheroscler. Rep.* **2015**, *17*, 491. [CrossRef]

9. Sturm, A.C.; Knowles, J.W.; Gidding, S.S.; Ahmad, Z.S.; Ahmed, C.D.; Ballantyne, C.M.; Baum, S.J.; Bourbon, M.; Carrié, A.; Cuchel, M.; et al. Convened by the Familial Hypercholesterolemia Foundation. Clinical Genetic Testing for Familial Hypercholesterolemia: JACC Scientific Expert Panel. *J. Am. Coll. Cardiol.* **2018**, *72*, 662–680. [CrossRef]
10. Motazacker, M.M.; Pirruccello, J.; Huijgen, R.; Do, R.; Gabriel, S.; Peter, J.; Kuivenhoven, J.A.; Defesche, J.C.; Kastelein, J.J.; Hovingh, G.K.; et al. Advances in genetics show the need for extending screening strategies for autosomal dominant hypercholesterolaemia. *Eur. Heart J.* **2012**, *33*, 1360–1366. [CrossRef]
11. van der Graaf, A.; Avis, H.J.; Kusters, D.M.; Vissers, M.N.; Hutten, B.A.; Defesche, J.C.; Huijgen, R.; Fouchier, S.W.; Wijburg, F.A.; Kastelein, J.J.; et al. Molecular basis of autosomal dominant hypercholesterolemia: Assessment in a large cohort of hypercholesterolemic children. *Circulation* **2011**, *123*, 1167–1173. [CrossRef] [PubMed]
12. Di Taranto, M.D.; Giacobbe, C.; Fortunato, G. Familial hypercholesterolemia: A complex genetic disease with variable phenotypes. *Eur J. Med. Genet.* **2020**, *63*, 103831. [CrossRef]
13. Berberich, A.J.; Hegele, R.A. The complex molecular genetics of familial hypercholesterolaemia. *Nat. Rev. Cardiol.* **2019**, *16*, 9–20. [CrossRef] [PubMed]
14. Abul-Husn, N.S.; Manickam, K.; Jones, L.K.; Wright, E.A.; Hartzel, D.N.; Gonzaga-Jauregui, C.; O'Dushlaine, C.; Leader, J.B.; Lester Kirchner, H.; Lindbuchler, D.M.; et al. Genetic identification of familial hypercholesterolemia within a single U.S. health care system. *Science* **2016**, *354*, aaf7000. [CrossRef] [PubMed]
15. Liu, D.J.; Peloso, G.M.; Yu, H.; Butterworth, A.S.; Wang, X.; Mahajan, A.; Saleheen, D.; Emdin, C.; Alam, D.; Alves, A.C.; et al. Exome-wide association study of plasma lipids in >300,000 individuals. *Nat. Genet.* **2017**, *49*, 1758–1766. [CrossRef]
16. Peloso, G.M.; Auer, P.L.; Bis, J.C.; Voorman, A.; Morrison, A.C.; Stitziel, N.O.; Brody, J.A.; Khetarpal, S.A.; Crosby, J.R.; Fornage, M.; et al. Association of low-frequency and rare coding-sequence variants with blood lipids and coronary heart disease in 56,000 whites and blacks. *Am. J. Hum. Genet.* **2014**, *94*, 223–232. [CrossRef]
17. van der Laan, S.W.; Harshfield, E.L.; Hemerich, D.; Stacey, D.; Wood, A.M.; Asselbergs, F.W. From lipid locus to drug target through human genomics. *Cardiovasc. Res.* **2018**, *114*, 1258–1270. [CrossRef]
18. Leren, T.P.; Finborud, T.H.; Manshaus, T.E.; Ose, L.; Berge, K.E. Diagnosis of familial hypercholesterolemia in general practice using clinical diagnostic criteria or genetic testing as part of cascade genetic screening. *Community Genet.* **2008**, *11*, 26–35. [CrossRef]
19. Sambrook, J.; Russell, D.W. Purification of nucleic acids by extraction with phenol: Chloroform. *CSH Protoc.* **2006**, *2006*, pdb.prot4455. [CrossRef]
20. Fouchier, S.W.; Dallinga-Thie, G.M.; Meijers, J.C.; Zelcer, N.; Kastelein, J.J.; Defesche, J.C.; Hovingh, G.K. Mutations in STAP1 are associated with autosomal dominant hypercholesterolemia. *Circ. Res.* **2014**, *115*, 552–555. [CrossRef]
21. Cao, Y.X.; Wu, N.Q.; Sun, D.; Liu, H.H.; Jin, J.L.; Li, S.; Guo, Y.L.; Zhu, C.G.; Gao, Y.; Dong, Q.T.; et al. Application of expanded genetic analysis in the diagnosis of familial hypercholesterolemia in patients with very early-onset coronary artery disease. *J. Transl. Med.* **2018**, *16*, 345. [CrossRef]
22. Fouchier, S.W.; Defesche, J.C. Lysosomal acid lipase A and the hypercholesterolaemic phenotype. *Curr. Opin. Lipidol.* **2013**, *24*, 332–338. [CrossRef] [PubMed]
23. Vinje, T.; Wierød, L.; Leren, T.P.; Strøm, T.B. Prevalence of cholesteryl ester storage disease among hypercholesterolemic subjects and functional characterization of mutations in the lysosomal acid lipase gene. *Mol. Genet. Metab.* **2018**, *123*, 169–176. [CrossRef] [PubMed]
24. Lamiquiz-Moneo, I.; Baila-Rueda, L.; Bea, A.M.; Mateo-Gallego, R.; Pérez-Calahorra, S.; Marco-Benedí, V.; Martín-Navarro, A.; Ros, E.; Cofán, M.; Rodríguez-Rey, J.C.; et al. ABCG5/G8 gene is associated with hypercholesterolemias without mutation in candidate genes and noncholesterol sterols. *J. Clin. Lipidol.* **2017**, *11*, 1432–1440. [CrossRef]
25. Richards, S.; Aziz, N.; Bale, S.; Bick, D.; Das, S.; Gastier-Foster, J.; Grody, W.W.; Hegde, M.; Lyon, E.; Spector, E.; et al. Standards and guidelines for the interpretation of sequence variants: A joint consensus recommendation of the American College of Medical Genetics and Genomics and the Association for Molecular Pathology. *Genet. Med.* **2015**, *17*, 405–423. [CrossRef]
26. Zakharova, F.M.; Damgaard, D.; Mandelshtam, M.Y.; Golubkov, V.I.; Nissen, P.H.; Nilsen, G.G.; Stenderup, A.; Lipovetsky, B.M.; Konstantinov, V.O.; Denisenko, A.D.; et al. Familial hypercholesterolemia in St-Petersburg: The known and novel mutations found in the low-density lipoprotein receptor gene in Russia. *BMC Med. Genet.* **2005**, *6*, 6. [CrossRef] [PubMed]
27. Shakhtshneider, E.; Orlov, P.; Ivanoshchuk, D.; Makarenkova, K.; Ragino, Y.; Voevoda, M. Analysis of the *LDLR* gene variability in patients with familial hypercholesterolemia in Russia using targeted high throughput resequencing. *Atherosclerosis* **2017**, *263*, e227. [CrossRef]
28. Shakhtshneider, E.; Ivanoshchuk, D.; Orlov, P.; Timoshchenko, O.; Voevoda, M. Analysis of the *LDLR*, *APOB*, *PCSK9* and *LDLRAP1* genes variability in patients with familial hypercholesterolemia in West Siberia using targeted high throughput resequencing. *Atherosclerosis* **2019**, *287*, e285. [CrossRef]
29. Vasilyev, V.; Zakharova, F.; Bogoslovskay, T.; Mandelshtam, M. Familial Hypercholesterolemia in Russia: Three Decades of Genetic Studies. *Front. Genet.* **2020**, *11*, 550591. [CrossRef]
30. Miroshnikova, V.V.; Romanova, O.V.; Ivanova, O.N.; Fedyakov, M.A.; Panteleeva, A.A.; Barbitoff, Y.A.; Muzalevskaya, M.V.; Urazgildeeva, S.A.; Gurevich, V.S.; Urazov, S.P.; et al. Identification of novel variants in the LDLR gene in Russian patients with familial hypercholesterolemia using targeted sequencing. *Biomed. Rep.* **2021**, *14*, 15. [CrossRef]

31. Semenova, A.E.; Sergienko, I.V.; García-Giustiniani, D.; Monserrat, L.; Popova, A.B.; Nozadze, D.N.; Ezhov, M.V. Verification of underlying genetic cause in a cohort of Russian patients with familial hypercholesterolemia using targeted next generation sequencing. *J. Cardiovasc. Dev. Dis.* **2020**, *7*, 16. [CrossRef]
32. Meshkov, A.N.; Malyshev, P.P.; Kukharchuk, V.V. Familial hypercholesterolemia in Russia: Genetic and phenotypic characteristics. *Ter. Arkh.* **2009**, *81*, 23–28. [PubMed]
33. Voevoda, M.; Shakhtshneider, E.; Orlov, P.; Ivanoshchuk, D.; Ivanova, M.; Nikitin, Y.; Malyutina, S. The mutation R3500Q of apolipoprotein B in caucasian population of west Siberia and in patients with highest total cholesterol level. *Atherosclerosis* **2014**, *235*, e100. [CrossRef]
34. Pamplona-Cunha, H.; Medeiros, M.F.; Sincero, T.C.M.; Back, I.C.; Silva, E.L.D. Compound Heterozygous Familial Hypercholesterolemia Caused by LDLR Variants. *Arq. Bras. Cardiol.* **2020**, *115*, 587–589. [CrossRef]
35. Shakhtshneider, E.V.; Ivanoshchuk, D.E.; Makarenkova, K.V.; Orlov, P.S.; Timoshchenko, O.V.; Bazhan, S.S.; Nikitin, Y.P.; Voevoda, M.I. Cascade genetic screening in diagnostics of heterozygous familial hypercholesterolemia: Clinical case. *Russ. J. Cardiol.* **2017**, *6*, 178–179. [CrossRef]
36. Shakhtshneider, E.; Ivanoshchuk, D.; Makarenkova, K.; Orlov, P.; Timoshchenko, O.; Bazhan, S.; Voevoda, M. Clinical case: The development of heterozygous familial hypercholesterolemia in a patient with rs879255191 in LDLR gene. *Atherosclerosis* **2018**, *275*, e179. [CrossRef]
37. Marduel, M.; Carrié, A.; Sassolas, A.; Devillers, M.; Carreau, V.; Di Filippo, M.; Erlich, D.; Abifadel, M.; Marques-Pinheiro, A.; Munnich, A.; et al. Molecular spectrum of autosomal dominant hypercholesterolemia in France. *Hum. Mutat.* **2010**, *31*, E1811–E1824. [CrossRef]
38. Koivisto, P.V.; Koivisto, U.M.; Miettinen, T.A.; Kontula, K. Diagnosis of heterozygous familial hypercholesterolemia. DNA analysis complements clinical examination and analysis of serum lipid levels. *Arterioscler. Thromb.* **1992**, *12*, 584–592. [CrossRef]
39. Available online: https://www.ncbi.nlm.nih.gov/clinvar/variation/17890/ (accessed on 1 October 2021).
40. Available online: https://gnomad.broadinstitute.org/variant/2-44059195-G-C?dataseT=gnomad_r2_1 (accessed on 1 October 2021).
41. Helgadottir, A.; Thorleifsson, G.; Alexandersson, K.F.; Tragante, V.; Thorsteinsdottir, M.; Eiriksson, F.F.; Gretarsdottir, S.; Björnsson, E.; Magnusson, O.; Sveinbjornsson, G.; et al. Genetic variability in the absorption of dietary sterols affects the risk of coronary artery disease. *Eur. Heart J.* **2020**, *41*, 2618–2628. [CrossRef] [PubMed]
42. Jorgensen, A.B.; Frikke-Schmidt, R.; Nordestgaard, B.G.; Tybjorg-Hansen, A.; Tybjorg-Hansen, A. Loss-of-Function Mutations in APOC3 and Risk of Ischemic Vascular Disease. *N. Engl. J. Med.* **2014**, *371*, 32–41. [CrossRef] [PubMed]
43. Surendran, R.P.; Visser, M.E.; Heemelaar, S.; Wang, J.; Peter, J.; Defesche, J.C.; Kuivenhoven, J.A.; Hosseini, M.; Péterfy, M.; Kastelein, J.J.; et al. Mutations in LPL, APOC2, APOA5, GPIHBP1 and LMF1 in patients with severe hypertriglyceridaemia. *J. Intern. Med.* **2012**, *272*, 185–196. [CrossRef] [PubMed]
44. Ma, Y.; Liu, M.S.; Chitayat, D.; Bruin, T.; Beisiegel, U.; Benlian, P.; Foubert, L.; De Gennes, J.L.; Funke, H.; Forsythe, I.; et al. Recurrent missense mutations at the first and second base of codon Arg243 in human lipoprotein lipase in patients of different ancestries. *Hum. Mutat.* **1994**, *3*, 52–58. [CrossRef]
45. Neuner, J.; Dimmock, D.; Kirschner, A.P.; Beaudry, H.; Paradowski, J.; Orlando, L. Results and Lessons of a Pilot Study of Cascade Screening for Familial Hypercholesterolemia in US Primary Care Practices. *J. Gen. Intern. Med.* **2020**, *35*, 351–353. [CrossRef] [PubMed]
46. Moldovan, V.; Banescu, C.; Dobreanu, M. Molecular diagnosis methods in familial hypercholesterolemia. *Anatol. J. Cardiol.* **2020**, *23*, 120–127. [CrossRef]
47. McGowan, M.P.; Cuchel, M.; Ahmed, C.D.; Khera, A.; Weintraub, W.S.; Wilemon, K.A.; Ahmad, Z. A proof-of-concept study of cascade screening for Familial Hypercholesterolemia in the US, adapted from the Dutch model. *Am. J. Prev. Cardiol.* **2021**, *11*, 100170. [CrossRef]
48. Peterson, A.L.; Bang, M.; Block, R.C.; Wong, N.D.; Karalis, D.G. Cascade Screening and Treatment Initiation in Young Adults with Heterozygous Familial Hypercholesterolemia. *J. Clin. Med.* **2021**, *10*, 3090. [CrossRef]
49. Truong, T.H.; Do, D.L.; Kim, N.T.; Nguyen, M.T.; Le, T.T.; Le, H.A. Genetics, Screening, and Treatment of Familial Hypercholesterolemia: Experience Gained From the Implementation of the Vietnam Familial Hypercholesterolemia Registry. *Front. Genet.* **2020**, *14*, 914. [CrossRef]
50. Garrahy, E.; Heal, C.; Hespe, C.M.; Radford, J.; Watts, G.F.; Brett, T. Familial hypercholesterolaemia and cascade testing in general practice: Lessons from COVID-19. *Aust J. Gen. Pract.* **2020**, *49*, 859–860. [CrossRef] [PubMed]
51. Kastelein, J.J.P.; Reeskamp, L.F.; Hovingh, G.K. Familial Hypercholesterolemia: The Most Common Monogenic Disorder in Humans. *J. Am. Coll. Cardiol.* **2020**, *26*, 2567–2569. [CrossRef] [PubMed]
52. Talmud, P.J.; Shah, S.; Whittall, R.; Futema, M.; Howard, P.; Cooper, J.A.; Harrison, S.C.; Li, K.; Drenos, F.; Karpe, F.; et al. Use of low density lipoprotein cholesterol gene score to distinguish patients with polygenic and monogenic familial hypercholesterolaemia: A case-control study. *Lancet* **2013**, *381*, e1293–e1301. [CrossRef]
53. Masana, L.; Ibarretxea, D.; Rodríguez-Borjabad, C.; Plana, N.; Valdivielso, P.; Pedro-Botet, J.; Civeira, F.; López-Miranda, J.; Guijarro, C.; Mostaza, J.; et al. Toward a new clinical classification of patients with familial hypercholesterolemia: One perspective from Spain. *Atherosclerosis* **2019**, *287*, 89–92. [CrossRef] [PubMed]

54. Mach, F.; Baigent, C.; Catapano, A.L.; Koskinas, K.C.; Casula, M.; Badimon, L.; Chapman, M.J.; De Backer, G.G.; Delgado, V.; Ference, B.A.; et al. 2019 ESC/EAS guidelines for the management of dyslipidaemias: Lipid modification to reduce cardiovascular risk. *Atherosclerosis* **2019**, *290*, 140–205. [CrossRef] [PubMed]
55. Sharma, K.; Baliga, R.R. Genetics of Dyslipidemia and Ischemic Heart Disease. *Curr. Cardiol. Rep.* **2017**, *19*, 46. [CrossRef] [PubMed]
56. Medeiros, A.M.; Alves, A.C.; Bourbon, M. Mutational analysis of a cohort with clinical diagnosis of familial hypercholesterolemia: Considerations for genetic diagnosis improvement. *Genet. Med.* **2016**, *18*, 316–324. [CrossRef]
57. Meshkov, A.; Ershova, A.; Kiseleva, A.; Zotova, E.; Sotnikova, E.; Petukhova, A.; Zharikova, A.; Malyshev, P.; Rozhkova, T.; Blokhina, A.; et al. The LDLR, APOB, and PCSK9 Variants of Index Patients with Familial Hypercholesterolemia in Russia. *Genes* **2021**, *12*, 66. [CrossRef]
58. Averkova, A.O.; Brazhnik, V.A.; Speshilov, G.I.; Rogozhina, A.A.; Koroleva, O.S.; Zubova, E.A.; Koroleva, O.S.; Zubova, E.A.; Galyavich, A.S.; Tereshenko, S.N.; et al. Target sequencing in patients with clinically diagnosed hereditary lipid metabolism disorders and acute coronary syndrome. *Bull. Russ. State Med. Univ.* **2020**, *5*, 93–99. [CrossRef]
59. Vlad, C.-E.; Foia, L.G.; Popescu, R.; Popa, I.; Aanicai, R.; Reurean-Pintilei, D.; Toma, V.; Florea, L.; Kanbay, M.; Covic, A. Molecular Genetic Approach and Evaluation of Cardiovascular Events in Patients with Clinical Familial Hypercholesterolemia Phenotype from Romania. *J. Clin. Med.* **2021**, *10*, 1399. [CrossRef]

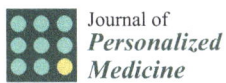

Article

Plateletworks® as a Point-of-Care Test for ASA Non-Sensitivity

Hamzah Khan [1], Shubha Jain [1], Reid C. Gallant [2], Muzammil H. Syed [1], Abdelrahman Zamzam [1], Mohammed Al-Omran [1,2,3], Margaret L. Rand [4,5,6], Heyu Ni [2,4], Rawand Abdin [7] and Mohammad Qadura [1,2,3,*]

1. Division of Vascular Surgery, St. Michael's Hospital, Toronto, ON M4B 1B3, Canada; hamzah.khan@mail.utoronto.ca (H.K.); jains@ucalgary.ca (S.J.); muzammil.syed@mail.utoronto.ca (M.H.S.); abdelrahman.zamzam@unityhealth.to (A.Z.); mohammed.al-omran@unityhealth.to (M.A.-O.)
2. Keenan Research Centre for Biomedical Science, Li Ka Shing Knowledge Institute of St. Michael's Hospital, Toronto, ON M4B 1B3, Canada; reid.gallant@mail.utoronto.ca (R.C.G.); Heyu.Ni@unityhealth.to (H.N.)
3. Department of Surgery, University of Toronto, Toronto, ON M4B 1B3, Canada
4. Department of Laboratory Medicine & Pathobiology, University of Toronto, Toronto, ON M4B 1B3, Canada; margaret.rand@sickkids.ca
5. Departments of Biochemistry and Pediatrics, University of Toronto, Toronto, ON M4B 1B3, Canada
6. Translational Medicine, Research Institute, Division of Haematology/Oncology, The Hospital for Sick Children, Toronto, ON M4B 1B3, Canada
7. Department of Medicine, McMaster University, Hamilton, ON L8N 3Z5, Canada; rawand.abdin@medportal.ca
* Correspondence: mohammad.qadura@utoronto.ca; Tel.: +1-416-864-6047

Abstract: Aspirin (ASA) therapy is proven to be effective in preventing adverse cardiovascular events; however, up to 30% of patients are non-sensitive to their prescribed ASA dosage. In this pilot study, we demonstrated, for the first time, how ASA non-sensitivity can be diagnosed using Plateletworks®, a point-of-care platelet function test. Patients prescribed 81 mg of ASA were recruited in a series of two successive phases—a discovery phase and a validation phase. In the discovery phase, a total of 60 patients were recruited to establish a cut-off point (COP) for ASA non-sensitivity using Plateletworks®. Each sample was simultaneously cross-referenced with a light transmission aggregometer (LTA). Our findings demonstrated that >52% maximal platelet aggregation using Plateletworks® had a sensitivity, specificity, and likelihood ratio of 80%, 70%, and 2.67, respectively, in predicting ASA non-sensitivity. This COP was validated in a secondary cohort of 40 patients prescribed 81 mg of ASA using Plateletworks® and LTA. Our data demonstrated that our established COP had a 91% sensitivity and 69% specificity in identifying ASA non-sensitivity using Plateletworks®. In summary, Plateletworks® is a point-of-care platelet function test that can appropriately diagnose ASA non-sensitive patients with a sensitivity exceeding 80%.

Keywords: aspirin; resistance; non-sensitivity; antiplatelet; atherosclerosis; light transmission aggregometry; Plateletworks®

Citation: Khan, H.; Jain, S.; Gallant, R.C.; Syed, M.H.; Zamzam, A.; Al-Omran, M.; Rand, M.L.; Ni, H.; Abdin, R.; Qadura, M. Plateletworks® as a Point-of-Care Test for ASA Non-Sensitivity. *J. Pers. Med.* **2021**, *11*, 813. https://doi.org/10.3390/jpm11080813

Academic Editor: Yuliya I. Ragino

Received: 12 July 2021
Accepted: 18 August 2021
Published: 20 August 2021

Publisher's Note: MDPI stays neutral with regard to jurisdictional claims in published maps and institutional affiliations.

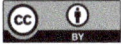

Copyright: © 2021 by the authors. Licensee MDPI, Basel, Switzerland. This article is an open access article distributed under the terms and conditions of the Creative Commons Attribution (CC BY) license (https://creativecommons.org/licenses/by/4.0/).

1. Introduction

Low-dose Aspirin (ASA), at 81 mg per day, is commonly prescribed for the secondary prevention of atherosclerotic/thrombotic adverse events such as myocardial infarction, cerebrovascular accidents, chronic limb threatening ischemia, and death [1–4]. It serves as first-line antiplatelet therapy among patients with coronary artery disease, carotid artery stenosis, and peripheral arterial disease [2–5]. The Antithrombotic Trialists Collaboration demonstrated that ASA is effective in reducing adverse cardiovascular events by approximately 20% [6]. However, an alarming 20–30% of patients with atherosclerotic disease suffer from ASA non-sensitivity, where ASA fails to prevent adverse cardiovascular events [7–12].

Plateletworks® is a point-of-care platelet function test that measures platelet aggregation in response to specific platelet activators [13]. In this point-of-care test, citrated-whole blood is incubated in pre-prepared tubes containing different platelet agonists, specifically arachidonic acid (AA), adenosine 5′-diphosphate (ADP), and collagen. A control ethylenediaminetetraacetic acid (EDTA) tube establishes a baseline platelet count to which all other platelet counts are compared. After platelet aggregation is induced with a particular agonist, whole-blood hematology analyzers are used to determine the platelet count in each tube and calculate the percent maximal platelet aggregation.

Plateletworks® has a number of appealing strengths and features. First, it is an efficient test that can be completed within 10 min and that can simultaneously provide a complete blood count (CBC). Second, minimal training is required to conduct a platelet function test with Plateletworks®. Third, previous studies have utilized it in a variety of settings, fortifying its legitimacy and appeal [13–16]. With these strengths, Plateletworks® is a potential point-of-care test that is easy, quick, and can readily be utilized in a variety of clinical settings. However, a cut-off point (COP) for ASA non-sensitivity using Plateletworks® needs to be established before it becomes common practice in these settings. Therefore, the aim of this pilot study was to determine and validate the optimal COP to detect ASA non-sensitivity using Plateletworks® in patients with established cardiovascular disease.

2. Materials and Methods

2.1. Ethics Approval

This study was performed in accordance with the Declaration of Helsinki and was approved by the Unity Health Toronto Research Ethics Board at St Michael's Hospital in Toronto, ON, Canada. Informed consent was obtained from each participant before enrolment in the study.

2.2. Patient Selection

A total of 100 patients were investigated in two successive phases: a discovery phase ($n = 60$) and a validation phase ($n = 40$). Patients with established cardiovascular disease presenting between September of 2019 and September of 2020 were recruited from St Michael's Hospital's outpatient vascular surgery clinic. Patients were eligible for inclusion if they were taking low-dose ASA (81 mg per day) for at least 14 days prior to recruitment. Patients that met any of the following criteria were excluded: (1) prior history of bleeding disorder, gastrointestinal bleeding, hemorrhagic stroke, thrombocytopenia, anemia, or leukopenia; (2) use of oral anticoagulants or antiplatelet medication other than ASA; (3) consumption of alcohol and/or another NSAID within the past 24 h and 3 days, respectively; (4) patients who are pregnant or nursing; (5) patients younger than 18 years of age. A negative control group, composed of patients with established atherosclerotic disease who had not yet been prescribed ASA or patients with venous disease not taking ASA, was also recruited.

2.3. Baseline Measurements

A complete medical history and physical exam were performed on each patient. Medical history included details of any previous coronary artery disease, hyperlipidemia, hypertension, renal disease, congestive heart failure, diabetes, history of stroke or transient ischemic attacks, and smoking status. Baseline variables were defined as previously described [17]. Patients with a glycosylated hemoglobin A1c $\geq 6.5\%$ or using anti-diabetic medication were classified as having diabetes mellitus (DM). Patients on anti-hyperlipidemic medication or having a total cholesterol > 5.2 mmol/L or triglyceride > 1.7 mmol/L were classified as having hyperlipidemia. Patients using antihypertensive medication or with a systolic blood pressure ≥ 130 mmHg or a diastolic pressure ≥ 80 mm Hg were classified as hypertensive. Renal disease was defined as an estimated glomerular filtration rate of less than 60 mL/min/1.73 m^2 [17].

2.4. Specimen Collection

Whole blood samples were drawn from the antecubital vein using a 21-gauge needle into 3.2% sodium citrate tubes to investigate ASA sensitivity immediately after collection.

2.5. Gold Standard Light Transmission Aggregometry-Aspirin Sensitivity Testing

Light transmission aggregometry (LTA) is the gold-standard test for ASA non-sensitivity testing. To establish a COP for ASA non-sensitivity with Plateletworks®, each patient's platelets were simultaneously tested with both Plateletworks® and LTA using arachidonic acid (AA) activation to determine their ASA non-sensitivity status. LTA was conducted according to previously published protocols [11,18]. In short, platelet-rich plasma (PRP) was prepared by the centrifugation of citrated blood at $300\times g$ for 7 min at room temperature, with deceleration set to 0. For PRP collection, 2 mm was cut off from the pipette tip to prevent the shear activation of platelets. Platelet-poor plasma (PPP) was prepared by centrifugation at $1200\times g$ for 10 min at room temperature. PRP and PPP were transferred to fresh tubes and kept at 37 °C until testing. Platelet counts in PRP were collected using a Mindray BC-3600 21-parameter hematology analyzer (Mindray, Shenzhen, China) and adjusted to $2\text{--}3 \times 10^8$ platelets/mL using autologous PPP. Platelet aggregation was performed with the stir bar speed set to 1000 rpm at 37 °C using a computerized aggregometer (Chrono-Log Corp, Havertown, PA, USA), with activation initiated with 0.5 mg/mL AA (101297, Bio/Data Corporation, Horsham, PA, USA). Patients were considered ASA non-sensitive if they had a residual maximal platelet aggregation $\geq 20\%$ after induction with AA, as per previous studies [19–23].

2.6. Plateletworks® Testing

Plateletworks® was conducted as per the manufacturer's protocol [13]. A total of 1 mL of citrated-whole blood was aliquoted into each Plateletworks® tube containing either EDTA, collagen, AA, or ADP. Each tube was inverted gently 20 times to ensure the adequate mixing of the agonists. Platelet counts were obtained by running each tube on a Mindray BC-3600 21-parameter hematology analyzer (Mindray, Shenzhen, China). First, a baseline single platelet count was obtained by running the EDTA tube on the hematology analyzer. Immediately following the baseline platelet count, the ADP Plateletworks® tube was gently inverted 5 times and a single platelet count was obtained. The collagen tube was gently mixed 5 times every 1 min for 4 min, after which a single platelet count was obtained. At the same time, the AA tube was gently inverted 5 times every 10 s for 2 min. The AA tube was then left at room temperature for 8 min, after which a single platelet count was obtained. The percentage of platelet activation by each agonist was then recorded using the following formula:

$$\text{Aggregation}\,(\%) = 100\,\frac{\text{Baseline Platelet Count} - \text{Platelet Count After Activation}}{\text{Baseline Platelet Count}}$$

2.7. Statistical Analysis

Demographics and clinical characteristics were expressed as means and standard deviations, or frequencies with percentages. Normality for continuous variables was assessed using normality plots and the Shapiro–Wilk test. Normally distributed continuous variables were reported with means and standard deviations. Median and interquartile ranges (IQR) were calculated for non-normally distributed data. Categorical variables were reported as counts and percentages. Pearson's correlation coefficient was calculated to compare the percent of maximal platelet aggregation by LTA and Plateletworks®, with $p < 0.05$ considered statistically significant. We calculated the diagnostic performance of Plateletworks® in detecting ASA non-sensitivity (i.e., sensitivity, specificity, positive predictive value and negative predictive value, and likelihood ratios) to determine the cut-off point for ASA non-sensitivity. All hypothesis testing was carried out at the 5% (2-sided) significance level. Statistical analysis was conducted using the GraphPad Prism software, version 8.4.2.

2.8. Optimal Cut-Off Point Selection for Predicting ASA Non-Sensitivity

To measure the sensitivity and specificity of Plateletworks® in detecting ASA sensitivity at different cut-off values, a conventional receiver-operating characteristic (ROC) curve was generated. We calculated the area under the curve (AUC) to ascertain the quality of Plateletworks® as a point-of-care test for ASA sensitivity. From the ROC analysis, the first identified maximal platelet aggregation value with a corresponding sensitivity of >80% was selected as a cut-off point to ensure a low rate of false negatives for ASA non-sensitivity.

3. Results

3.1. ASA Non-Sensitivity Cut-Off Point Discovery

3.1.1. Patient Characteristics

In the discovery phase, a total of 60 patients were recruited, comprising 20 control patients not taking ASA and 40 patients on 81 mg of ASA daily. The median age for the discovery cohort was 67 years and the majority were male patients (72%). Noticeably, 62% of the discovery phase cohort were smokers, 66% suffered from hyperlipidemia, and 60% had hypertension. No recruited patients had thrombocytopenia, anemia, leukopenia, or any other blood disorders. Comparing these characteristics showed that patients taking 81 mg of ASA had significantly higher cardiovascular risk factors, such as hypertension, hyperlipidemia, and diabetes, compared to the control group not taking 81 mg of ASA (Table 1).

Table 1. Baseline characteristics of patients recruited to the discovery phase.

	Discovery Phase	
	Control Cohort (n = 20)	Patients on 81 mg ASA (n = 40)
		Mean (SD)
Age (yrs)	58 (19)	68 (9)
Platelet Count (10^8/mL)	186 (62)	209 (70.47)
WBC (10^8/mL)	6.2 (2.0)	6.8 (1.7)
HCT	0.380 (0.04)	0.384 (0.03)
		Frequency (%)
Sex (male)	15 (75)	28 (70) *
Hypertension	8 (40)	28 (70) *
Hyperlipidemia	8 (40)	32 (80) *
Diabetes	2 (10)	15 (37) *
Smoking	7 (35)	30 (75) *
CAD	0 (0)	12 (30) *
PAD	5 (13)	24 (60) *
		Medication (%)
Statin	9 (45)	33 (83) *
ACEi/ARB	6 (30)	21 (53) *
B-blockers	1 (5)	9 (23) *

Acetylsalicylic acid, ASA; white blood cells, WBC; hematocrit, HCT; angiotensin-converting enzyme inhibitors ACEi/Arb; coronary artery disease, CAD; peripheral arterial disease, PAD. Continuous variables are shown as mean (standard deviation). Categorical variables are shown as frequency (%). * represents significant difference ($p < 0.05$) between controls not taking ASA and patients on 81 mg of ASA.

3.1.2. Plateletworks® Analysis

To investigate if Plateletworks® could be utilized to distinguish patients on ASA from controls not taking ASA, Plateletworks® analysis was conducted on all 60 patients recruited to the discovery phase. Relative to the controls, patients taking 81 mg of ASA had a significantly lower maximal platelet aggregation in response to activation with arachidonic acid (AA) and collagen (difference between means of 34 ± 4%, 95% CI: 26–43% and 29 ± 5%, 95% CI: 17–40%, respectively). We did not observe any significant difference in the maximal platelet aggregation between both groups post activation with ADP (Figure 1).

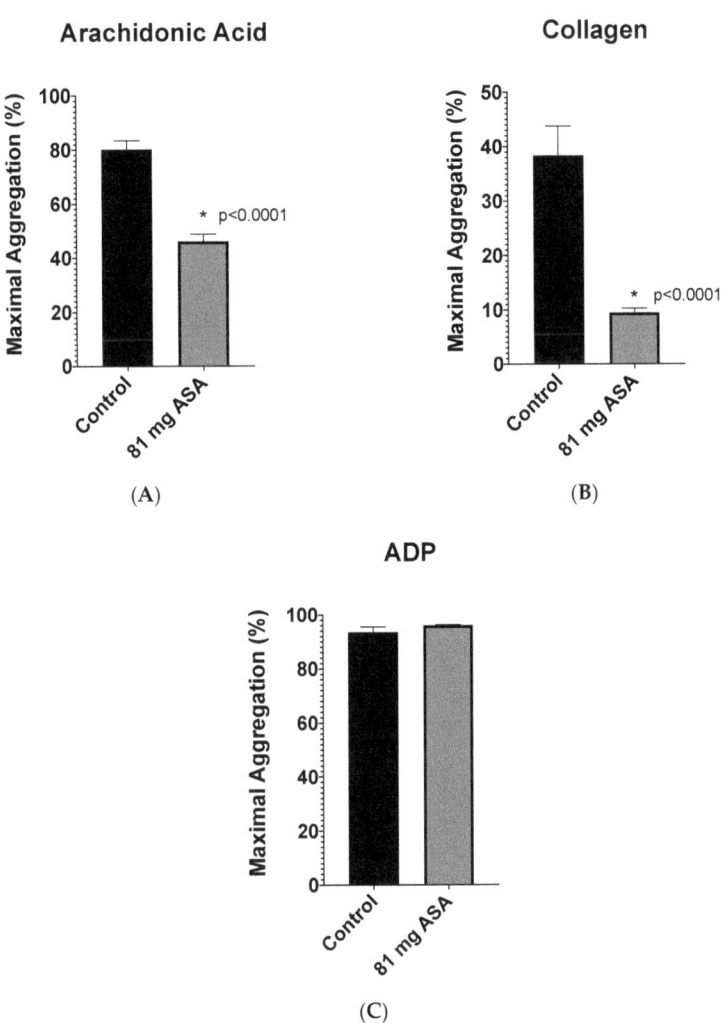

Figure 1. Plateletworks® analysis between patients not on ASA (control, $n = 20$) and patients taking 81 mg aspirin (81 mg ASA, $n = 40$) using platelet activation agonists (**A**) arachidonic acid, (**B**) collagen, and (**C**) adenosine 5′-diphosphate (ADP). Error bars represent standard error of the mean. * represents significant difference between control and 81 mg ASA patients.

To establish ASA sensitivity, the gold-standard LTA was utilized. All patients on 81 mg of ASA underwent LTA analysis with AA-induced platelet activation. LTA analysis demonstrated that 10 patients on ASA (25%) had a $\geq 20\%$ maximal platelet aggregation, suggesting ASA non-sensitivity. As anticipated, all control patients who were not prescribed ASA had a maximal platelet aggregation $\geq 20\%$ (Figure 2).

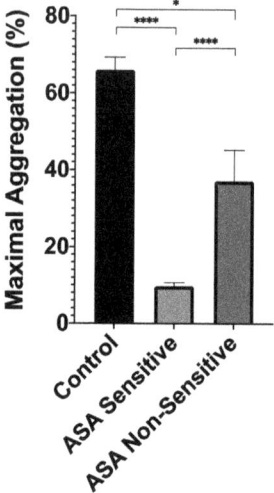

Figure 2. Light transmission aggregometry analysis between ASA sensitive patients ($n = 30$), ASA non-sensitive patients ($n = 10$), and controls not taking ASA ($n = 20$) with platelet activation using arachidonic acid. Error bars represent standard error of the mean. * represents $p < 0.05$, **** represents $p < 0.0001$.

Next, patients prescribed ASA were categorized into two groups based on their ASA sensitivity: patients who were sensitive to 81 mg of ASA ($n = 30$) and those who were non-sensitive to the prescribed 81 mg of ASA ($n = 10$). To assess Plateletworks® ability to detect a difference between ASA sensitive and non-sensitive patients, the Plateletworks® results of both groups were compared (Figure 3). Relative to ASA sensitive patients, the ASA non-sensitive patients had a significantly higher response to AA, with a difference between means of $23 \pm 5\%$ (95% CI: 12–35%, $p < 0.001$). We did not observe any difference in response to collagen and ADP while comparing ASA non-sensitive to ASA sensitive patients (Figure 3).

Next, we studied the correlation between maximal platelet aggregation in response to AA by LTA, with maximal platelet aggregation in response to AA by Plateletworks® (Figure 4). Our analysis yielded a correlation coefficient of 0.75, suggesting a high correlation between Plateletworks® and the gold-standard LTA ($p < 0.0001$) [24].

3.1.3. Cut-Off Point Discovery

An ROC analysis was conducted that compared the percent maximal platelet aggregation in response to AA in Plateletworks® between both ASA-sensitive and non-sensitive patients (Figure 4). Our data demonstrated that ASA non-sensitive patients had an area under the curve (AUC) of 0.89 (95% CI: 0.77 to 0.99, p-value = 0.0003) (Figure 5). Extrapolating the data from the ROC analysis, the first COP with a corresponding sensitivity of at least 80% was chosen. This value was identified to be >52% maximal platelet aggregation in response to AA, and hence was chosen as a diagnostic COP to distinguish ASA non-sensitive patients using Plateletworks®. This cut-off point had a sensitivity, specificity, and likelihood ratio of 80%, 70%, and 2.67, respectively.

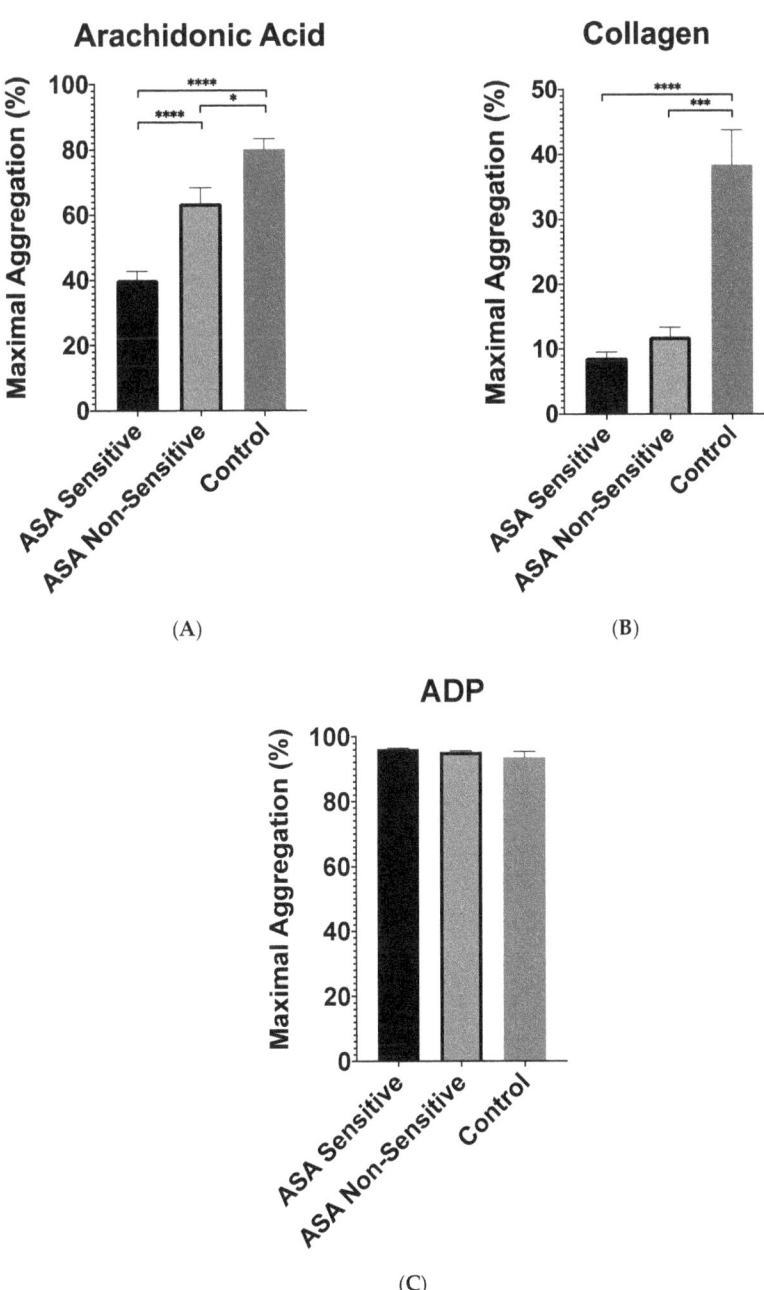

Figure 3. Plateletworks® analysis between patients sensitive to 81 mg of ASA ($n = 30$), and ASA non-sensitive ($n = 10$) using platelet activation agonists (**A**) arachidonic acid, (**B**) collagen, and (**C**) adenosine 5'-diphosphate (ADP). Error bars represent standard error of the mean. Dotted line represents maximal aggregation in control patients not taking 81 mg of ASA. * represents $p < 0.05$; *** represents $p < 0.001$; and **** represents $p < 0.0001$.

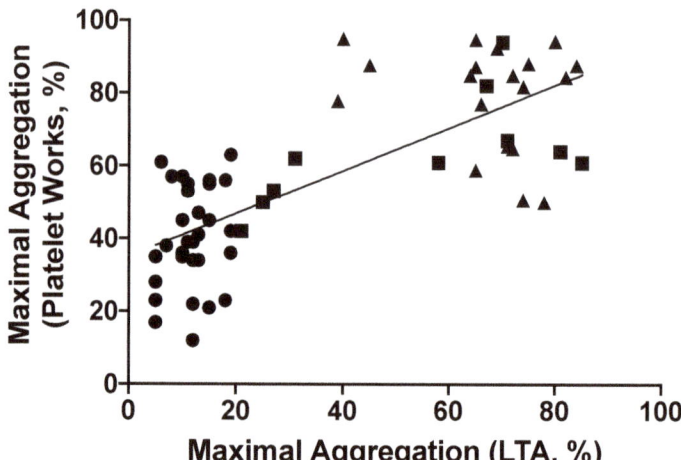

Figure 4. Pearson correlation between maximal platelet aggregation in response to Arachidonic acid using Plateletworks® and light transmission aggregometry (n = 60). There is a good correlation between the two methods of platelet aggregation testing (r = 0.749, 95% CI: 0.6096 to 0.8432, $p < 0.0001$). Triangles represent patients not taking ASA (n = 20), circles represent ASA-sensitive patients (n = 30), and squares represent ASA non-sensitive patients (n = 10).

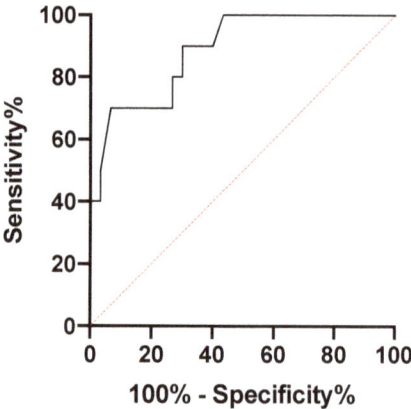

Figure 5. Receiver operating characteristics curve comparing ASA-sensitive patients (n = 30) to ASA non-sensitive patients (AUC = 0.89, 95%CI 0.78–0.99, $p = 0.0003$).

3.2. ASA Non-Sensitivity Cut-Off Point Validation

3.2.1. Patient Characteristics

A validation phase was conducted to confirm the COP of >52% maximal platelet aggregation using Plateletworks® in predicting ASA non-sensitivity determined in the discovery phase. An additional 40 patients on 81 mg of ASA were recruited for the validation phase. Patients in the validation phase cohort had median age of 69 years, and primarily comprised males (63%). Notably, 75% of our study cohort were smokers, 85% suffered from hyperlipidemia, and 70% had hypertension (Table 2). No significant differences were noted between the patients on 81 mg of ASA in the discovery and validation cohorts in terms of all measured baseline demographics and clinical characteristics.

Table 2. Baseline characteristics of patients recruited for the validation phase of the study.

	Validation Phase	
Patient Demographics		Patients on 81 mg ASA (n = 40)
	Mean (SD)	
Age (yrs)		68 (11)
Platelet Count (10^8/mL)		185.3 (48)
WBC (10^8/mL)		6.8 (1.9)
HCT		0.3832 (0.03)
	Frequency (%)	
Sex (male)		24 (60)
Hypertension		27 (68)
Hyperlipidemia		33 (83)
Diabetes		20 (50)
Smoking		29 (73)
CAD		13 (33)
PAD		22 (55)
	Medications (Frequency, %)	
Statin		34 (85)
ACEi/ARB		20 (50)
B-blockers		9 (23)

Acetylsalicylic acid, ASA; white blood cells, WBC; hematocrit, HCT; angiotensin-converting enzyme inhibitors/angiotensin receptor blocker ACEi/Arb; coronary artery disease, CAD; peripheral arterial disease, PAD. Continuous variables are shown as means (and standard deviations). Categorical variables are shown as frequencies (%).

3.2.2. Cut-Off Point Validation

To investigate the diagnostic performance of the established COP, platelet aggregation post-AA stimulation was investigated using Plateletworks®. Each sample was simultaneously investigated and cross referenced with LTA. LTA analysis of the 40 patients showed that 11 patients (28%) were non-sensitive to 81 mg ASA. Our data demonstrated that the COP for Plateletworks® of >52% maximal platelet aggregation post-AA stimulation has a sensitivity and specificity of 91% and 69%, respectively. This COP value was determined to have negative and positive predictive values of 95% and 53%, respectively, and a diagnostic accuracy of 75%.

4. Discussion

In this study, we demonstrated that Plateletworks® was able to distinguish between patients who were non-sensitive to 81 mg ASA therapy from patients who are sensitive to 81 mg ASA. Using Plateletworks®, our results suggest a COP of >52% maximal platelet aggregation in response to AA has good sensitivity in identifying ASA non-sensitivity. We were also able to demonstrate that Plateletworks® has a good correlation with LTA, the current gold standard.

ASA non-sensitivity has become a well-known and prevalent issue, with anywhere between 20 and 30% of patients at risk of further adverse cardiovascular events due to the failure of ASA to completely inhibit platelet aggregation. Previous studies have reported that 15% of patients with atherosclerotic vascular disease were non-sensitive to their prescribed 81 mg ASA therapy, and a further 32% of patients with cardiovascular risk factors were also non-sensitive to ASA [11,12]. There are two main mechanisms of ASA non-sensitivity: (1) pharmacokinetic variability in patients' response to ASA—for example reduced absorption within the gastrointestinal tract, higher ASA metabolism, or increased platelet turnover; (2) pharmacodynamic differences such as genetic polymorphisms leading to structural changes in the COX enzyme [25]. A third reason why patients may be identified as non-sensitive is if patients are non-compliant with their ASA therapy.

In this study, 21 of our 80 patients (26%) were non-sensitive to their therapy. This is a significant number, as these ASA non-sensitive patients have a ~6 fold increase odds of cardiovascular related death when compared to ASA sensitive patients [26]. Collectively, these data highlight the urgent need of a quick and easy, point-of-care test for ASA non-sensitivity that is not only available in hospitals, but also smaller clinical settings to allow for routine ASA non-sensitivity testing.

LTA is the current gold standard for platelet function and ASA non-sensitivity testing [27–29]. It has a well-established COP for ASA non-sensitivity testing, specifically with patients with $\geq 20\%$ maximal platelet aggregation in response to AA being considered ASA non-sensitive. Several studies have used this method for determining ASA non-sensitivity in both vascular and cardiac disease patients [19–23]. However, LTA can be time consuming, requires specialized equipment, and needs highly trained staff. LTA is not feasible for widespread use as a clinical ASA non-sensitivity test. There remains a need for a suitable quick, point-of-care test for ASA non-sensitivity, which can potentially be met by Plateletworks®.

There are several point-of-care platelet function test currently available, however many have not been optimized to accurately detect ASA non-sensitivity. One such platelet function test is the Platelet Function Analyzer (PFA) 100/200. Citrated-whole blood is aspirated at high shear through a membrane coated with platelet agonists to mimic the in vivo environment of an injury. PFA-100/200, however, is an expensive test, has poor agreement with LTA, and the collagen/epinephrine cartridge (which is recommended for ASA non-sensitivity testing), and has shown to overestimate the prevalence of ASA non-sensitivity. One study demonstrated a sensitivity and specificity of 75% and 40%, respectively [20]. Another platelet function test that is becoming more commonly used in cardiac patients is the VerifyNow Aspirin test. In this assay, citrated whole blood is placed within cuvettes containing AA and microbeads coated with fibrinogen. Platelet aggregation is initiated and is recorded in Aspirin Reaction Units (ARU). A cut-off of >550 ARU has been recommended by the manufacturer as a cut-off for ASA non-sensitivity [30,31]. VerifyNow has been shown to be a good contender for ASA non-sensitivity testing in cardiac patients, with a high sensitivity and specificity demonstrated by several studies (100% and 96% respectively) [32–34]. However, some studies have shown a specificity as low as 35% [20]. There is a paucity of data regarding the use of VerifyNow within patients with vascular disease.

Plateletworks® is a platelet function test that has potential to accurately detect antiplatelet non-sensitivity testing. The good correlation with LTA; its ability to be used on any hematology analyzer; its fast processing times (ASA non-sensitivity tests are run within 10 min); and the minimal training required for use are major strengths that suggest potential as an ideal point-of-care screening test for ASA non-sensitivity [13,15,35]. If more robustly proven, Plateletworks® would enable physicians to conduct routine ASA non-sensitivity screening and inform physicians if further testing is required. Ultimately, by ensuring that patients are responding to their antiplatelet therapy, this test can help reduce the adverse cardiovascular events and intervention failures that occur due to ASA non-sensitivity. A potential COP for Plateletworks® has also been suggested, with its feasibility demonstrated as an ASA non-sensitivity screening test. Our study demonstrates that Plateletworks® has a comparable sensitivity and specificity to current point-of-care ASA non-sensitivity test frontrunners such as VerifyNow, and it shows a good correlation with the gold standard LTA.

This study has some limitations. First, a relatively small sample size was used; however, this study was designed to be a pilot that assesses the potential of Plateletworks® as a point-of-care test for ASA non-sensitivity testing. In the future, larger studies need to be conducted to verify our COP for ASA non-sensitivity. Second, while patients were asked about ASA compliance, this was not formally assessed. Therefore, the non-compliance of patients nonetheless remains as a possibility. Despite this, Plateletworks® still provides physicians with vital information about patients' platelet activity, allowing physicians to further investigate the cause of their patients' ASA non-sensitivity.

5. Conclusions

In conclusion, we demonstrated that Plateletworks® may potentially be useful as a point-of-care screening test for ASA non-sensitivity using our validated COP in patients taking low-dose ASA (81–325 mg). While Plateletworks® may not replace LTA as a gold-standard test for ASA sensitivity, Plateletworks® can be utilized as a diagnostic screening tool or "pre-test" for ASA non-sensitivity, which could then be confirmed by LTA. It can also be helpful where LTA analysis is not available, such as in outpatient clinics in primary care or in resource-limited settings. Further clinical studies with larger sample sizes are required for validating this COP. With Plateletworks®, physicians will have easy access to point-of-care platelet function testing in a variety of clinical settings, allowing for fast and convenient ASA non-sensitivity testing. Additional research studies may use Plateletworks® for investigating non-sensitivity to other antiplatelet agents that have also been found to be prevalent within the vascular population, such as clopidogrel [9]. The effective non-sensitivity testing of antiplatelet agents that can be performed with a point-of-care test such as Plateletworks® will help to reduce the high risk of adverse cardiovascular events.

Author Contributions: Conceptualization, R.A. and M.Q.; data curation, H.K.; formal analysis, H.K., S.J., R.C.G., A.Z., M.A.-O., M.L.R. and M.Q.; funding acquisition, R.A. and M.Q.; investigation, H.K., S.J., R.C.G., H.N. and M.Q.; methodology, H.K., S.J., M.L.R., H.N., M.A.-O., R.A. and M.Q.; project administration, M.Q.; resources, H.N., M.A.-O. and M.Q.; supervision, M.L.R., M.A.-O. and M.Q.; visualization, H.K. and M.Q.; writing—original draft, H.K., S.J., R.C.G., A.Z., M.H.S., R.A. and M.Q.; writing—review and editing, H.K., S.J., R.C.G., A.Z., M.H.S., M.L.R., H.N., M.A.-O., R.A. and M.Q. All authors have read and agreed to the published version of the manuscript.

Funding: This research received no external funding.

Institutional Review Board Statement: The study was conducted according to the guidelines of the Declaration of Helsinki, and approved by the Unity Health Toronto Research Ethics Board of St. Michaels Hospital (REB #16-375).

Informed Consent Statement: Informed consent was obtained from all subjects involved in the study.

Data Availability Statement: The data presented in this study are available on request from the corresponding author.

Acknowledgments: We would like to thank Helena Laboratories for supplying the Plateletworks® Kits, and Canadian Hospital Specialties Ltd. for the BC3600 Mindray Analyzer and supplies.

Conflicts of Interest: The authors declare no conflict of interest. The funders had no role in the design of the study; in the collection, analysis, or interpretation of data; in the writing of the manuscript; or in the decision to publish the results.

References

1. Ittaman, S.V.; VanWormer, J.J.; Rezkalla, S.H. The Role of Aspirin in the Prevention of Cardiovascular Disease. *Clin. Med. Res.* **2014**, *12*, 147–154. [CrossRef]
2. Ricotta, J.J.; Aburahma, A.; Ascher, E.; Eskandari, M.; Faries, P.; Lal, B.K. Updated Society for Vascular Surgery guidelines for management of extracranial carotid disease: Executive summary. *J. Vasc. Surg.* **2011**, *54*, 832–836. [CrossRef] [PubMed]
3. 2019 ACC/AHA Guideline on the Primary Prevention of Cardiovascular Disease: A Report of the American College of Cardiology/American Heart Association Task Force on Clinical Practice Guidelines. Available online: https://pubmed.ncbi.nlm.nih.gov/30879355/ (accessed on 30 March 2021).
4. Society for Vascular Surgery Practice Guidelines for Atherosclerotic Occlusive Disease of the Lower Extremities: Management of Asymptomatic Disease and Claudication. Available online: https://pubmed.ncbi.nlm.nih.gov/25638515/ (accessed on 30 March 2021).
5. Bachert, C.; a, A.; Eisebitt, R.; Netayzhenko, V.Z.; Voelker, M. Aspirin Compared with Acetaminophen in the Treatment of Feverand OtherSymptoms of Upper Respiratory Tract Infection in Adults: A Multicenter, Randomized, Double-Blind, Double-Dummy, Placebo-Controlled, Parallel-Group, Single-Dose, 6-Hour Dose-Ranging Study. *Clin. Ther.* **2005**, *27*, 993–1003. [CrossRef] [PubMed]

6. Group BMJP. Collaborative meta-analysis of randomised trials of antiplatelet therapy for prevention of death, myocardial infarction, and stroke in high risk patients. *BMJ* **2002**, *324*, 71–86. [CrossRef] [PubMed]
7. Schwartz, K.A. Aspirin Resistance. *Neurohospitalist* **2011**, *1*, 94–103. [CrossRef]
8. Clavijo, L.C.; Al-Asady, N.; Dhillon, A.; Matthews, R.V.; Caro, J.; Tun, H.; Rowe, V.; Shavelle, D.M. Prevalence of high on-treatment (aspirin and clopidogrel) platelet reactivity in patients with critical limb ischemia. *Cardiovasc. Revascularization Med.* **2018**, *19*, 516–520. [CrossRef] [PubMed]
9. Guirgis, M.; Thompson, P.; Jansen, S. Review of aspirin and clopidogrel resistance in peripheral arterial disease. *J. Vasc. Surg.* **2017**, *66*, 1576–1586. [CrossRef]
10. Pasala, T.; Hoo, J.S.; Lockhart, M.K.; Waheed, R.; Sengodan, P.; Alexander, J.; Gandhi, S. Aspirin Resistance Predicts Adverse Cardiovascular Events in Patients with Symptomatic Peripheral Artery Disease. *Tex. Heart Inst. J.* **2016**, *43*, 482–487. [CrossRef]
11. Khan, H.; Gallant, R.C.; Zamzam, A.; Jain, S.; Afxentiou, S.; Syed, M.; Kroezen, Z.; Shanmuganathan, M.; Britz-McKibbin, P.; Rand, M.L.; et al. Personalization of Aspirin Therapy Ex Vivo in Patients with Atherosclerosis Using Light Transmission Aggregometry. *Diagnostics* **2020**, *10*, 871. [CrossRef]
12. Khan, H.; Gallant, R.; Jain, S.; Al-Omran, M.; De Mestral, C.; Greco, E.; Wheatcroft, M.; Alazonni, A.; Abdin, R.; Rand, M.; et al. Ticagrelor as an Alternative Antiplatelet Therapy in Cardiac Patients Non-Sensitive to Aspirin. *Medicina* **2020**, *56*, 519. [CrossRef]
13. Campbell, J.; Ridgway, H.; Carville, D. Plateletworks®. *Mol. Diagn. Ther.* **2008**, *12*, 253–258. [CrossRef] [PubMed]
14. Karkouti, K.; Callum, J.; Wijeysundera, D.; Rao, V.; Crowther, M.; Grocott, H.P.; Pinto, R.; Scales, D.C.; Achen, B.; Brar, S.; et al. Point-of-Care Hemostatic Testing in Cardiac Surgery. *Circulation* **2016**, *134*, 1152–1162. [CrossRef] [PubMed]
15. van Werkum, J.W.; Kleibeuker, M.; Postma, S.; Bouman, H.J.; Elsenberg, E.H.; Berg, J.M.T.; Hackeng, C.M. A comparison between the Plateletworks™-assay and light transmittance aggregometry for monitoring the inhibitory effects of clopidogrel. *Int. J. Cardiol.* **2010**, *140*, 123–126. [CrossRef]
16. White, M.M.; Krishnan, R.; Kueter, T.J.; Jacoski, M.V.; Jennings, L.K. The Use of the Point of Care Helena ICHOR/Plateletworks® and the Accumetrics Ultegra® RPFA for Assessment of Platelet Function with GPIIb-IIIa Antagonists. *J. Thromb. Thrombolysis* **2004**, *18*, 163–169. [CrossRef]
17. Syed, M.H.; Zamzam, A.; Khan, H.; Singh, K.; Forbes, T.L.; Rotstein, O.; Abdin, R.; Eikelboom, J.; Qadura, M. Fatty acid binding protein 3 is associated with peripheral arterial disease. *JVS Vasc. Sci.* **2020**, *1*, 168–175. [CrossRef]
18. Xu, X.R.; Wang, Y.; Adili, R.; Ju, L.; Spring, C.M.; Jin, J.W.; Yang, H.; Neves, M.A.; Chen, P.; Yang, Y.; et al. Apolipoprotein A-IV binds αIIbβ3 integrin and inhibits thrombosis. *Nat. Commun.* **2018**, *9*, 1–18. [CrossRef]
19. Gum, P.A.; Kottke-Marchant, K.; Poggio, E.D.; Gurm, H.; Welsh, P.A.; Brooks, L.; Sapp, S.K.; Topol, E.J. Profile and prevalence of aspirin resistance in patients with cardiovascular disease. *Am. J. Cardiol.* **2001**, *88*, 230–235. [CrossRef]
20. Lordkipanidze, M.; Pharand, C.; Schampaert, E.; Turgeon, J.; Palisaitis, D.A.; Diodati, J.G. A comparison of six major platelet function tests to determine the prevalence of aspirin resistance in patients with stable coronary artery disease. *Eur. Heart J.* **2007**, *28*, 1702–1708. [CrossRef]
21. Maree, A.; Curtin, R.; Dooley, M.; Conroy, R.; Crean, P.; Cox, D.; Fitzgerald, D.J. Platelet Response to Low-Dose Enteric-Coated Aspirin in Patients with Stable Cardiovascular Disease. *J. Am. Coll. Cardiol.* **2005**, *46*, 1258–1263. [CrossRef]
22. Pedersen, S.B.; Grove, E.; Nielsen, H.L.; Mortensen, J.; Kristensen, S.D.; Hvas, A.-M. Evaluation of aspirin response by Multiplate® whole blood aggregometry and light transmission aggregometry. *Platelets* **2009**, *20*, 415–420. [CrossRef]
23. Tantry, U.S.; Bliden, K.P.; Gurbel, P.A. Overestimation of Platelet Aspirin Resistance Detection by Thrombelastograph Platelet Mapping and Validation by Conventional Aggregometry Using Arachidonic Acid Stimulation. *J. Am. Coll. Cardiol.* **2005**, *46*, 1705–1709. [CrossRef]
24. Mukaka, M.M. A guide to appropriate use of Correlation coefficient in medical research. *Malawi Med. J.* **2012**, *24*, 69–71.
25. Westphal, E.S.; Rainka, M.; Amsler, M.; Aladeen, T.; Wisniewski, C.; Bates, V.; Gengo, F.M. Prospective Determination of Aspirin Sensitivity in Patients Resistant to Low Dose Aspirin: A Proof of Concept Study. *J. Clin. Pharmacol.* **2018**, *58*, 1157–1163. [CrossRef] [PubMed]
26. Krasopoulos, G.; Brister, S.J.; Beattie, W.S.; Buchanan, M.R. Aspirin "resistance" and risk of cardiovascular morbidity: Systematic review and meta-analysis. *BMJ* **2008**, *336*, 195–198. [CrossRef] [PubMed]
27. Frontroth, J.P. Light Transmission Aggregometry. *Adv. Struct. Saf. Stud.* **2013**, *992*, 227–240. [CrossRef]
28. Hvas, A.-M.; Favaloro, E.J. Platelet Function Analyzed by Light Transmission Aggregometry. *Methods Mol. Biol.* **2017**, *1646*, 321–331. [CrossRef]
29. Sun, P.; McMillan-Ward, E.; Mian, R.; Israels, S.J. Comparison of light transmission aggregometry and multiple electrode aggregometry for the evaluation of patients with mucocutaneous bleeding. *Int. J. Lab. Hematol.* **2019**, *41*, 133–140. [CrossRef]
30. Van Werkum, J.W.; Harmsze, A.M.; Elsenberg, E.H.A.M.; Bouman, H.J.; Berg, J.M.T.; Hackeng, C.M. The use of the VerifyNow system to monitor antiplatelet therapy: A review of the current evidence. *Platelets* **2008**, *19*, 479–488. [CrossRef]
31. Chung, Y.H.; Lee, K.A.; Cho, M.; Shin, S.; Lee, B.K. Performance comparison of platelet function analyzers in cardiology patients: VerifyNow and Anysis-200 aspirin assays. *Clin. Hemorheol. Microcirc.* **2020**, *76*, 33–42. [CrossRef]
32. Nielsen, H.L.; Kristensen, S.D.; Thygesen, S.S.; Mortensen, J.; Pedersen, S.B.; Grove, E.L.; Hvas, A.-M. Aspirin response evaluated by the VerifyNow™ Aspirin System and Light Transmission Aggregometry. *Thromb. Res.* **2008**, *123*, 267–273. [CrossRef]
33. Nielsen, H.L.; Kristensen, S.D.; Hvas, A.-M. Is the New Point-of-Care Test VerifyNow® Aspirin Able to Identify Aspirin Resistance Using the Recommended Cut-Off? *Blood* **2007**, *110*, 3896. [CrossRef]

34. Pharand, C.; Lordkipanidzé, M.; Sia, Y.K.; Merhi, Y.; Diodati, J.G.; Blais, N. Response to aspirin in healthy individuals. Cross-comparison of light transmission aggregometry, VerifyNow system, platelet count drop, thromboelastography (TEG) and urinary 11-dehydrothromboxane B(2). *Thromb. Haemost.* **2009**, *102*, 404–411. [CrossRef] [PubMed]
35. Koltai, K.; Kesmarky, G.; Feher, G.; Tibold, A.; Toth, K. Platelet Aggregometry Testing: Molecular Mechanisms, Techniques and Clinical Implications. *Int. J. Mol. Sci.* **2017**, *18*, 1803. [CrossRef]

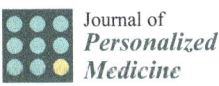

Article

Association of Matrix Metalloproteinases with Coronary Artery Calcification in Patients with CHD

Yana V. Polonskaya [1,*], Elena V. Kashtanova [1], Ivan S. Murashov [2], Evgenia V. Striukova [1], Alexey V. Kurguzov [2], Ekaterina M. Stakhneva [1], Viktoria S. Shramko [1], Nikolay A. Maslatsov [1], Aleksandr M. Chernyavsky [2] and Yulia I. Ragino [1]

1. Research Institute of Internal and Preventive Medicine—Branch of the Institute of Cytology and Genetics, Siberian Branch of Russian Academy of Sciences (IIPM–Branch of IC&G SB RAS), 175/1 B. Bogatkova Str., 630089 Novosibirsk, Russia; elekastanova@yandex.ru (E.V.K.); stryukova.j@mail.ru (E.V.S.); stahneva@yandex.ru (E.M.S.); nosova@211.ru (V.S.S.); maslatsoff@mail.ru (N.A.M.); ragino@mail.ru (Y.I.R.)
2. The Federal State Budgetary Institution "National Medical Research Center Named Academician E.N. Meshalkin" of the Ministry of Health of the Russian Federation, Rechkunovskaya Str., 15, 630055 Novosibirsk, Russia; ivmurashov@gmail.com (I.S.M.); aleksey_kurguzov@mail.ru (A.V.K.); amchern@mail.ru (A.M.C.)
* Correspondence: yana-polonskaya@yandex.ru

Abstract: This work is aimed at studying the relationship of matrix metalloproteinases with calcification of the coronary arteries. The study included 78 people with coronary heart disease (CHD) and 36 without CHD. Blood and samples of coronary arteries obtained as a result of endarterectomy were examined. Serum levels of metalloproteinases (MMP) MMP-1, MMP-2, MMP-3, MMP-7, MMP-9, MMP-10, MMP-12, and MMP-13 were determined by multiplex analysis. In blood vessel samples, MMP-1, MMP-3, MMP-7, and MMP-9 were determined by enzyme immunoassay; MMP-9 expression was evaluated by immunohistochemistry. Patients with CHD had higher serum levels of MMP-1, MMP-7, and MMP-12. Blood levels of MMP-1 and MMP-3 were associated with calcium levels, MMP-9 with osteoprotegerin and osteonectin, MMP-7 and MMP-10 with osteoprotegerin, MMP-12 with osteocalcin, and MMP-13 with osteopontin. Calcified plaques had higher levels of MMP-1 and MMP-9 compared to plaques without calcification. The relative risk of coronary arteries calcification was associated with MMP-9, which is confirmed by the results of immunohistochemistry. The results obtained indicate the participation of some MMPs, and especially MMP-9, in the calcification processes. The study can serve as a basis for the further study of the possibility of using MMP-1, MMP-7 and MMP-12 as potential biomarkers of CHD.

Keywords: metalloproteinases; calcification; atherosclerosis; multiplex assay; coronary heart disease

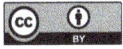

1. Introduction

Cardiovascular diseases (CVD) are considered the leading causes of morbidity and mortality worldwide [1]. Calcification of the vascular wall, which contributes to a decrease in vascular elasticity, is one of the leading factors in CVD. The initial stages of calcification are partly related to elastin degradation with the formation of mineral deposits. Metalloproteinases (MMP) play a significant role in the degradation of elastin; MMP-2 and MMP-9 bind to insoluble elastin and break it down to soluble elastin peptides, which bind to receptors on the surface of vascular smooth muscle cells [2], contributing to their osteogenic differentiation. There is an increase in the expression of MMP in smooth muscle cells and macrophages in atherosclerosis, which leads to the destabilization of the atherosclerotic process in the vascular wall. A particularly high level of MMP is observed in the accumulation of foam cells area and the area of the shoulder of the plaque [3–6]. MMPs are involved in the development and progression of atherosclerosis, and changes in their level are associated with an increased risk of cardiovascular morbidity and mortality [7–9].

Studies on the relationship of MMPs with the calcification process are few. Therefore, according to Gaubatz J. W. et al. [10], the positive association of MMP-7 with the calcification of the carotid arteries was revealed. Experimental studies in mice have shown that MMP-2 deficiency contributes to atherosclerotic calcification development [11]. A study on cell cultures showed that gelatinases promote calcification by stimulating osteoblastic differentiation of vascular smooth muscle cells [12]. Extracellular vesicles, secreted by various cells, have been shown to transport and activate MMP and promote vascular microcalcification. The cellular and molecular mechanisms of MMP's effect on atherosclerotic plaque calcification require further study, which will improve the possible therapy aimed at stabilizing the plaque by reducing the level of its calcification. Therefore, our work aimed to study the relationship of matrix metalloproteinases with coronary arteries calcification.

2. Materials and Methods

The study was conducted jointly with the E.N. Meshalkin National Medical Research Center of the Ministry of Health of the Russian Federation and approved by the Ethical Committees of both institutions. The study included 114 people. All patients completed an Informed Consent form.

The core group included 78 men admitted to the National Medical Research Center named after academician E.N. Meshalkin for coronary bypass surgery. The excluding criteria were myocardial infarction less than six months, acute and exacerbation of chronic infections and inflammatory diseases, renal failure, active liver diseases, oncological diseases, hyperparathyroidism. Blood sampling was performed 12 h after the meal, before the operation. During the surgical procedure, according to intraoperative indications, an endarterectomy was performed from the coronary artery (s), after which the surgical material delivered to the histological laboratory within 30 min was divided longitudinally and transversely into fragments for histological and biochemical studies. Macro- and micro-histological analyses of 156 samples of intima/media of the coronary arteries were performed using an Axiostar Plus binocular microscope (C. Zeiss, Munich, Germany) with digital photo output. Fixed tissue samples were dehydrated and embedded in paraffin by means of an automatic embedding device. Serial histological sections (4 μm) were either stained with hematoxylin and eosin (H&E) or were used for immunohistochemistry. Immunohistochemical staining was performed in a LabVision Autostainer 720 (Thermo Scientific, Verona, Fitchburg, MA, USA) according to the UltraVision Quanto HRP DAB protocol with primary polyclonal antibody (Thermo Scientific, Fremont, CA, USA) to MMP-9 (rabbit, polyclonal, ready-to-use) conjugated with horseradish peroxidase. All atherosclerotic plaques samples, depending on calcium deposits presence according to histological analysis results, were divided into (1) samples without calcifications-53, (2) samples with calcifications-103.

As a control group, 36 men were taken from a population sample of Novosibirsk without CHD, comparable to the core group in terms of age and body mass index. Blood sampling was performed 12 h after the meal before the operation.

In the blood we determined the following biochemical calcification factors: (osteoprotegerin (Bender MedSystems, Vienna, Austria), osteocalcin (Immunodiagnostic Systems Ltd., Bensheim, Germany), osteopontin (Bender MedSystems, Vienna, Austria), osteonectin (Immunodiagnostic Systems Ltd., Bensheim, Germany), calcitonin (Biomerica). We did this using the enzyme immunoassay method on a Multiscan analyzer (Finland).

The analysis of MMP concentrations in blood serum was carried out by multiplex analysis on a Luminex MAGPIX flow fluorimeter using two panels (Millipore) manufactured by Merck KGaA (Darmstadt, Germany):

- Panel Milliplex Catalog ID. HMMP1MAG-55K-03, including the determination of matrix metalloproteinase 3 (MMP-3), matrix metalloproteinase 12 (MMP-12) and matrix metalloproteinase 13 (MMP-13);
- Panel Milliplex Catalog ID. HMMP2MAG-55K-05, including the determination of matrix metalloproteinase 1 (MMP-1), matrix metalloproteinase 2 (MMP-2), matrix

metalloproteinase 7 (MMP-7), matrix metalloproteinase 9 (MMP-9) and matrix metalloproteinase 10 (MMP-10).

For biochemical analyses, the vessel samples obtained during the surgery were frozen in liquid nitrogen and homogenized in a phosphate–salt buffer solution, with the resulting 1% homogenates divided into aliquots. The protein in the homogenates of the samples was measured using the Lowry method. In the homogenates, we calculated the biochemical parameters relative to the protein.

MMP-9 (RD), MMP-3 (Biosource), MMP-1 (RayBiotech), and MMP-7 (BCM Diagnostics kits) were determined in the homogenates of intima/copper samples of coronary arteries by enzyme immunoassay.

We used the licensed version of the SPSS program (13.0) to perform the statistical processing of the results. The normality of the distribution of biomarkers was determined using the Kolmogorov–Smirnov test. Under normal distribution, the data were presented as M ± SD. Since most biomarkers did not have a normal distribution, we used nonparametric criteria. The results are presented as the 25th, 50th, and 75th percentiles. The significance of the differences was evaluated using the Mann–Whitney test and the chi-square test for categorical variables. We carried out one-factor correlation analysis (Spearman's method). We used multivariate logistic regression analysis to determine independent predictors of coronary artery calcification. The differences were considered statistically significant at $p < 0.05$.

3. Results

Table 1 presents the initial characteristics of patients in the core group.

Table 1. Characteristics of patients of the core group.

Parameters	Meaning
Clinical and anamnestic characteristics	
Age, years (M ± SD)	60.4 ± 6.3
Body mass index, kg/m2 (M ± SD)	29.3 ± 4.7
Systolic pressure, mmHg (M ± SD)	137.7 ± 12.8
Diastolic pressure, mmHg (M ± SD)	84.9 ± 7.3
Heart rate, beats per minute (M ± SD)	69.7 ± 6.81
The history of heart attack (absolute in %)	69.2
The history of type II diabetes (absolute in %)	11.5
The family history of CHD (absolute in %)	41.3
Smoking (absolute in %)	15.4
Angina pectoris	
Functional Class I	0%
Functional Class II	10.3%
Functional Class III	83.3%
Functional Class IV	6.4%
Multivessel atherosclerotic lesion	
of coronary arteries (more than two vessels)	92.3%

Table 1. Cont.

Parameters	Meaning
Biochemical parameters, Me (25%; 75%)	
Calcitonin, (pg/mL)	1.86 (0.02; 2.98)
Osteoprotegerin, (pg/mL)	52.99 (35.43; 79.95)
Osteopontin, (ng/mL)	27.05 (17.62; 39.61)
Osteocalcin, (ng/mL)	13.26 (8.46; 16.63)
Osteonectin, (µg/mL)	8.96 (7.74; 10.72)
Ca (mol/L)	2.3 (2.22; 2.43)

Table 2 and Figures 1 and 2 present the data of the multiplex analysis on the metalloproteinases level for the control group and the group with verified coronary atherosclerosis.

Table 2. The level of destruction markers in the blood of patients. Me (25%; 75%).

Parameters	Control $n = 36$	Group with CHD $n = 78$	p
MMP-2 (ng/mL)	111.68 (89.14; 126.89)	104.28 (78.71; 120.04)	0.422
MMP-3 (ng/mL)	47.1 (28.4; 66.5)	33.44 (21.11; 63.65)	0.311
MMP-9 (ng/mL)	228.0 (130.18; 354.96)	276.01 (151.31; 327.58)	0.342
MMP-10 (ng/mL)	0.62 (0.52; 0.82)	0.68 (0.51; 0.82)	0.785
MMP-13 (pg/mL)	30.35 (17.56; 71.9)	36.37 (17.28; 58.16)	0.739

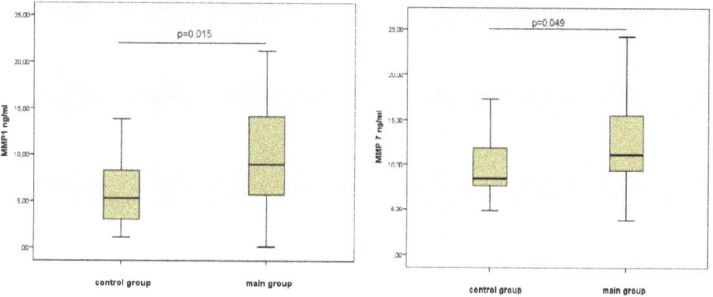

Figure 1. The concentration of MMP-1 and MMP-7 in the studied group, Me (25%; 75%).

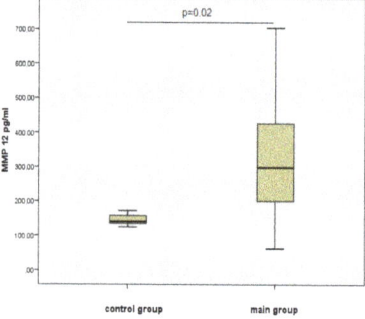

Figure 2. The level of MMP-12 in the studied groups, Me (25%; 75%).

For MMP-1, MMP-7, and MMP-12, we obtained significant differences (Figures 1 and 2). Thus, the level of MMP-1, which is involved in the degradation of collagen in inflammatory diseases and activates MMP-2 and MMP-9, was 1.7 times higher in men of the core group. The content of MMP-7, secreted by epithelial cells and involved in the utilization of extracellular matrix proteins and the activation of pro-MMP-1, -2, and -9, in the serum of men in this group was also 1.3 times higher (Figure 1).

The level of MMP-12, which can hydrolyze elastin and intercellular matrix proteins, as well as activating MMP-3 and MMP-2, was statistically significantly higher in the group of men with atherosclerosis—2.1 times compared to the control group (Figure 2).

At the next stage, we analyzed the relationships of the most significant metalloproteinases with risk factors for cardiovascular diseases. The results are presented in Table 3.

Table 3. The level of metalloproteinases, depending on the risk factors for cardiovascular diseases in men with CHD.

Parameters		MMP-1 (ng/mL)	p	MMP-7 (ng/mL)	p	MMP-12 (pg/mL)	p
BMI	<25	7.96 (4.61; 15.78)	0.97	9.36 (8.25; 12.31)	0.65	218.7 (116.9; 338.5)	0.10
	>25	7.74 (5.49; 11.84)		11.07 (9.36; 15.86)		233.6 (149.6; 382.8)	
Smoking	no	9.22 (6.18; 18.37)	0.52	11.48 (9.36;15.09)	0.08	299.5 (208.6; 513.6)	0.67
	yes	8.37 (2.11; 20.29)		15.09 (8.92; 17.36)		200.8 (101.2; 354.5)	
Family history of CHD	no	10.71 (7.64; 22.78)	0.04	12.72 (9.36; 16.05)	0.53	298.7 (205.3; 554.9)	0.19
	yes	7.41 (5.36; 13.26)		10.22 (9.36; 15.09)		301.4 (174.0; 393.2)	

To assess the relationship of metalloproteinases with calcification, we performed correlation analyses with the biochemical factors of calcification and with the presence of calcified plaques in the coronary arteries. There was no association with the presence of plaques, but there was an association of MMP-1 and MMP-3 levels in the blood with calcium levels ($r = -0.438$; $p = 0.005$ and $r = -0.345$; $p = 0.034$, respectively); MMP-7 with osteoprotegerin ($r = 0.337$; $p = 0.019$); MMP-9 with osteoprotegerin ($r = -0.414$; $p = 0.001$) and with osteonectin ($r = 0.409$; $p = 0.011$); MMP-10 with osteoprotegerin ($r = 0.366$; $p = 0.011$); MMP-12 with osteocalcin ($r = 0.354$; $p = 0.032$); MMP-13 with osteopontin ($r = 0.661$; $p = 0.0001$).

In the next stage of our study, we examined some of the studied metalloproteinases in atherosclerotic plaques with and without calcifications. Table 4 presents the results.

Table 4. The level of metalloproteinases in atherosclerotic foci.

Parameters	With Calcification n = 103	Without Calcification n = 53	p
MMP-9 (ng/mg of protein)	3.61 (1.62; 5.08)	2.24 (1.22; 4.16)	0.017
MMP-3 (ng/mg of protein)	2.05 (1.52; 3.3)	2.00 (1.24; 4.38)	0.881
MMP-7 (ng/mg of protein)	0.78 (0.27; 2.41)	0.62 (0.29; 1.56)	0.6
MMP-1 (ng/mg of protein)	71.37 (21.09;154.99)	49.21 (6.05;299.3)	0.048

In calcified plaques, the levels of MMP-9 and MMP-1 were significantly higher by 1.61 and 1.45 times, respectively, compared to plaques without calcification.

When performing a multivariate logistic regression analysis, where the presence/absence of calcification in the atherosclerotic plaque is taken as a dependent variable and the studied MMPs are taken as independent variables, the relative risk of calcification formation in the coronary artery was associated with MMP-9 (Exp (B) = 1.458; 95% CI 1.049–2.027; p = 0.025).

The obtained results have been confirmed by immunohistochemical analysis (Figure 3).

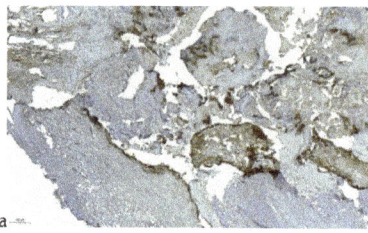 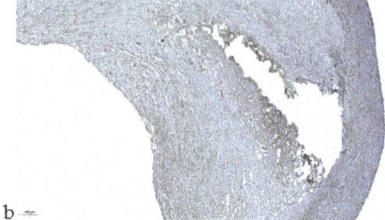

Figure 3. Atherosclerotic plaques of coronary arteries. (**a**) The unstable atherosclerotic plaque with calcification (magnification 100×; MMP9 immunostaining). MMP-9 expression in necrotic areas in the extracellular matrix along the periphery of the calcification core, and in thinned and damaged parts of the fine fibrous cap. (**b**) The stable atherosclerotic plaque without calcification (magnification 100×; MMP9 immunostaining). Lacks MMP-9 expression both in the atheromatous core and in the fibrous cap.

The immunohistochemical investigation of unstable atherosclerotic plaques with calcification showed MMP-9 expression in the necrotic areas in the extracellular matrix along the periphery of the calcification core, and also in thinned and damaged parts of the fine fibrous cap (Figure 3a). The stable atherosclerotic plaque without calcification lacks MMP-9 expression both in the atheromatous core and in the fibrous cap (Figure 3b).

4. Discussion

According to the multiplex analysis, the blood levels of MMP-1, MMP-7 and MMP-12 were higher in patients with CHD, which is consistent with the data in the literature. Thus, according to Kondapalli MS et al., elevated levels of MMP-1 in the blood were observed in patients with CHD [13]. The study by Lehrke M. et al., showed that the circulating MMP-1 level may be a possible prognostic marker of the presence of the atherosclerotic plaques, but not a marker of calcification [14]. In the work of Gaubatz J. W. et al., plasma MMP-1 levels were positively associated with carotid artery calcification [10]. In our study, the level of MMP-1 was higher in calcified plaques, although the subsequent logistic regression analysis did not show the effect of MMP-1 on the formation of calcified foci. Since most of the calcified plaques in our study were unstable, this suggests that MMP-1 may play a role in the destabilization of the atherosclerotic plaque. These findings are consistent with those of Cavusoglu E. et al., who found that elevated blood levels of MMP-1 are associated with an increased risk of all-cause mortality in the long-term in patients with CHD. This association was independent of other clinical, angiographic, and laboratory variables [15].

In the literature, there are data on the association of MMP-3 with vascular calcification [16]. According to our data, there was no association of MMP-3 with vascular calcification, but MMP-3 showed an inverse relationship with the level of calcium in the blood. We found no association of MMP-3 with osteopontin, although, according to Fedarko NS et al., osteopontin binds proMMP-3 and active MMP-3 [17].

Goncalves I et al., have demonstrated an association between CVD and increased circulating MMP-7 and -12 levels [18]. According to other authors, patients with carotid artery atherosclerosis had increased plasma levels of MMP-7 compared to healthy people [19]. In our study, MMP-7 and MMP-12 levels were also significantly higher in patients with CHD and verified coronary artery atherosclerosis than in the control group. In a Gaubatz J. W. et al., study, plasma MMP-1 levels were positively associated with carotid artery calcification [10]. The authors found a significant relationship between the MMP-7 level in plasma and the area of carotid artery calcification, which suggests a possible role of MMP-7 in vascular calcification [10]. We obtained data on the relationship of MMP-7 and MMP-12 levels in the blood with calcification factors. Thus, the serum level of MMP-7 showed an association with osteoprotegerin and MMP-12-with osteocalcin.

In terms of serum levels of MMP-9 and MMP-3, we did not find a statistically significant difference between patients with CHD and the control group. Although, according to Ben Braiek A et al., blood levels of MMP-3 and MMP-9 in patients with CHD were significantly higher [20]. In the study by Wu HD et al., and Moradi N et al., elevated serum levels of MMP-9 were also associated with CHD [21,22]. When studying MMP-9 in samples of atherosclerotic plaques, we found that the relative risk of calcification in the coronary artery was associated with MMP-9. This is consistent with the data of Yajie Chen et al., which indicated an association of MMP-9 with vascular calcification [23]. The mechanisms of influence of MMP-9 on calcification can be different. The increased expression of MMP-9 may lead to an osteogenic transformation of smooth muscle cells and macrophages, and may increase the infiltration of monocytes/macrophages into the affected area of the vessel, promoting calcification through secreted microvesicles [23–25].

The level of MMP-12, an elastolytic metalloproteinase, in our study was higher in patients with CHD. MMP-12 is activated in atherosclerotic lesions and aneurysms and can promote the activation of other MMPs, which, in turn, destroy other proteins of the extracellular matrix [26].

Thus, the broad and diverse function of these destructive MMPs underscores the importance of expanding our understanding of the role of these destructive proteinases in cardiovascular diseases, which will significantly expand our understanding of the pathogenetic mechanisms of the development of coronary atherosclerosis and, in particular, the calcification of atherosclerotic plaques.

5. Conclusions

The results obtained indicate the involvement of some MMPs, especially MMP-9, in the processes of calcification, which requires additional research on the role of MMPs in vascular calcification and atherosclerosis development. The study can serve as a basis for the further study of the possibility of using MMP-1, MMP-7 and MMP-12 as potential CHD biomarkers.

Author Contributions: Conceptualization, Y.V.P. and E.V.K.; methodology, Y.I.R.; validation, E.M.S. and N.A.M.; formal analysis, E.V.S. and V.S.S.; investigation, I.S.M.; resources, A.V.K.; data curation, A.M.C.; writing—review and editing, Y.V.P. and E.V.K.; final approval of the manuscript for publication, Y.I.R. All authors have read and agreed to the published version of the manuscript.

Funding: The study was supported by state assignment № AAAA-A17-117112850280-2, Russian Foundation for Basic Research grant № 19-015-00055a, "The role of vascular calcification in the stability and instability of atherosclerotic plaques," and the study involved materials from the "Collection of human biomaterials at the Institute of Internal and Preventive Medicine—a branch of ICG SB RAS" (№ 0324-2017-0048).

Institutional Review Board Statement: This study was approved by the local Ethics Committee of the Research Institute of Internal and Preventive Medicine—Branch of the Institute of Cytology and Genetics, Siberian Branch of Russian Academy of Sciences (protocol № 2, approval on 3 July 2017).

Informed Consent Statement: Informed consent was obtained from all subjects involved in the study.

Data Availability Statement: The datasets before and after analysis in this study are available from the corresponding author on reasonable request.

Conflicts of Interest: The authors declare no conflict of interest. The funders had no role in the design of the study; in the collection, analyses, or interpretation of data; in the writing of the manuscript, or in the decision to publish the results.

References

1. Roth, G.A.; Johnson, C.; Abajobir, A.; Abd-Allah, F.; Abera, S.F.; Abyu, G.; Ahmed, M.; Aksut, B.; Alam, T.; Alam, K.; et al. Global, Regional, and National Burden of Cardiovascular Diseases for 10 Causes, 1990 to 2015. *J. Am. Coll. Cardiol.* **2017**, *70*, 1–25. [CrossRef]
2. Lee, J.S.; Basalyga, D.M.; Simionescu, A.; Isenburg, J.C.; Simionescu, D.T.; Vyavahare, N.R. Elastin calcification in the rat subdermal model is accompanied by up-regulation of degradative and osteogenic cellular responses. *Am. J. Pathol.* **2006**, *168*, 490–498. [CrossRef]
3. Beaudeux, J.-L.; Giral, P.; Bruckert, E.; Foglietti, M.-J.; Chapman, M.J. Matrix metalloproteinases, inflammation and atherosclerosis: Therapeutic perspectives. *Clin. Chem. Lab. Med.* **2004**, *42*, 121–131. [CrossRef] [PubMed]
4. Kadoglou, N.P.; Daskalopoulou, S.S.; Perrea, D.; Liapis, C. Matrix Metalloproteinases and Diabetic Vascular Complications. *Angiology* **2005**, *56*, 173–189. [CrossRef] [PubMed]
5. Uzui, H.; Harpf, A.; Liu, M.; Doherty, T.M.; Shukla, A.; Chai, N.N.; Tripathi, P.V.; Jovinge, S.; Wilkin, D.J.; Asotra, K.; et al. Increased expression of membrane type 3-matrix metalloproteinase in human atherosclerotic plaque: Role of activated macrophages and inflammatory cytokines. *Circulation* **2002**, *106*, 3024–3030. [CrossRef] [PubMed]
6. Johnson, J.L. Matrix metalloproteinases: Influence on smooth muscle cells and atherosclerotic plaque stability. *Expert Rev. Cardiovasc. Ther.* **2007**, *5*, 265–282. [CrossRef]
7. Hopps, E.; Caimi, G. Matrix metalloproteases as a pharmacological target in cardiovascular diseases. *Eur. Rev. Med. Pharm. Sci.* **2015**, *19*, 2583–2589.
8. Cuvelliez, M.; Vandewalle, V.; Brunin, M.; Beseme, O.; Hulot, A.; De Groote, P.; Amouyel, P.; Bauters, C.; Marot, G.; Pinet, F. Circulating proteomic signature of early death in heart failure patients with reduced ejection fraction. *Sci. Rep.* **2019**, *9*, 1–12. [CrossRef]
9. Vacek, T.; Rehman, S.; Yu, S.; Neamtu, D.; Givimani, S.; Tyagi, S. Matrix metalloproteinases in atherosclerosis: Role of nitric oxide, hydrogen sulfide, homocysteine, and polymorphisms. *Vasc. Health Risk Manag.* **2015**, *11*, 173–183. [CrossRef]
10. Gaubatz, J.W.; Ballantyne, C.M.; Wasserman, B.A.; He, M.; Chambless, L.E.; Boerwinkle, E.; Hoogeveen, R.C. Association of Circulating Matrix Metalloproteinases With Carotid Artery Characteristics: The Atherosclerosis Risk in Communities Carotid MRI Study. *Arter. Thromb. Vasc. Biol.* **2010**, *30*, 1034–1042. [CrossRef]
11. Sasaki, T.; Nakamura, K.; Sasada, K.; Okada, Y.; Cheng, X.W.; Suzuki, T.; Murohara, T.; Sato, K.; Kuzuya, M. Matrix metalloproteinase-2 deficiency impairs aortic atherosclerotic calcification in ApoE-deficient mice. *Atherosclerosis* **2013**, *227*, 43–50. [CrossRef] [PubMed]
12. Zhao, Y.-G.; Meng, F.-X.; Li, B.-W.; Sheng, Y.-M.; Liu, M.-M.; Wang, B.; Li, H.-W.; Xiu, R.-J. Gelatinases promote calcification of vascular smooth muscle cells by up-regulating bone morphogenetic protein-2. *Biochem. Biophys. Res. Commun.* **2016**, *470*, 287–293. [CrossRef]
13. Kondapalli, M.S.; Galimudi, R.K.; Gundapaneni, K.K.; Padala, C.; Cingeetham, A.; Gantala, S.; Ali, A.; Shyamala, N.; Sahu, S.K.; Nallari, P.; et al. MMP 1 circulating levels and promoter polymorphism in risk prediction of coronary artery disease in asymptomatic first degree relatives. *Gene* **2016**, *595*, 115–120. [CrossRef] [PubMed]
14. Lehrke, M.; Greif, M.; Broedl, U.C.; Lebherz, C.; Laubender, R.P.; Becker, A.; Von Ziegler, F.; Tittus, J.; Reiser, M.; Becker, C.; et al. MMP-1 serum levels predict coronary atherosclerosis in humans. *Cardiovasc. Diabetol.* **2009**, *8*, 50. [CrossRef] [PubMed]
15. Cavusoglu, E.; Marmur, J.D.; Hegde, S.; Yanamadala, S.; Batuman, O.A.; Chopra, V.; Ay, G.; Eng, C. Relation of baseline plasma MMP-1 levels to long-term all-cause mortality in patients with known or suspected coronary artery disease referred for coronary angiography. *Atherosclerosis* **2015**, *239*, 268–275. [CrossRef] [PubMed]
16. Aloui, S.; Zidi, W.; Ouali, S.; Guizani, I.; Hadj-Taieb, S.; Mourali, M.S.; Feki, M.; Allal-Elasmi, M. Association of matrix metalloproteinase 3 and endogenous inhibitors with inflammatory markers in mitral valve disease and calcification. *Mol. Biol. Rep.* **2018**, *45*, 2135–2143. [CrossRef]
17. Fedarko, N.S.; Jain, A.; Karadag, A.; Fisher, L.W. Three small integrin-binding ligand N-linked glycoproteins (SIBLINGs) bind and activate specific matrix metalloproteinases. *FASEB J.* **2004**, *18*, 734–736. [CrossRef]
18. Goncalves, I.; Bengtsson, E.; Colhoun, H.M.; Shore, A.C.; Palombo, C.; Natali, A.; Edsfeldt, A.; Dunér, P.; Fredrikson, G.N.; Björkbacka, H.; et al. Elevated Plasma Levels of MMP-12 Are Associated With Atherosclerotic Burden and Symptomatic Cardiovascular Disease in Subjects With Type 2 Diabetes. *Arter. Thromb. Vasc. Biol.* **2015**, *35*, 1723–1731. [CrossRef]
19. Abbas, A.; Aukrust, P.; Russell, D.; Krohg-Sørensen, K.; Almås, T.; Bundgaard, D.; Bjerkeli, V.; Sagen, E.L.; Michelsen, A.E.; Dahl, T.B.; et al. Matrix Metalloproteinase 7 Is Associated with Symptomatic Lesions and Adverse Events in Patients with Carotid Atherosclerosis. *PLoS ONE* **2014**, *9*, e84935. [CrossRef]
20. Ben Braiek, A.; Chahed, H.; Dumont, F.; Abdelhak, F.; Hichem, D.; Gamra, H.; Baudin, B. Identification of biomarker panels as predictors of severity in coronary artery disease. *J. Cell. Mol. Med.* **2021**, *25*, 1518–1530. [CrossRef]
21. Wu, H.-D.; Bai, X.; Chen, D.-M.; Cao, H.-Y.; Qin, L. Association of Genetic Polymorphisms in Matrix Metalloproteinase-9 and Coronary Artery Disease in the Chinese Han Population: A Case–Control Study. *Genet. Test. Mol. Biomarkers* **2013**, *17*, 707–712. [CrossRef]
22. Moradi, N.; Fadaei, R.; Ahmadi, R.; Mohammad, M.H.; Shahmohamadnejad, S.; Tavakoli-Yaraki, M.; Aghajani, H.; Fallah, S. Role of serum MMP-9 levels and vitamin D receptor polymorphisms in the susceptibility to coronary artery disease: An association study in Iranian population. *Gene* **2017**, *628*, 295–300. [CrossRef]

23. Chen, Y.; Waqar, A.B.; Nishijima, K.; Ning, B.; Kitajima, S.; Matsuhisa, F.; Chen, L.; Liu, E.; Koike, T.; Yu, Y.; et al. Macrophage-derived MMP-9 enhances the progression of atherosclerotic lesions and vascular calcification in transgenic rabbits. *J. Cell. Mol. Med.* **2020**, *24*, 4261–4274. [CrossRef] [PubMed]
24. Hecht, E.; Freise, C.; Websky, K.V.; Nasser, H.; Kretzschmar, N.; Stawowy, P.; Hocher, B.; Querfeld, U. The matrix metalloproteinases 2 and 9 initiate uraemic vascular calcifications. *Nephrol. Dial. Transplant.* **2016**, *31*, 789–797. [CrossRef] [PubMed]
25. Freise, C.; Kretzschmar, N.; Querfeld, U. Wnt signaling contributes to vascular calcification by induction of matrix metalloproteinases. *BMC Cardiovasc. Disord.* **2016**, *16*. [CrossRef] [PubMed]
26. Liang, J.; Liu, E.; Yu, Y.; Kitajima, S.; Koike, T.; Jin, Y.; Morimoto, M.; Hatakeyama, K.; Asada, Y.; Watanabe, T.; et al. Macrophage Metalloelastase Accelerates the Progression of Atherosclerosis in Transgenic Rabbits. *Circulation* **2006**, *113*, 1993–2001. [CrossRef] [PubMed]

MDPI
St. Alban-Anlage 66
4052 Basel
Switzerland
Tel. +41 61 683 77 34
Fax +41 61 302 89 18
www.mdpi.com

Journal of Personalized Medicine Editorial Office
E-mail: jpm@mdpi.com
www.mdpi.com/journal/jpm

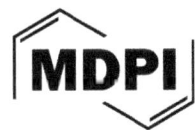